HEAD INJURIES

HEAD INJURIES

PROCEEDINGS OF THE SECOND CHICAGO SYMPOSIUM ON NEURAL TRAUMA

Edited by

ROBERT L. McLAURIN, M.D.
Neurosurgical Division
Department of Surgery
University of Cincinnati Medical Center
Cincinnati, Ohio

GRUNE & STRATTON, INC.
A Subsidiary of Harcourt Brace Jovanovich, Publishers
New York   San Francisco   London

Proceedings of the Second Chicago Conference on Neural Trauma
University of Chicago, Center for Continuing Education
Chicago, Illinois
March 21–23, 1975

This conference was supported by Grant NS 12146-01
Institute of Neurologic Disease and Stroke
National Institutes of Health
Bethesda, Maryland

Library of Congress Cataloging in Publication Data

Chicago Symposium on Neural Trauma, 2d, 1975.
  Head injuries.

  Bibliography: p.
  Includes index.
  1. Head—Wounds and injuries—Congresses.
2. Prognosis—Congresses. 3. Brain—Wounds and
injuries—Congresses. 4. Intracranial pressure—
Congresses. I. McLaurin, Robert L. II. Title.
[DNLM: 1. Head injuries—Congresses. W3 C155E 1975h/
WE705 C532 1975h]
RD521.C42 1975   617'.1   76-12968
ISBN 0-8089-0938-X

Grune & Stratton, Inc.
111 Fifth Avenue
New York, New York 10003

Distributed in the United Kingdom by
Academic Press, Inc. (London) Ltd.
24/28 Oval Road, London NW 1

Library of Congress Catalog Number 76-12968
International Standard Book Number 0-8089-0938-X
Printed in the United States of America

CONTENTS

IV CEREBRAL MICROCIRCULATION

V PRESSURE-VOLUME RELATIONSHIPS

PREFACE

The first Head Injury Conference was held at the University of Chicago Center for Continuing Education, February 6–9, 1966. Dr. Joseph P. Evans was the host. The conference was organized in response to an increasing awareness of the importance of head injury as a cause of death and disability in our society. It was attended by approximately 50 scientists from the United States and abroad, to review the current state of knowledge regarding this facet of bodily trauma and to make recommendtions for the future.

At the end of that conference a resolution was adopted which included the following recommendation:

Establishment of specialized facilities with integrated services for the treatment and investigation of head injuries, which will include sequential studies and rehabilitation, and multidisciplinary research programs.

One of the consequences of this resolution was the establishment of several "head injury centers," funded by the National Institute of Neurologic Disease and Stroke, for the pursuit of basic and clinical research. On two occasions, the centers have held workshops, and on numerous other occasions the principal investigators have assembled to review and plan for further studies. In 1974, it was agreed that a second major conference was needed to permit broader discussion and integration of several areas of current research relating to head injury. The principal investigators acted as an organizing committee and selected five topics for review: (1) prognostic considerations, (2) blood-brain barrier, (3) respiratory pathophysiology, (4) cerebral microcirculation, and (5) pressure-volume relationships. Participants were invited to make specific presentations of ongoing research and to participate in the open discussion.

The proceedings of the Second Chicago Conference on Neural Trauma, held at the University of Chicago Center for Continuing Education, March 21–23, 1975, are being published as a report of the progress that has been made and as a basis for continuing efforts to minimize the morbidity and mortality accompanying head injury.

Robert L. McLaurin, M.D.

PARTICIPANTS

Dr. William Adams
Medical College of Virginia
Richmond, Virginia

Dr. Donald Becker
Medical College of Virginia
Richmond, Virginia

Dr. Michael Behbehani
University of Cincinnati
Cincinnati, Ohio

Dr. Robert Berne
University of Virginia
Charlottesbille, Virginia

Dr. Byron Bloor
Loyola Univerity
Maywood, Illinois

Dr. Charles Brackett
E. University of Kansas
Kansas City, Kansas

Dr. Milton Brightman
Department of Health, Education and Welfare
National Institutes of Health
Bethesda, Maryland

Dr. Derek Bruce
Hospital of the University of Pennsylvania
Philadelphia, Pennsylvania

Dr. Gleb Budzilovich
New York University
New York, New York

Dr. William F. Collins, Jr.
Yale University
New Haven, Connecticut

Dr. Allen Crockard
University of Chicago
Chicago, Illinois

Dr. Jack de la Torre
University of Chicago
Chicago, Illinois

Dr. Carl Dila
Montreal Neurological Institute
Montreal, Quebec, Canada

Dr. Thomas Ducker
Medical College of South Carolina
Charleston, South Carolina

Dr. Eduardo Eidelburg
The Barrow Neurological Institute
Phoenix, Arizona

Dr. M. Feinsod
Hadassah University
Jerusalem, Israel

Dr. Eugene Flamm
New York University
New York, New York

Dr. Alan Fleischer
Emory University
Atlanta, Georgia

Dr. Edward Ganz
University of Chicago
Chicago, Illinois

Dr. Thomas Gennarelli
Department of Health, Education and Welfare
National Institutes of Health
Bethesda, Maryland

Dr. Murray Goldstein
Department of Health, Education and Welfare
National Institutes of Health
Bethesda, Maryland

Dr. Stanley J. Goodman
Harbor General Hospital
Torrance, California

Dr. Robert Greenberg
Medical College of Virginia
Richmond, Virginia

Dr. Robert Grossman
University of Texas
Galveston, Texas

Dr. Neal Gunby
Armed Forces Radiobiology Research Institute
Department of Health, Education and Welfare
Bethesda, Maryland

Dr. William K. Hass
New York University
New York, New York

Dr. Javad Hekmatpanah
University of Chicago
Chicago, Illinois

Dr. Gerald Hochwald
New York University
New York, New York

Dr. Julian Hoff
University of California
San Francisco, California

Dr. William Hunt
Ohio State University
Columbus, Ohio

Dr. Bryan Jennett
Killearn Hospital
Killearn, Stirlingshire, Scotland

Dr. Glenn Kindt
University of Michigan
Ann Arbor, Michigan

Dr. Arthur Kobrine
Walter Reed Army Hospital
Washington, D.C.

Dr. Theodore Kurze
University of Southern California
Los Angeles, California

Dr. Thomas Langfitt
Hospital of the University of Pennsylvania
Philadelphia, Pennsylvania

Dr. Robert Loudon
University of Cincinnati
Cincinnati, Ohio

Dr. Anthony Marmarou
Albert Einstein College of Medicine
New York, New York

Dr. Julio Martinez
Medical College of Virginia
Richmond, Virginia

Dr. Robert McLaurin
University of Cincinnati
Cincinnati, Ohio

Dr. J. Douglas Miller
Institute of Neurological Sciences
Glasgow, Scotland, United Kingdom

Dr. John D. Mitchenfelder
Mayo Clinic
Rochester, Minnesota

Dr. Robert Moody
Cook County Hospital
Chicago, Illinois

Dr. Gerald Moss
Polytechnical Institute
Rensselaer, New York

Dr. James Mosso
University of Cincinnati
Cincinnati, Ohio

Dr. Sean Mullan
University of Chicago
Chicago, Illinois

Dr. Walter Obrist
Duke University
Durham, North Carolina

Dr. Michael O'Connor
University Hospital of Pennsylvania
Philadelphia, Pennsylvania

Dr. Ayub Ommaya
Department of Health, Education and Welfare
National Institutes of Health
Bethesda, Maryland

Dr. Jorn Overgaard
Odense University
Odense, Denmark

Mr. John Overman
Kansas City Medical Center
Kansas City, Kansas

Dr. Phanor Perot, Jr.
Medical College of South Carolina
Charleston, South Carolina

Dr. John Pickard
University of Pennsylvania Hospital
Philadelphia, Pennsylvania

Dr. Fred Plum
Cornell University
New York, New York

Dr. Joseph Ransohoff
New York University
New York, New York

Dr. Stanley Rapoport
Department of Health, Education and Welfare
National Institutes of Health
Bethesda, Maryland

Dr. Harry Rappaport
New York University
New York, New York

Dr. W. Rosenblum
Medical College of Virginia
Richmond, Virginia

Dr. Romas Sakalas
Medical College of Virginia
Richmond, Virginia

Dr. Harvey Shapiro
Hospital of University of Pennsylvania
Philadelphia, Pennsylvania

Dr. Samuel Shelburne
University of Cincinnati
Cincinnati, Ohio

Dr. Ken Shulman
Albert Einstein College of Medicine
New York, New York

Dr. Humbert Sullivan
Medical College of Virginia
Richmond, Virginia

Dr. Lindsay Symon
National Hospital
London, England

Dr. Aubrey Taylor
University of Mississippi
Jackson, Mississippi

Dr. George Tindall
Emory University
Atlanta, Georgia

Dr. Patricia Tornheim
University of Cincinnati
Cincinnati, Ohio

Dr. John Vries
Medical College of Virginia
Richmond, Virginia

Dr. Alvin Wald
New York University
New York, New York

Dr. Earl Walker
Baltimore, Maryland

Dr. Frank Yatsu
University of California
San Francisco, California

HEAD INJURIES

Prognostic Considerations

John J. Caronna, M.D.
Fred Plum, M.D.

1

Prognosis and Medical Coma

Prognosis is of particular importance when coma complicates acute medical illness. If the eventual outcome of subjects in coma could be predicted within hours of onset, expensive, emotionally draining, and time-consuming therapeutic measures could be concentrated on patients with a genuine possibility of recovery. Furthermore, the efficacy of new treatments can be assessed only if the natural outcome of the disease is accurately known.

As yet, no clear prognostic scheme has been devised for medical (i.e., nontraumatic) coma because so many factors seem likely to influence outcome. Previous studies of outcome of non-drug-induced medical coma have identified general factors which improve or worsen the outlook. The following paragraphs review those studies of coma resulting from anoxia-ischemia, where sufficient information is given to suggest a conclusion about prognosis.

COMA DUE TO ANOXIA-ISCHEMIA

It has sometimes been considered that survivors of cardiac arrest either die or have complete neurological recovery, but this is surely too great a simplification. Every hospital has patients who survive with permanent brain damage after cardiac arrest. Furthermore, neurological recovery is particularly in doubt during the early postarrest state when important management decisions must be made. The prognostic criteria

Aided by Contract #N01-NS-4-2328 and Grant #NS-03346 from NINDS.

used to gauge outcome have been:

Duration of anoxia;[1]
Age of patient and duration of postanoxic coma;[2]
Systemic acid base status after resuscitation;[3]
Cardiac rhythm after resuscitation;[4]
EEG;[5]
Pupillary light reaction and size;[6]
Motor response to stimulation;[7]

Each of these schemes has merits but perhaps even greater limitations. Duration of anoxia-ischemia or duration of circulatory arrest is rarely known with precision.

The outcome of severe brain damage of whatever etiology has been related to age and duration of coma.[8,9,10] In fact, unconsciousness per se is an important and unfavorable sign in older people.[11]

Bokonjic and Buchthal[2] reported that 90 percent of patients in coma less than 48 hours made a complete recovery. However, the findings of Willoughby and Leach[7] directly contradict this assertion; anyway, one would prefer to know outcome within 12 hours of cardiac arrest.

In cases of cerebral anoxia-ischemia due to stroke, both Rout et al.[12] and Mazzara et al.[3] have related breathing pattern and $PaCO_2$ to survival. None of Mazzara's 7 patients with severe hyperventilation survived. Patients with a $PaCO_2$ of less than 35 mm Hg had a 70 percent mortality. Vapalahti and Troup[13] associated the presence of respiratory alkalosis and hypocapnia in the first 48 hours after head injury with survival in the persistent vegetative state, rather than death or recovery. Recently, North and Jennett[14] found that abnormal breathing patterns, especially tachypnea (f > 25/min), combined with $PaCO_2$ values less than 30 mm Hg were indicative of a poor prognosis. This combination and the fact that such hyperpnea occurs without respect to neurological disease[3,15] suggests that overwhelming and possible independently fatal pulmonary infection or microembolism governed these results.

Recently, Liberthson et al.[4] have pointed out that of 101 patients resuscitated after cardiac arrest, 59 who had a bradycardia, a junctional or an indioventricular rhythm died compared to 42 patients with normal sinus rhythm and a pulse of 100 beats per minute or greater who survived. Of the 42 patients leaving the hospital, 60 percent (25) returned to their previous way of life, 12 percent (5) were institutionalized because of neurological deficit, and a further 28 percent had some neurological deficit. The frequency of neurological injury is higher than is usual in hospital coronary-care units and reflects the duration of hypoxemia; these patients were resuscitated outside hospital by the Miami paramedic team.

The problem with the methods of appraisal described above stems from the fact that many of these methods depend on respiratory and circulatory data and fail to consider the primary role of the brain as the organ integrating body homeostasis. While these methods are of value in predicting extremes of outcome, death or survival, their published correlations with outcome indicate that they are subject to error and exceptions and are insufficiently discriminating to allow a decision for management. Recently, attention has been directed to the prediction of outcome in terms of the assessment of neurological function.

Prior[5] has used the EEG to predict death or survival in 115 postcardiorespiratory arrest patients. A visual rating system (Grade 1-alpha rhythm; Grade 2-rare alpha; Grade 3-continuous delta; Grade 4-isoelectric intervals of 1 second or more; Grade 5-isoelectric) was used to predict outcome. The rating system was most accurate if Grades 4 or 5 were present, and confusion and inaccuracy were more prevalent with records showing milder grades of abnormality. An overall accuracy of the order of 80 to 85 percent was possible as early as 6 to 12 hours after resuscitation. EEG assessment, when inaccurate, generally gave a more hopeful estimate of prognosis than was justified. Nevertheless, false positive results suggesting irreversible brain damage when there

was none were encountered in instances of drug overdose, hypothermia, trauma, and encephalitis. Although a somewhat improved accuracy was reported obtained with the use of a linear discriminant score based on 36 variables or an adaptive discriminant score using 13, the presence of overly pessimistic prognostic errors would appear substantially to weaken the value of any prognostic scheme based on EEG.

Two problems surround the use of pupillary reactivity to predict outcome of medical coma. One is that the significance of unreactive pupils apparently differs in different diseases. Thus, in coma following cardiac arrest, fixed dilated pupils do not always have a fatal prognosis. There are numerous reports of patients recovering after demonstrating such a pupillary condition. In these cases, pupillary dilation may indicate anoxia or even hyperepinephrinemia rather than irreversible structural damage. The second problem is that observers often record pupillary reactions incorrectly. When testing the accuracy of different observers on the same patient, we find that reports of unreactive pupils are frequently incorrect due to observer inexperience or failure to use a sufficiently strong light and magnifying glass to make the observation.

Motor response of the extremities has been used for an estimate of prognosis in coma. Jennett[16] and Overgaard et al.[11] emphasized that the motor response to noxious stimulation was an important guide to prognosis during the early days of coma after head injury. Brendler and Selverstone,[17] however, noted that in 16 patients with coma due to brain lesions, the clinical state of motor decerebration was potentially reversible if the corneal and one or more deep tendon reflexes were preserved and if hypotension was absent. In a series of patients in coma due to anoxia-ischemia, Willoughby and Leach[7] stated that all patients unresponsive or showing only reflex movement to a noxious stimulus within the first hour following cardiac arrest either died or survived with neurological damage.

Other approaches, mainly in the evaluation of coma following head injury, have included determination of the oculovestibular response to ice water,[18,19,20] measurement of CBF, $CMRO_2$, and measurements of intraventricular pressure. In general, such studies have accurately predicted the extremes of outcome (death and survival) but by themselves have failed to provide sufficient documentation to allow the physician accurately and confidently to predict degree of recovery in the individual patients.

THE PRESENT STUDY

The present report represents an exploration of three questions: Does medical coma lend itself to a predictive scheme based on the early bedside assessment of central nervous system function? If so, what clinical features (indicants) are of predictive value? And finally, can a protocol enable physicians and nurses to obtain and record accurate clinical data on the depth and duration of coma? What we will describe has been collected as part of a larger collaborative study on outcome of severe neurological injury being conducted at the Universities of Glasgow, Newcastle-upon-Tyne, Southern California, and Cornell. This report deals only with patients in medical coma studies thus far at Cornell and must be regarded as no more than a description of how we are approaching the problem.

There is ready agreement among neurosurgeons that the severity of a head injury is reflected in the immediately observed clinical neurological dysfunction. In medical coma, particularly that following cardiac arrest, there is no agreement as to whether the heart or the brain has been the crucial watershed organ for recovery. This ambiguity has led several investigators, particularly Hossmann and his colleagues,[21] to challenge the long-held belief that severe hypoxia-ischemia of no more than a few minutes duration irreversibly damages cerebral neurons. The findings will not be reviewed in detail but they can be classified as generating two postulates:

1. Cerebral ischemia can be greatly prolonged perhaps to as much as 60 minutes without producing permanent brain damage if post-ischemic abnormalities can be prevented in the systemic circulation.
2. Abnormalities in the cerebral microcirculation are an early consequence of cerebral ischemia and, by interfering with tissue perfusion ("no reflow"), prevent the recovery of potentially viable brain tissue when an effective systemic circulation is restored.

Both these postulates imply that the neuroglial elements of the brain are much more resistant to hypoxic-ischemic insult than previously believed on the basis of classical clinical and neuropathologic studies. The first postulate can be largely dismissed on the basis of recent experimental studies. Levy et al.,[22] in our laboratory, have investigated the question of neuronal versus vascular damage in rats with anoxic-ischemic injury. The experiments show that extensive functional and histological evidence of irreversible damage to cerebral neurons can occur during anoxia-ischemia without any evidence of injury or obstruction to the cerebral microcirculation. In other words, no-reflow is neither a necessary nor a frequent precursor to experimental ischemic cerebral infarction.

To examine whether neurological recovery is possible after prolonged cerebral ischemia, we have gone to the bedside to find out whether any clinical factors observable at admission to hospital or within the first 24 hours of anoxic-ischemic coma could provide accurate indicants to the neurological outcome. We reasoned that neurological findings present on admission to the study (within from minutes to as much as 6 hours after anoxic-ischemic coma) reflected primarily the intensity of initial cerebral anoxic-ischemic injury rather than complicating systemic problems. Once admitted to the hospital or cardiac unit, most subjects had treatment aimed at supporting blood pressure, blood volume, and blood gases at physiological levels. Accordingly, if the conditions of systemic circulation blood gases and electrolytes were the main factors determining the degree of neurological recovery, outcome should correlate poorly with neurological signs on admission but should correlate highly with subsequent general medical difficulties. Conversely, if degree of initial neurological anoxic-ischemic injury largely determined neurological recoverability, it should be possible to find indicants of that outcome almost immediately after injury.

METHODS

Patients admitted to the New York Hospital and Memorial Hospital who were in coma for more than 6 hours were followed prospectively by the authors (see Table 1). Only adults with acute or subacute medical, i.e., nontraumatic, coma of known cause were included: cases of narcotic and nonnarcotic drug overdose as well as patients in

Table 1
Criteria for Entry into Study

1. Age > 10 years.
2. Acute medical illness with unresponsiveness (nontraumatic, non-drug intoxication).
3. Persistence of unresponsiveness and survival for 6 hours or more.

Table 3
Best Motor Response

Score	Upper Limbs
1	Nil
2	Abnormal extensor
3	Abnormal flexor
4	Withdrawing—localizing
5	Obeys commands

terminal comas were excluded. Children were excluded because their number would be small and their prognosis is generally believed to be better and yet more difficult to predict than that of adults.[23] The investigators were not responsible for the care of the patients and tried not to transmit notions of prognosis to the medical staff. Neither prolongation nor discontinuation of life support therapy was affected by the conduct of this study.

Assessment of coma (see Table 2) was carried out according to a clinical coma profile which included a modification of the "practical scale" developed in Glasgow for use in head injured subjects,[24] supplemented by a specific appraisal of brain stem function. For the practical scale, eye opening and motor and verbal responses were recorded after supraorbital pressure or compression of a distal interphalangeal joint. The upper extremities were used to assess motor function and the motor score was that determined in the best limb (see Table 3). All patients were deeply comatose on admission to the study, i.e., they had less than normal scores in all three categories scored. Brain stem function was assessed according to the principles outlined by Plum and Posner.[25] Oculocephalic responses were elicited by raising the head from the pillow and moving it to-and-fro in horizontal and vertical planes. Oculovestibular responses were determined using 5 ml or 20 ml of ice water to irrigate the external auditory canal and tympanum.

Table 2
Assessment of Coma

A. Verbal response 1–4
B. Eye opening 1–4
C. Pupils 1–3
D. Oculocephalic-oculovestibular responses 1–4
E. Motor response 1–5
F. Respiration 1–4

Where appropriate, alcohol and barbiturate levels in blood were determined to rule out any contributory drug depression. Some patients received anticonvulsant medications. Patients on respirators were examined at least 2 hours after any dose of paralyzing drug, at which time skeletal muscle movement had returned.

The following outcomes were identified: death, persistent vegetative state (PVS), severe disability (dependent but conscious), moderate disability (independent but disabled), and good recovery.

RESULTS

Sixty-three patients in medical coma have been followed prospectively and the outcome determined. There were 24 men and 39 women. Medical coma carried a poor prognosis: 51 percent of the subjects died and only 19 percent made a good or moderate recovery.

Because of the small number of subjects, particularly in the subgroups, the results must be considered as preliminary and no more than trends. For that reason, no attempt has been made to assign significance or percentages to any of the numbers.

The subjects were allotted to one of nine diagnostic categories, and the best outcome at any time up to 3 months after the onset of coma was determined (see Table 4). The category "mass lesions" included 2 patients with brain tumors with reversible cerebral edema producing acute transtentorial herniation and coma who recovered consciousness but died subsequently, and one patient with a chronic subdural hematoma who died at 1 month postoperatively without recovering consciousness. One patient in the category "cardiac arrest" was alert several hours after the hypoxic insult but without further circulatory difficulty lapsed into coma on the fourth day, presumably as a result of a delayed postanoxic encephalopathy.[26]

Table 4
Best Outcome at 3 Months

Diagnosis	N	Died	PVS	SD	MD	GR
Cardiac arrest	12	6	1	3	0	2
Cerebral hemorrhage	11	8	1	2	0	0
Subarachnoid hemorrhage	10	4	2	1	2	1
Anoxia-ischemia	8	2	1	2	0	3
Ischemic stroke	6	3	0	3	0	0
Liver failure	5	3	0	1	0	1
Multiple—other	5	3	0	1	0	1
Pulmonary failure	3	3	0	0	0	0
Mass lesion	3	0	0	1	0	2
Total	63	32	5	14	2	10

Indicants Not Predictive of Coma

Age at onset of coma bore no relation to outcome. The mean age for subjects who died was 59 ± 3 years (S.E.M.), while for good recovery it was 64 ± 4 years. The presence or absence of pupillary responses, spontaneous eye movements, and oculocephalic responses thus far appear to have no specific predictive value, but numbers may be too small to tell. The potential significance of $PaCO_2$ could not be assessed in seriously ill patients because of the frequent use of mechanical ventilation with a resultant respiratory alkalosis. Blood pressure and heart rate if abnormal were regulated to normal.

Indicants Predictive of Coma

On the basis of the practical scale motor score on admission, i.e., less than 12 hours after onset of coma, it was not possible to distinguish among the possible outcomes (see Table 5). On admission, the total coma score and the motor score had an identical correlation with outcome because in every case eye opening and verbal responses to stimulation were nil.

Table 5
Motor Score <12 H

Outcome	1	2	3	≥ 4
Death	13	11	1	7
PVS	0	2	2	1
Severe disab	2	2	3	7
Mod disab	0	1	0	1
Good recov	2	2	0	6
Total	17	18	6	22

Examinations of oculovestibular (OV) responses appeared to provide useful information (see Table 6). Even if the motor score was ignored, absent OV responses on admission were never associated with good recovery, and at 24 hours absent OV responses were never associated with survival. If one combined oculovestibular responses with the motor score, it enhanced the apparent predictive ability (see Table 7).

Thus, on admission at a minimal coma score, absent OV responses always were associated with death and even at higher practical scores, absent OV responses implied an outcome no better than severe disability.

The present early results in patients with coma associated with medical disease appear to justify the following conclusions.

1. The immediate and acute degree of brain damage is the major factor governing outcome from anoxic-ischemic coma. This study does not support the theoretical position that the intensity of ischemic insult is not correlated with survival.

Table 6
Oculovestibular Response

Outcome	<12 H		24 H	
	Absent	*Present*	*Absent*	*Present*
Death	11	21	14	18
PVS	0	5	0	5
Severe disab	1	13	0	14
Mod disab	0	2	0	2
Good recov	0	10	0	10
Total	12	51	14	49

Table 7
Oculovestibular Response Present

Outcome	Best Motor Score < 12 H		
	1	2–3	4
Death	7	9	5
PVS	0	4	1
Severe disability	2	4	7
Mod. disability	0	1	1
Good recovery	2	2	6

2. One can predict from early neurological findings alone the general probability of survival and the likelihood of residual damage in patients with anoxic-ischemic coma. Since humanitarian medicine requires that such predictions have an extremely high statistical accuracy, however, the results cannot yet be applied to therapy.

3. It remains to be seen whether it will be possible to give an accurate prognosis before 24 hours.

This study is continuing to determine whether present trends accurately reflect the universal experience of such patients. The clinical coma profile is still being evaluated to determine the consistency with which different observers record similar findings, and which functions are truly independent of each other so that they are of cardinal importance in diagnosis. Although more subjects must be evaluated before absolute criteria can be established, the preliminary results indicate that clinical assessment can yield accurate predictive information about the potential for recovery from medical coma.

REFERENCES

1. Bell JA, Hodgson HJF: Coma after cardiac arrest. Brain 97:361–372, 1974
2. Bokonjic N, Buchthal F: Postanoxic unconsciousness as related to clinical and EEG recovery in stagnant anoxia and carbon monoxide poisoning, in Gastaut H, Meyer, JS (eds): Cerebral Anoxia and the Electroencephalogram. Springfield, Ill, Thomas, 1961, pp 118–125
3. Mazzara JT, Ayres SM, Grace WJ: Extreme hypocapnia in the critically ill patient. Am J Med 58:450–456, 1974
4. Liberthson RR, Nagel EL, Hirschman JC, Nussenfeld SR: Prehospital ventricular defibrillation: prognosis and followup. N Engl J Med 291:317–321, 1974
5. Prior PF: The EEG In Acute Cerebral Anoxia. Amsterdam, Excerpta Medica, 1973
6. Plum F: Brain swelling and edema in cerebral vascular disease. Cerebrovasc Dis 41:318–348, 1966
7. Willoughby JO, Leach BG: Relation of neurological findings after cardiac arrest to outcome. Br Med J 3:437–439, 1974
8. Marquardsen J: The natural history of cerebrovascular disease. Acta Neurol Scand Suppl. 38, 45:1–192, 1969
9. McKissock W, Richardson A, Walsh L: Posterior communicating aneurysms: A controlled trial of the conservative and surgical treatment of ruptured aneurysms of the internal carotid artery at or near the point of origin of the posterior communicating artery. Lancet 1:1203–1206, 1960
10. Carlsson CA, von Essen C, Lofgren J: Factors affecting the clinical course of patients with severe head injuries. J Neurosurg 29:242–251, 1968
11. Overgaard J, Hvid-Hansen O, Land AM, et al: Prognosis after head injury based on early clinical examination. Lancet 2: 631–635, 1973
12. Rout MW, Lane DJ, Wallner L: Prognosis in acute cerebrovascular accidents in relation to respiratory pattern and blood gas tensions. Br Med J 3:7–9, 1971
13. Vapalahti M, Troup H: Prognosis for patients with severe brain injuries. Br Med J 3:404–407, 1971
14. North JB, Jennett S: Abnormal breathing patterns associated with acute brain damage. Arch Neurol 31:338–344, 1974
15. Plum F: Hyperpnea, hyperventilation and brain dysfunction. Ann Intern Med 76:328, 1972
16. Jennett B: Prognosis after severe head injury, in Clinical Neurosurgery, vol. 21. Baltimore, Williams & Wilkins, 1972, chap 11, pp. 200–207.
17. Brendler SJ, Selverstone B: Recovery from decerebration. Brain 93:381–392, 1970
18. Poulsen J, Zilstorff K: Prognostic value of the caloric-vestibular test in the unconscious patient with cranial trauma. Acta Neurol Scand 48:282, 1972
19. Tarkkanen J, Troup H: Letter to the editor. Laryngoscope 31:1741, 1971

20. Jadhav WR, Sinha A, Tandon PN, Kacker SK, Banerji AK: Cold caloric test in altered states of consciousness. Laryngoscope 81:391–402, 1971

21. Hossmann KA, Kleihues P: Reversibility of ischemic brain damage. Arch Neurol 29:375–384, 1973

22. Levy DE, Brierley JB, Silverman DG, Plum F: Brief hypoxia-ischemia initially damages cerebral neurons. Arch Neurol (in press)

23. Brown JK, Ingram TTS, Seshia SS: Pattern of decerebration in infants and children. Defects in homeostasis and sequelae. J Neurol Neurosurg Psych 36:431–444, 1973

24. Teasdale G, Jennett B: Assessment of coma and impaired consciousness. Lancet 2:81–84, 1974

25. Plum F, Posner JB: Diagnosis of Stupor and Coma (ed 2). Philadelphia, Davis, 1972

26. Plum F, Posner JB, Hain RF: Delayed neurological deterioration after anoxia. Arch Intern Med 110:56–63, 1962

Jorn Overgaard, M.D.

2

Reflections on Prognostic Determinants in Acute Severe Head Injury

The conditions for recovery following acceleration-deceleration head injury brain damage depend on at least five phenomena: (1) the parenchymal lesion, (2) the vascular lesion, (3) the possible aggravation of both, (4) the management of the patient, and (5) a genetic factor. The last mentioned is mainly unknown but may have relationship to the finding that age over 20 years has an unfavorable influence on outcome in traumatic coma and may also in part be responsible for an unexpected rapid recovery in a few seriously ill patients.[1,2]

All the involved people wish to know prognosis as early as possible, and the close relatives hope for affirmative information within a few hours after the accident. Are we able to present reliable predictions for this outcome at an earlier date than nonprofessionals? It is not to be forgotten that many patients who finally make a good recovery have taken the last steps toward this rare occurrence months or even years after leaving our care.[3]

Computer storage of clinical information may in the near or distant future reveal its superiority to expert clinical intuition, for the clinician cannot predict a patterned recovery. He can only treat the patient to prevent death, including living

death, apallic syndrome, and persistent vegetative state. He must then fear that survival will include disturbing mental deficiencies and only as a gift learn that the patient has recovered.[1,4]

Is it at all possible to find at an early date differences which are determinative for the final outcome? The complexities of prognostic forecasting are so difficult to deal with that a core of simplified concepts concerning brain injury is necessary.

A HYPOTHESIS FOR THE LOCATION AND SEVERITY OF BRAIN INJURY AND ITS RELATION TO OUTCOME

Despite intensive theoretical and experimental research, a simple clinical concept of the relationship between injury and prognosis has not been established. Certain lesions, such as the laceration of the language area in the cerebral cortex, are never followed by a complete recovery. Apart from such examples, caused by loss of brain substance, it may be that no simple relationship exists. How can one determine which part of the brain has suffered most injury? The brain stem or perhaps the centrum semiovale? A hypothesis has been presented by Ommaya and Gennarelli.[5] It is convincing in that it is founded on different experimental approaches and also includes a noninvasive technique for patient investigation. These concepts have assisted my deductions, based on clinical findings and CBF studies.

In acceleration-deceleration head injury unconsciousness (coma and semicoma) occurs due to abolition of mesencephalic reticular formation

Neurokirurgisk afdeling, Odense Amts og Bys sygehus, 5000 Odense, Denmark.

This work was supported by the Board of the Odense County Hospital. The author also gratefully acknowledges the inspiration of Dr. M. Hjelm and Dr. E. Sindrup as well as the staff of the Neurosurgical Clinic. Mrs. B. Tang and L. Bruus prepared the figures and the typewriting.

Table I

	GR	Sl. Def.	Sev. Def.	Died	Apallic
Class A	9 Patients				8	1
Class B	45 Patients	4	9	20	4	8
Class C	20 Patients	9	6	4	1	
Class D	2 Patients	1		1		

Key:
  GR = Good recovery
  Sl. Def. = Slight deficit
  Sev. Def. = Severe deficits
  Died = Lethal outcome in the clinic
  Apallic = Persistent vegetative state
  Good recovery + slight deficits = Recovery

pacemaker activity projecting to cortical fields. If the impairment of brain stem function is reversible, one can expect the extremity motor pattern associated with the coma state to depend on the severity of cortical injury and especially on the integrity of the cortical fields pertaining to the extrapyramidal motor system. According to this reasoning, the finding of a normal flexor and avoidance motor pattern (Class C patients) is tantamount to a less severe cortical injury as compared to the finding of an extensor response with rigidity (Class B patients). A symmetrically abnormal motor response was not required for inclusion in the latter patient class. In cases of irreversible damage to brain stem functions, neither extensor rigidity nor a normal motor pattern is to be expected. The extremities are mostly hypotonic, the tendon reflexes are not elicitable, the oculomotor activity is extincted, and the pupils are dilated and nonreactive (Class A patients). It was further assumed that most or all brain injury in patients with contusion had occurred within a few minutes of injury. Thus the on-admission classification could inform with regard to the severity of traumatic brain injury.[6]

The outcome for 76 recently studied young patients with head injury from traffic accidents has supported earlier findings (Table 1). In 10 Class B patients and 2 from Class C, the follow-up interval was too short for final assessment. Consequently, they were called severe deficits.

The completely different outcome patterns in these three patient classes carried the following tentative conclusions. (1) Primary brain stem lesion is a rare occurrence in traffic accident

patients who are alive on arrival. (2) In all survivors, mesencephalic pacemaker activity is resumed, but the quality of survival depends on cortical neuronal recovery. When this recovery rate is minimal, an apallic condition is present. When recovery is complete, clinical recovery is also without deficits. Between these extremes the outcome condition is often mainly determined by severe mental disturbances which possibly are caused by impairment of the highest integrative cortical functions.

The functional reconnection of reticular formation pacemaker activity and cortical function is difficult to determine. Spoken intelligible language seems impossible without cortical activity and was therefore chosen as an indication of reawakening. In 33 patients surviving from Class B, the first day of intelligible speech was recorded (n = 33 patients): max. 39, mean 2 $\pm$ 21, av. 8 days, postinjury and for 19 Class C patients these figures were (n = 19): 12, 4 $\pm$ 11, 3 days. The difference was striking and significant $(0,001 > p)$.

The differences in neurological condition on admission in the two patient classes B and C is consequently not only in projection to final outcome pattern but also in recognizing one of the important steps in the recovery phase. Although supplying useful information about outcome in patient classes, the weakness of the system is that it does not permit reliable prognostic forecasting in the individual patient allocated to Class B or C. The patient may, however, benefit from the fact that his severity classification can be determined immediately on admission. This is especially important for patients in Class B, as it may possibly prevent an expectant attitude created by the futile supposition—"he will awaken by morning."

Why do a few of these patients recover from a severe traumatic brain injury? It is probably more favorable to sustain an impact causing immediate coma with extensor response (Class B) than a light injury followed by later deterioration to this condition, as none of the 4 patients with epidural hematoma survived to a better category than "severe deficits." This is further supported by the finding that 10 of the 13 patients who recovered from the Class B condition had a cerebral contusion, not a surgical lesion.

In comatose patients apparently identical with regard to motor pattern, neurophthalmological findings, spontaneous hyperventilation, and arterial hypertension, the possible differences with regard to cerebral (cortical ?) damage are difficult to detect. The ideal technique would be noninvasive, applicable at the bedside, and repeatable at reasonable intervals.[5]

Changes in cerebral blood flow (CBF) affecting the whole hemisphere or only focally may reflect degrees of damage. The relative amounts of neuronal and cerebral vessel damage responsible for the clinical findings is now known. CBF findings may be caused by neuronal damage, uncoupling of the oxygen uptake/function relationship (cytotoxic edema), lactic acidosis (luxury perfusion), and vascular lesion paralysis of arteriolar myotactic reflexes (impaired autoregulation and reduced CO_2 reactivity) and opening of capillary endothelial tight junctions (vasogenic edema). Based on biochemical findings in experimental head injury, it has recently been assumed "that the brain tissue itself is rather resistant to trauma, but that secondary ischemic and hypoxic changes of complex pathophysiology and probably a very inhomogenous flow are responsible for much of the brain damage, even in the acute phase."[2,7]

CEREBRAL BLOOD FLOW—CLINICAL OBSERVATIONS

For clinical use the method should be applicable to emergency situations and prestudy preparations should be minimal, so that the staff on duty can perform the investigations as a routine procedure, with no greater difficulty than making burr holes or angiography.

The method of choice is the intraarterial Xenon-133 bolus injection through a catheter placed in the internal carotid artery.[8] Clearance of the tracer should be displayed as the logarithmic conversion of the initial part of the curve (CBFinit) as this mainly represents gray matter perfusion (cortex). Using a commercially available machine with 35 individual detectors* each looking at its own cortical region, our normal values for hemispheric mean flow was CBFinit 58.7 ± 6.7 ml/100 g/min at an average $PaCO_2$ of 37.5 torr.[9,10,11] Multiple injections are often

*Meditronic Cerebrograph 35
Meditronic a/s—Smedevaenget 12—DK 9560 Hadsund, Denmark.

necessary to get a reliable picture of the flow situation. At least in the acute stage, flow studies without simultaneously monitoring the intracranial pressure are not of much value. Both of these parameters are in part dependent on the $PaCO_2$, and the perfusion pressure (CPP) cannot be determined by monitoring the arterial blood pressure alone.

Impaired autoregulation and reduced CO_2 reactivity following severe head injury have been reported and may be regarded as inevitable consequences of acute brain damage.[11-14]

Classification based on flow findings is doubtful because CBF pathophysiology is dependent on multiple factors.[15] Moreover, a limiting circumstance in severe head injury is that blood flow in the brain stem cannot be included as a parameter. It seems proven that extremely low hemispheric flow values at normocapnia and normothermia, lasting more than a few minutes, are incompatible with survival of brain function,[16,17] as well as that hyperemia reflects uncoupling of homeostatic mechanisms.[8,18] A normal flow is not an indication of normal brain function.

The flow findings in the 76 young patients were classified in accordance with the following criteria. Ischemia = hemispheric flow lower than 20 ml/100 g/min (7 patients); hyperemic flow = hemispheric flow over 65 ml/100 g/min (20 patients); oligonormemic flow = hemispheric flow 21–65 ml/100 g/min. All values are expressed as CBFinit. The third group contained 49 patients. Based on some striking differences of clinical importance—arrival time after injury, aggravation factors, and management, they were divided into two groups: (1) initial oligonormemic hemispheric perfusion (12 patients), and (2) subacute oligonormemic perfusion (37 patients). The first flow study determined allocation to a group.

ISCHEMIC HEMISPHERIC PERFUSION (Fig. 1)

In Class A, of 4 patients, 4 died. In Class B, of 3 patients, 1 died and 2 remained apallic. The ages ranged from 3 to 45 years with an average of 19 years.

The clinical condition and the flow measured in this group indicates that the cerebral hemispheres had suffered a very severe injury and the

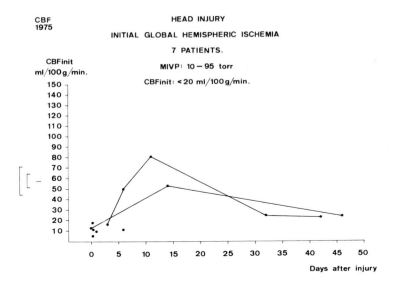

Fig. 1. CBFinit. in 7 patients in whom the first study revealed an ischemic perfusion of the studied cerebral hemisphere.

outcome showed that the lesions were irreversible. This is valid also for the two survivors, who had transient hyperemia following the initial cortical ischemia.

It may be postulated that the Class B condition is impossible without at least some degree of brain stem function, whereas the more serious condition, typical for Class A, is caused by an additional failure of brain stem activity. The impairment of mesencephalic and pontine function may be elicited by a short-lived ischemia or primary injury, but this initial lesion is sublethal as the patient is "alive" on admission.

When the brain stem lesion is developing slowly relative to the impact as in neglected epidural hematoma, the surgical evacuation of the hematoma may be followed by hemispheric cortical hyperemia. However, the potential for survival is dependent on the rapid recovery of brain stem function. The quality of survival, however, depends on restitution of hemispheric cortical activity.

These considerations are based on the experiences with 9 Class A patients. Only one survived—but in an apallic state—following evacuation of an epidural hematoma. With the above exception, the apallic outcome was exclusively related to the Class B condition, from which 18 percent survived to this state. This was never seen in association with patient Classes C and D.

HYPEREMIC HEMISPHERIC PERFUSION (Fig. 2)

In Class A, 1 patient died. Of 13 Class B patients, 4 remained with severe deficits, 1 was apallic, and 2 died. There were 3 good recoveries and 3 recoveries with slight deficits. In 6 Class C patients, there were 2 with severe deficits, 1 with a slight deficit, and 3 recovered completely. The age range was 6 to 33 years with an average age of 18 years.

Although most of these 20 patients arrived within 6 hours following injury and had excellent transportation management, the outcome in 4 patients may have been partly determined by treatment delay. Three survived with severe deficits and 1 died following evacuation of an epidural hematoma; this was the Class A patient. The two other deaths occurred in the ward some weeks after injury and were both caused by tracheostomy complications.

Thirteen patients had cerebral contusions. The intracranial pressure was monitored in 14 patients in the first week ($n = 14$; mean intraventricular pressure – MIVP: 16.67 ± 5.25 and $PaCO_2$: 36.00 ± 4.95).

Traumatic arterial hypertension (systolic blood pressure >160 torr) was obtained in 13 patients.

Focal hyperemia represented by tissue

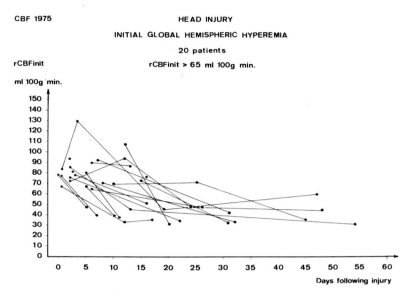

Fig. 2. CBFinit. in 20 patients in whom the first study revealed a hemispheric blood flow over 65 ml/100 g/min. (Hyperemia).

peaks[9] were never seen before the third day, but they occurred especially in the third week and at that time often revealed persisting focally impaired autoregulation. They were disclosed in 15 patients, 12 of which had cerebral contusions without a surgical brain lesion. They were seen in 12 of the 13 Class B patients and in 3 of the 6 patients from Class C. These hyperemic foci had no relation to outcome.

The flow pattern observed in these patients probably represents an initial severe diffuse vascular and neuronal cortical injury associated with a strong capacity for recovery. Clinical criteria could not have predicted that approximately half of the patients from Class B would recover.

INITIAL OLIGONORMEMIC HEMISPHERIC PERFUSION (Fig. 3)

Both Class A patients died. In 6 Class B patients, there were 2 patients with severe deficits, 3 with slight deficits, and 1 with good recovery. Of 4 Class C patients, 1 had a slight deficit and 3 had good recoveries. The age range was 13 to 36 years, averaging 19 years.

These 12 patients had excellent preadmission management and arrived early to the clinic. The two exceptions had huge epidural hematomas and both were in Class A condition on admission. The early precautions may in part, explain that high intracranial pressures (45 and 55 torr) were only monitored in 2 patients. In the other cases, the highest measured pressure under normocapnia was 24 torr.

Tissue peaks were observed as early as 2 hours following injury and within the first 24 hours following injury they were seen in 5 patients. In another 5 patients, they appeared during later studies, mainly indicating focally impaired autoregulation. Early posttraumatic arterial hypertension was measured in 9 patients.

Although the CBFinit in 8 of these patients was in the range of 22–48 ml/100 g/min and therefore was called oligemic, these values hardly represent tissue underperfusion. The normal values in four patients may indicate an intact coupling between flow and metabolism, but in 2 of these patients, the $CMRO_2$ at day zero was 2.14 ml/100 g/min and 1.18 ml/100 g/min. Relative to these values for oxygen uptake the flow may be regarded as high.

Only 2 patients had remarkable increase of flow within the next 7 to 20 days and both made fast and good recoveries as expected in young patients from Class C. It was, however, surprising that 4 of the 6 patients in Class B recovered.

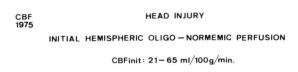

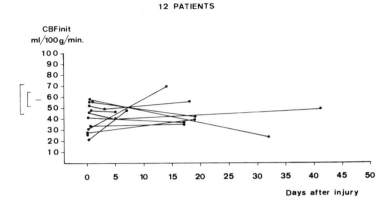

Fig. 3. CBFinit. in 12 patients who had their first study within 24 hours following injury, with hemispheric perfusion in the range of 21–65 ml/100 g/min. (Initial oligonormemic perfusion).

SUBACUTE OLIGONORMEMIC HEMISPHERIC PERFUSION (Fig. 4)

Of 2 Class A patients, 1 died and 1 was apallic. Of 23 Class B patients, 1 died, 5 were apallic, 14 remained with severe deficits, and 3 with slight deficits. Of 10 Class C patients, 1 died, 2 had severe deficits, 4 had slight deficits, and 3 patients had good recoveries. Of 2 Class D patients, 1 had a severe deficit and 1 had a good recovery. The age range was 3 to 45 years, averaging 19 years.

Only 9 of the 37 patients in this group arrived shortly after the accident, and on admission they were all allocated to Class B. Another 9 patients had very late arrivals, between 1 day and 1 week,

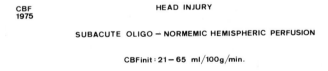

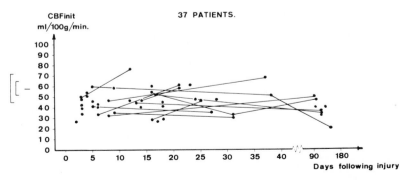

Fig. 4. CBFinit. in 37 patients in whom the first study was done later than the first 24 hours. The hemispheric perfusion range at the first study was 21–65 ml/100 g/min. (Subacute oligo-normemic perfusion).

and 7 belonged to Class C, 5 of whom had surgical lesions. The remaining 19 patients arrived from 2 to 10 hours following injury and included 13 belonging to Class B and 3 to Class C. Intermittent arterial hypertension was recorded in 17 patients. The intracranial pressure as well as the CBF was completely unknown within the first 24 hours. The highest intracranial pressures were recorded in this group—in 3 patients, 44–88–95 torr at a $PaCO_2$ of 31–35 torr. Only a total of 16 patients had MIVP measurements within the first week after admission and, excluding the above-mentioned 3 patients, the figures were (n = 3; MIVP: 17.33 ± 7.50 and $PaCO_2$: 34.17 ± 6.15).

Tissue peaks were seen on the flow curves of 19 patients, occurring in 8 of 15 with surgical lesions and in 11 of 22 with contusions. In a few they persisted until 2 months following injury.

The flow pattern in this group of patients had no discriminative value for prognostic considerations. The study practice was unsatisfactory and this is only in part explicable by inexperience during the early period of these studies. It cannot be excluded that the 23 Class B patients represent a borderline fraction of this clinical picture, but if so, this may be explained by a combination of late arrival, bad transportation management, and too much delay following admission. In no less than 15 patients the immediate management problems on admission were determined by lesion aggravating circumstances: respiratory arrest, occluded airways, neglected thoracic lesions, and intracranial hematomas. Three patients had been transported despite an episode of cardiac arrest. The extremely bad outcome for Class B patients may be associated with such hypoxia-producing phenomena, as none of the 3 patients who recovered to slight deficits had such complications, and 2 had been admitted shortly after injury.

COMMENTS OF THE CBF FINDINGS

The wide variation of cerebral blood flow is a reflection of the initial brain damage, secondary influences, and study practice. It was expected that these values were powerful indicators of brain damage, but they have not contributed to facilitate the understanding of severe traumatic brain injury. Their value is probably foremost related to the fact that flow findings may indicate extremes of cerebral injury: irreversible damage,

as occurred when the hemispheric flow is under 20 ml/g/min., provided normocapnia and normothermia is present. The hemispheric hyperemia is more difficult to evaluate with regard to prognosis for the diseased cerebral tissue. It may be caused by neuronal injury, but it cannot be excluded that primary vascular damage is of equal importance. The clinical experience of the patient with the highest flow value measured in this series also being among the few who had a fast reawakening and recovery from the Class B condition, can certainly not be interpreted as favoring an isolated vascular injury without neuronal damage or vice versa. Although these high flow values may be compared with the flow found in patients with pure anoxic brain injury, our experience is that the anoxic patient never recovers hemispheric cortical function.

The findings of recoveries among the Class B patients in two flow groupings was not expected. The most favorable flow finding for recovery was the initial oligonormemic perfusion. The patients in this group had the best preadmission management and arrived early after injury. Do they represent the "pure" traumatic brain injury only complicated with a minimal degree of aggravation? The reestablishment of intelligible language occurred earlier in this group of patients (Fig. 5), and it may be relevant to conclude that the cortical injury was of less severity.

The extremely bad outcome pattern in the third group may be related to a heavy contamination with aggravation factors, an insufficient study practice, as well as to more severe primary brain injury. However, the question remains of why these patients reestablished intelligible language just as fast as the patients in the hyperemia group. The answer does not seem to be related to episodic ischemic flow as this is not compatible with recovery of cortical function. It is probably more reasonable to assume that the highest integrative cortical functions cannot recover unless the cortical tissue pressure is kept very close to the normal range.

TRAUMATIC BRAIN EDEMA

Reliable clinical criteria for assessment of brain edema do not exist. The hemodynamics of this condition was investigated in 26 patients in the first 2 weeks following injury. The criterion for division into slight edema or severe edema was an

CBF   FIRST DAY OF SPEAKING
1975

FLOW PATTERN

N = 16	N = 10	N = 23
M : 37,64 ± 26,00	M : 18,60 ± 13,56	M : 31,73 ± 22,02
N.S.	0,05 < p < 0,01	N.S.
CLASS B : N = 10	CLASS B : N = 6	CLASS B : N = 15
M : 45,44 ± 27,70	M : 28,20 ± 11,10	M : 41,14 ± 22,35
CLASS C : N = 6	CLASS C : N = 4	CLASS C : N = 8
M : 21,80 ± 16,32	M : 6,25 ± 4,99	M : 15,71 ± 6,58
HYPEREMIA	INITIAL OLIGO – NORM-	SUBACUTE OLIGO–

Fig. 5. Pattern of reestablishment of intelligible language in three classes of hemispheric perfusion, expressed as CBFinit.

MIVP of 20 torr or less and over 20 torr, respectively, measured during CBF investigation. By definition, MIVP was different and also CPP was different, but in $PaCO_2$, CBFinit, and CVR there was no significant difference between the two groups.[19] Another criterion for hemispheric traumatic brain edema is a dislocation on angiograms or ventriculograms not caused by a hematoma. As all the CBF studies were followed by angiography and in most cases also ventriculography, the x-rays from the first 3 weeks were divided into two groups: (1) no dislocation of the midline or elevation of the sylvian vessels = no edema; (2) dislocation of the midline or elevation of the sylvian vessels = edema present. Thirty-five patients had edema according to these criteria and 41 patients did not. A good recovery was made by 10 of the patients with edema and by 4 of the patients without edema.

The following considerations concerning edema as a secondary lesion resulted from these findings: edema may be a result of the capacity of white matter to receive transudated fluid from cortical gray matter vessels, whose capillary tight junctions (blood brain barrier) are impaired. When this capacity is exhausted, intracranial pressure rises steeply, and when perfusion pressure has decreased below a level which is determined by the condition of the brain tissue, CBF will rapidly decrease, eventually reaching ischemic levels, which provoke irreversible cortical

damage. This point of view on vasogenic edema, of course, is hypothetical. It includes further the unproven assumption that within limits the mechanism of transferring surplus extravascular fluid from the cortical gray matter to the white substance interstitial fluid, is a mechanism which protects damaged cortical cells with cytotoxic edema from further injury. The acidic fluid is directed away from the neurones. As long as this mechanism operates, the neurones have the capability to recover and increase their oxydative metabolism. Tissue hyperemia may increase that this process operates.

Experimental observations indicate that cytotoxic edema is an immediate reaction to injury, whereas the vasogenic edema is a delayed response, starting a few hours later.[20–29] Both edema types increase brain volume, and intracranial content is further increased when the cerebral vessels are dilated, for example, during hypercapnia.[30] The rate of expansion of cerebral volume seems to be important for the development of elevated intracranial pressure. If volume is slowly increased, a pressure response may fail to appear and brain death may occur without significant increases of systemic blood pressure or intracranial pressure, that is, without a Cushing reflex.[31] Monitoring of intracranial pressure would not indicate this development, but testing intracranial compliance might reveal impending danger.[22,32,33] Some degree of edema formation seems to be obligatory in acute severe head injury. A condition for a good recovery is, however, that the intracranial pressure does not exceed the normal range.

This view is supported by the findings in 8 patients who made a good recovery: $n = 8$

PaCO$_2$ 38.71 ± 3.09

MIVP   13.71 ± 3.82

CPP   97.86 ± 17.99

CBFinit   71.71 ± 33.32

Day   6.00 ± 5.72

Included are all four Class B patients who made a good recovery. In 5 patients the angio- and ventriculograms made in connection with the study revealed dislocations indicating "edema." In 4 of the 8 patients, the intraventricular pressure promptly varied with blood pressure changes during test of autoregulation.

MANAGEMENT

Management starts principally at the site of the accident. The risk for hypoxia—or anoxia-producing events—is large on site and during transportation to the primary hospital, but should not occur during a second transportation to a neurosurgical clinic.[34] Intubation, assisted ventilation to moderate hypocapnic levels, and sedation were requested before transportation.

The importance of simple precautions is emphasized by the finding that among the 59 patients who had a second transportation period before arrival to the clinic, no less than 21 seems to have suffered complicating circumstances with anoxia-producing potentiality. This occurred only in 3 of the 17 patients who were admitted directly from the hospital's accident reception area. Even more striking is that 2 of these 17 patients died, whereas 11 of the 59 "late" arrivals had a lethal outcome. An apallic outcome occurred only among patients who had to travel a long distance, and when these 9 patients are included, 33 percent of the 59 patients had an outcome without survival of the brain.

These figures are not caused by a single factor, but I suggest that one of the important circumstances is related to geography: there was a long distance from the accident site to the ambulance garage and the first hospital.

These introductory remarks were necessary because without this knowledge it is difficult to understand that the very intensive treatment supplied at the specialist clinic could hardly be related to a favorable outcome. It included respirator-assisted or controlled ventilation for 40 patients, but only 8 of the 13 patients from Class B who recovered received this form of management. Since a total of 29 Class B patients were treated with respirator, the figure for recovery is not impressive. Well-oxygenated air plus a hypocapnic PaCO$_2$ level was used mainly to prevent a rise of the intracranial pressure caused by hypercapnia, but the level of PaCO$_2$ was also set according to the findings at the CBF studies. It was thought that hyperemia is harmful to the brain and hypocapnic vasoconstriction of benefit, and this is possibly true. It cannot be excluded that more patients would have recovered if respirator treatment had been applied. However, this treatment may be harmful if the hypocapnia produces ischemia in vasoreactive areas and further dilatation in vasoparalytic foci. Ventricular drainage lasting for some days combined with respirator treatment was possibly of importance in determining a favorable outcome among 7 patients in the group: initial oligonormemic perfusion. As only 2 of the 4 patients with recovery from Class B had this combination, no definite conclusion can be drawn. In the group subacute oligonormemic perfusion, neither respirator treatment nor ventricular drainage nor a combination of both was associated with a better outcome than no such treatment. It is surprising, however, that when respirator treatment is associated with arrival conditions, in early admissions the recovery rate becomes 40 percent (6/15) in 13 Class B patients and 2 Class C patients.

Steroids, mannitol, and furosemide may have saved a few from death but could not be correlated to the recovery outcome.

Shunting valves were applied to 9 patients because of ventricular dilatation. In 2 patients, an awake akinetic condition was replaced by rapid improvement in only 1, recovering to a level of slight deficit. Four have severe deficits and in 4 it should have been avoided as the apallic state remained unchanged.

The basic medication for all patients in the first 2 to 3 weeks was phenobarbital, but often supplemented with chlorpromazine. The conversion of a comatose patient with decerebrate rigidity, diverging eye axes, arterial hypertension and hyperthermia into a state dominated by flaccid extremities, normal blood pressure, and normothermia is most impressive but can only be conducted in association with respirator treatment. This is the only combination of possible methods of management that, I am convinced, can change an initial prediction of a bad outcome to a good recovery, provided no neglected hematoma caused the condition.

CONCLUSION

In patients with acute severe head injury, the clinical examination done immediately on admission to the neurosurgical clinic has a high potential for predicting outcome in three patient classes (A, B, and C). For the individual patient, however, the system is too uncertain if allocated as a result of this examination to Classes B and C. A patient who, on admission, belongs to Class A will never recover brain function.

The interval between trauma and admission is also of importance, as the rate of anoxia-producing circumstances increases with this parameter. The condition of coma with extensor response and rigidity may be followed by recovery if it is present immediately following the injury (contusio cerebri) but not if it develops due to an expanding surgical lesion.

CBF studies revealed that patients belonging to Classes B and C, especially Class B, who finally recovered were shown to have a hemispheric (cortical) hyperemia, often lasting more than a week. Another condition for recovery in this type of patients was an oligonormemic hemisphere perfusion within a few hours following injury; as these patients had excellent preadmission treatment, the flow finding may be a reflection of management, not of cerebral injury.

The CBF studies supported the assumption that cerebrovascular disturbances are elicited immediately following severe head injury—impaired autoregulation, reduced CO_2 reactivity and unstable intracranial pressure, often following blood pressure variations. The fluid movements (edema formation) into the interstitial brain tissue in the white substance seems to be a delayed phenomenon. It is postulated that reflectance of extravascular fluid in the cortex may be beneficial to the damaged neurones as long as the hemispheric white substance can accumulate the transudated fluid and its constituents. Conventional methods for monitoring intracranial pressure are thought to be incapable for the detection of critical pressure levels in the brain tissue. A good recovery was only found when the intracranial pressure did not exceed the normal range in the first 2 weeks.

The CBF studies did not answer the important question: Is the vascular reaction following severe head injury caused by neuronal or vascular damage? A hemispheric blood flow below 20 ml/100 g/min was, however, never associated with recovery of cortical neuronal function.

REFERENCES

1. Jennett WB, Plum F: Persistent vegetative state after brain damage. Lancet 734–737, April 1, 1972
2. Ponten U, Jagodzinski, Nilsson B: Brain energy metabolism in head injury. Recent Progress in Neurological Surgery. ICS 320, pp 300–309. Amsterdam, Excerpta Medica, 1974
3. Lewin W: Observations on prolonged unconsciousness after head injury, in Cumings JN, Kremer M (ed): Biochemical Aspects of Neurological Disorders. Second Series. Oxford, Blackwell, 1965, pp 182–198
4. Jennett WB, Plum F, Shaw D: Progress in coma. Lancet 1:100, 1975 (letter to the editor)
5. Ommaya AK, Gennarelli TA: Neural trauma: Correlations between the biomechanics and pathophysiology of head injury. Recent Progress in Neurological Surgery. ICS 320, pp 275–285. Amsterdam, Excerpta Medica, 1974
6. Overgaard J, et al: Prognosis after head injury based on early clinical examination. Lancet 631–635, Sept. 22, 1973
7. Ponten U: Cerebral energy metabolism. J Neurosurg Sci, vol. 17, nr. 4:213–216, 1973
8. Lassen NA, Ingvar DH: Radioisotopic assessment of regional cerebral blood flow. Prog Nucl Med 1:376–409, 1972
9. Olesen J, Paulson OB, Lassen NA: Regional cerebral blood flow in man determined by the initial

slope of the clearance of intraarterial injected 133 Xe. Stroke 2:519–540, 1971

10. Olessen J: Cerebral blood flow. Thesis, FADL forlag Kobenhavn-Arhus, Odense 1974, 134 pp

11. Overgaard J, Tweed WA: rCBF in acute severe head injury. J Neurosurg 41:531–541, 1974

12. Bruce DA, Langfitt TW, Miller D, et al: Regional cerebral blood flow, intracranial pressure and brain metabolism in comatose patients. J Neurosurg 38:144, 1973

13. Fieschi C, Beduschi A, Agnolli A, et al: Regional cerebral blood flow and intraventricular pressure in acute brain injuries. Eur Neurol 8:192–199, 1972

14. Tweed WA, Overgaard J: Cerebral hemodynamics and the effects of traumatic brain edema. Abstract, Lund Symposium, 1974

15. Langfitt TW: The pathophysiology of the cerebral circulation in head injury. Clin Neurosurg 19:84–97, 1972

16. Boysen G: Cerebral hemodynamics in carotid surgery. Acta Neurol Scand 49, Suppl. 52, 1973

17. Boysen G, Engell HC, Pistoless G, et al: On the critical lower level of cerebral blood flow in man with particular reference to carotid surgery. Circulation 49(6):1023–1025, 1974

18. Lassen NA, Wahl M, Deetjen P, et al: Regulation of cerebral arterilar diameter by extracellular pH variations in the perivascular fluid, in Ross RW (ed): Brain and Blood Flow. London, Pitman, 1971, pp 174–177

19. Tweed WA, Overgaard J: Cerebral hemodynamics and the effects of traumatic brain edema. Abstract, Lund Symposium, 1974

20. Frei HJ, Wallenfang T, Poll W, et al: Regional cerebral blood flow and regional metabolism in cold induced edema. Acta Neurochir 29:15–28, 1973

21. Go KG, Zijlstr WG, Flanderijn H, et al: Circulatory factors influencing exudation in cold induced cerebral edema. Exp Neurol 42:332–338, 1974

22. Johansson B, Choh-Luh L, Olsson Y, et al: The effect of acute arterial hypertension on the blood-brain barrier to protein tracers. Acta Neuropathol (Berl) 16:117–124, 1970

23. Klatzo I: Some early reactions of brain tissue to injury, in Head Injuries. Proceedings of the Int Symposium, held in Edinburgh and Madrid, April 1970, Churchill Livingstone, 1971, pp 214–221

24. Klatzo I: Pathophysiological aspects of brain edema, in Reulen HJ, Schurmann K (eds): New York, Springer-Verlag, 1972, pp 1–8

25. Klatzo I: Pathophysiology of brain edema—pathological aspect, in Schurmann K, Brock M, Reulen HJ, Voth D (eds): Advances in Neurosurgery 1. New York, Springer-Verlag, 1973, pp 1–4

26. Klatzo I: Neuropathological mechanisms in brain injury. Recent Progress in Neurosurgery. ICS 320, pp 310–311. Amsterdam, Excerpta Medica, 1974

27. Pappius HM: Biochemical studies on experimental brain edema, in Klatzo I, Seitelberger F (eds): Proceedings of the Symposium, September 11–13, 1965. Vienna, Springer, 1967, pp 445–460

28. Poll W, Brock M, Markakis E, et al: Brain tissue pressure, in Brock M, Dietz H (eds): Intracranial Pressure. New York, Springer, 1972, pp 188–194

29. Schutta HS, Kassell NF, Langfitt TW: Brain swelling produced by injury and aggravated by arterial hypertension. Brain 91:281–294, 1968

30. Crockard HA: Bullet injuries of the brain. Ann R Coll Surg Engl 55:111–123, 1974

31. Nakatani S, Ommaya AK: A critical rate of cerebral compression, in Broc M, Dietz H (eds): Intracranial Pressure. New York, Springer, 1972, pp 144–148

32. Jennett WB: Intracranial pressure measurements in clinical practice. Adv Neurosurg 1:52–56, 1973. Springer

33. Miller JD: Studies of intracranial pressure and volume in patients with head injury. J Neurosurg Sci, vol. 17, nr. 4: 217–223, 1973

34. Taylor AR: The immediate care of the acutely head injured. Recent Progress in Neurological Surgery. ICS 320, pp 312–315. Amsterdam, Excerpta Medica, 1974

Derek A. Bruce, M.D.
Thomas W. Langfitt, M.D.

3

The Prognostic Value of ICP, CPP, CBF, and CMRO$_2$ in Head Injury

This is a brief review of our data on intracranial pressure (ICP), cerebral profusion pressure (CPP), cerebral blood flow (CBF), and cerebral metabolic rate for oxygen (CMRO$_2$) in 35 comatose patients, most of them with head injuries.[1] We have reviewed the data to see if there are trends that will help us in deciding the ultimate prognosis for a given patient early in the course of head injury.

Patients with a mass lesion had a significantly higher ICP than those with no mass.[1] The CBF and CMRO$_2$ were not significantly different between the groups, although the mean values of both were lower in the former group. The mortality rate was 50 percent in the mass lesion group and 40 percent in those without a mass. The presence or absence of autoregulation had no prognostic significance nor did the response to mannitol.

Table 1 shows the initial measurements of CPP, CBF, and CMRO$_2$ as a function of the ICP at the time of the initial study. Note the similarity in results for the CBF (mean flow), f$_g$ (gray matter flow), and w$_g$ (gray matter weight) between the groups. The only parameter that shows a progressive change with rising ICP is the CMRO$_2$. The difference does not become statistically significant, but this may be because of the small number of patients in this group. It is interesting to speculate why the CMRO$_2$ should be so out of phase with the CBF in the over 35 mm Hg group. We found that it was the group with high ICP and low CMRO$_2$ who showed the greatest increase in CMRO$_2$ after mannitol administration. This may

Supported by NIH Grant NS 08803-05

suggest that edema, causing the high ICP, has a greater effect on oxygen extraction than on blood flow. No greater proportion of patients with ICP over 35 mm Hg died than with ICP under 35 mm Hg.

To see if we could identify which parameter had best prognostic value, we tabulated first studies of ICP, CPP, CBF, and CMRO$_2$ in 15 patients with severely disturbed consciousness from head injury without any history of hypoxia or shock. Table 2 shows the results. The difference in ICP between the two groups is striking although it just fails to reach statistical significance. Thus, our results tend to agree with those of Vapalhati et al.[2] In any individual patient, however, the trend was not helpful since the lowest ICP in the mortality group was 24 mm Hg and the highest in the survivors was 77 mm Hg. The CPP, CBF, and CMRO$_2$ were all lower in the group who died, but all of these failed to reach statistically significant levels of difference. The actual values were not helpful in any single patient. The highest CBF was 46 ml/100 g/min in the mortality group and the

Table 1
First Studies on 34 Comatose Patients

ICP	20	20–35	35
CPP	80	73	66
CBF	39	40	35
CMRO$_2$	2.06	1.65	1.40
f$_g$	57	59	58
w$_g$	49	46	45

Note: None of the parameters showed a significant difference.

Table 2
Acutely Head Injured Patients

	Lived	$n = 11$	Died	$n = 6$	p<
ICP	33 ± 7.9		68 ± 17		.10
CPP	68 ± 7.1		46 ± 8		n.s.
CBF	41 ± 2.5		31 ± 7.5		n.s.
$CMRO_2$	1.5 ± .20		1.09 ± .63		n.s.

Note: Initial studies in comatose or semicomatose patients: mean ±s.e..

lowest 32 ml/100 g/min in the survivors. Of perhaps greater importance are the findings related to $CMRO_2$. Shalit[3] has stated that the $CMRO_2$ of less than 1 ml/100 g/min is not compatible with survival. Two patients in the survival group had $CMRO_2$ of less than 1 (.76 ml/100 g/min and .87 ml/100 g/min). Two had $CMRO_2$ of 1.0 ml/100 g/min and 1.15 ml/100 g/min. In these patients, the mean ICP was 49 mm Hg and the mean CBF was 36 ml/100 g/min. We believe that these data plus the above suggest that the $CMRO_2$ is not a good indicator of survival potential, especially if the ICP is high.

It is not uncommon for us to be faced with a patient in a coma from a head injury who has also had either a cardiac arrest and resuscitation, severe hypoxia, or shock added to the injury. If there is no improvement over 24 hours, the question of primary injury due to trauma or secondary injury due to hypoxia, ischemia, or shock becomes important in deciding what supportive therapy should be continued. We have had the opportunity of studying 7 such patients. Table 3 shows the results of $CMRO_2$ and CBF measurements. We have calculated the ratio of $CMRO_2$ over CBF in each patient ($AVDO_2$). The ratio is not less than 50 percent of normal in the group of patients who either survived or at autopsy had a deep midline and brain stem hemorrhage but intact cortical structures. In both patients who had severe neocortical damage presumably secondary to ischemia rather than head injury, the ratio was less than 30 percent. The numbers are small, but we believe this flow metabolism mismatch is a useful sign of early diffuse neocortical damage and would like to see further patients studied to see if this trend is consistent. Unfortunately, these studies give us no information whether the brain stem lesion has caused irreversible damage or not.

In summary, ICP, CPP, CBF, and $CMRO_2$ may be useful in helping to predict outcome in a large group of patients. However, for any individual patient these studies do not help. The $CMRO_2$ has been shown to be the least useful parameter, especially when the ICP is high. It is suggested that the ratio of $CMRO_2$ to CBF ($AVDO_2$) is useful in distinguishing diffuse neocortical damage from brain stem damage.

Table 3
Cortical vs Brainstem Injury

	Patients with flow metabolism missmatch				Patients with flow metabolism match		
	$CMRO_2$	CBF	$\dfrac{CMRO_2}{CBF}$		$CMRO_2$	CBF	$\dfrac{CMRO_2}{CBF}$
1	1.32	77	.027	1	2.1	34	.062
2	1.42	114	.012	2	1.6	31	.052
				3	2.56	41	.062
				4	2.68	30	.089
				5	1.43	36	.040

Normal value for $\dfrac{CMRO_2}{CBF} = \dfrac{3.5}{50} = .07 (AVDO_2)$

Both patients with ratios of 50% of normal had diffuse cortical necrosis at autopsy. Three patients with ratio 50% died, all showed evidence of deep, thalamic, hypothalamic and brainstem petichiae with preservation of the cortex.

REFERENCES

1. Bruce DA, Langfitt TW, Miller JD, et al: Regional cerebral blood flow, intracranial pressure and brain metabolism in comatose patients. J Neurosurg 38:131–144, 1973
2. Vapalhati, M: Intracranial pressure, acid base status of blood and cerebrospinal fluid, and pulmonary function in the prognosis of severe head injury. Thesis, Melsinki, 1970
3. Shalit MN, Beller AJ, Feinsod NM, Zeigler M, Cotev S: Critical values for cerebral oxygen utilization in man, in Russel R (ed): Brain and Blood Flow. London, Pitman, 1971, pp 130–135

D. P. Becker, M.D., J. K. Vries, M.D.
R. Sakalas, M.D., H. F. Young, M.D.
J. Ward, M.D.

4

Early Prognosis in Head Injury Based on Motor Posturing, Oculocephalic Reflexes, and Intracranial Pressure

The ability to prognosticate ultimate outcome in severe head injury early after the injury is a prerequisite to evaluation of new therapies and determining proper management decisions in individual patients. If the location and extents (volume) of the injured brain can be defined early after injury, prognosis may be more simply defined.

Utilizing this concept we have evaluated the neurological examination and intracranial pressure (ICP) level as providers of predictive power. Concerning critical deep localization of injury, the motor exam (posturing) and neurophthalmological exam (oculocephalic reflexes) are important.[1,2] ICP may be an indicator of volume of supratentorial injury. Our study shows that early knowledge of these three bits of information can usually permit a reliable prediction of outcome in broad categories.

METHODS

This study includes 100 consecutive patients who fulfilled the following criteria. The patients were seen by us within 4 hours of severe head injury. They could not follow more than one-stage commands because of a disordered level of consciousness. Patients with multiple injuries were included. Patients who fulfilled the criteria of brain death in the emergency room were excluded.

These patients were managed in a standardized fashion. A twist drill ICP measurement and limited ventriculogram was performed after stabilization of vital signs and an adequate airway.

Intracranial masses were promptly treated surgically (elevated ICP, ventricular shift >0.4 cm). Controlled ventilation (rate 10–12/min, tidal volume 15 cc/kg) was utilized with PaO_2 maintained above 70 and $PaCO_2$ between 25 and 30 mm Hg. Patients were maintained in metabolic balance and at normothermia and steroids were administered. ICP was monitored chronically. Other therapy was added only for elevating ICP (over 25–40 mm Hg) associated with clear neurological deterioration. This therapy included, in usual order, increased hyperventilation, ventricular drainage, lowering of cerebral perfusion pressure, chronic mannitol, and hypothermia.

Outcome is defined in five broad categories as follows: excellent—return to premorbid level of socioeconomic performance; good—independent, but performing at downgraded level; poor—able to feed and clothe self but otherwise dependent; negative—totally or almost totally dependent for care; and dead. Outcome was determined from 4 months to $2\frac{1}{2}$ years after the injury, with most patients being at 1 to $2\frac{1}{2}$ years postinjury.

RESULTS

Diffuse Cerebral Injury

Ultimate result in two broad categories (excellent-good and poor-vegetative-dead) correlated well with information concerning two aspects of the neurological examination (posturing and integrity of oculocephalic reflexes) and ICP level

Table 1

Severe Mechanical Brain Injury Diffuse Cerebral Injury with normal ICP
(<11 mm Hg) at Admission

	Ultimate Result					
	Excellent	*Good*	*Poor*	*Veg*	*Dead*	*Total*
No posturing—O.C. intact	9	1				10
Posturing—O.C. intact	2	2				4
Posturing—O.C. impaired			2	1	1	4
Total						18

Key: Posturing = Decorticate or decerebrate rigidity.   O.C. = Oculocephalic reflex.

(Tables 1 and 2). Thus, in diffuse cerebral injury with no posturing and intact oculocephalic reflexes, patients all did well regardless of level of ICP. If posturing was present and oculocephalic reflexes impaired or absent, patients did poor or worse regardless of level of ICP.

It was in the group of patients with posturing and intact oculocephalic reflexes that ICP added predictive power. Thus, in this group, if ICP was normal (under 11 mm Hg), our patients ended up good or excellent. However, all patients with elevated ICP ended up poor, vegetative, or dead.

Acute Major Intracranial Mass
(36 Patients)

Patients in this group all had elevated ICP in the emergency room. In more than half, the ICP was over 30 mm Hg (see chapter by Becker et al., p. 157). All had midline shifts of 0.4 cm or more. Ultimate result correlated well with two aspects of the neurological examination, specifically motor posturing and oculocephalic reflexes. Examinations are reported as they appeared prior to surgical evacuation of masses.

In acute epidural hematoma (Table 3), acute subdural hematoma (Table 4), or acute major intracerebral hematoma or contusion (Table 5), a good result correlated with no posturing and intact oculocephalic reflexes. Likewise, if there was posturing present, but oculocephalic reflexes were *intact,* a good result could be expected if masses were promptly removed. In the group with posturing and impaired or absent oculocephalic reflexes, most patients ended up poor or worse. However, with prompt treatment, 3 out of 14 patients in this group had a good result. Table 6 summarizes the results in patients with acute intracranial mass lesions.

DISCUSSION

In patients with diffuse cerebral injury (no major focal mass) resulting in depression of level of consciousness, often the neurological examination alone could predict outcome. Patients with no posturing and oculocephalic reflexes intact should do well. Patients with posturing and oculocephalic reflexes impaired or absent almost always do poorly.

Table 2

Severe Mechanical Brain Injury
Diffuse Cerebral Injury with *Elevated* ICP (11 mm Hg or more) at Admission

	Ultimate Result					
	Excellent	*Good*	*Poor*	*Veg*	*Dead*	*Total*
No posturing—O.C. intact	18	2				20
Posturing—O.C. intact			5	2	4	11
Posturing—O.C. impaired		1	4	1	9	15
Total						46

Key: Posturing = Decorticate or decerebrate rigidity.   O.C. = Oculocephalic reflexes.

Table 3
Acute Epidural Hematoma
Result Related to Posturing and Oculocephalic Reflexes

	Excellent	Good	Poor	Veg	Dead	Total
No posturing—O.C. intact	4					4
Posturing—O.C. intact	1					1
Posturing—O.C. impaired					1	1
Totals	5				1	6

Table 4
Acute Subdural Hematoma
Result Related to Posturing and Oculocephalic Reflexes

	Excellent	Good	Poor	Veg	Dead	Total
No posturing—O.C. intact		1			1*	2
Posturing—O.C. intact	2	1				3
Posturing—O.C. impaired		2	1		8	11
No Posturing—O.C. impaired			1			1
Totals	2	4	2		9	17

*Error in therapy.

Table 5
Acute Major Intracerebral Hematoma—Contusion
Result Related to Posturing and Oculocephalic Reflexes

	Excellent	Good	Poor	Veg	Dead	Total
No posturing—O.C. intact	2	6			1*	9
Posturing—O.C. intact		1				1
Posturing—O.C. impaired		1			1	2
No posturing—O.C. impaired	1					1
Totals	3	8	0	0	2	13

*Error in therapy.

Table 6
Severe Mechanical Brain Injury
Acute Intracranial Major Mass—ICP > 11 mm Hg
(Subdural, Epidural, Intracerebral)

	Ultimate Result					
	Excellent	*Good*	*Poor*	*Veg*	*Dead*	*Total*
No posturing—O.C. intact	6	7			2*	15
Posturing—O.C. intact	3	2				5
Posturing—O.C. impaired		3	1		10	14
No posturing—O.C. impaired	1		1			2

Key: Posturing = Decorticate or decerebrate rigidity.
     O.C. = Oculocephalic reflexes.
     * = Errors in therapy.

However, in patients with posturing and intact oculocephalic reflexes, the result may be excellent to dead. But if one adds ICP information to this group, we find that normal ICP correlates with a good recovery and high ICP correlates with a poor recovery. We reason that ICP provides predictive power here as it yields some information concerning the volume of the supratentorial brain injury. Thus, patients in this group (posturing, intact oculocephalic reflexes), all have posterior diencephalic and/or upper brain stem injuries accounting for their motor pictures. This brain stem injury is limited in extent, as oculocephalic reflexes were intact. The patients with normal ICP have only a limited degree of supratentorial brain injury, without swelling or edema. Since their injury is limited in degree and extent, their recovery is good. The patients with elevated ICP have, in addition to their diencephalic upper brain stem injury, a rather extensive supratentorial brain injury causing increased ICP from increased intracranial volume. Since their brain injury is extensive in volume in addition to including a critical deep location, these patients end up poor or worse with present-day standard but intensive therapy.

All patients in our series with acute major intracranial masses had elevated ICP, many in the range of 50 to 70 mm Hg. However, result did not correlate here with ICP, but rather with the neurological examination. In this case, elevated ICP usually related to an extracerebral mass or a focal intracerebral mass. The neurological examination better defined the locus of the intrinsic injury. But even with elevated ICP, patients here did well with or without decorticate or decerebrate posturing as long as oculocephalic reflexes were intact. However, if oculocephalic reflexes were impaired or absent, patients tended to do poorly. Yet even in this group there were good results, so therapy must be aggressive. We feel the most important message here is that the earlier major masses are evacuated, the better will be the result. It is undesirable to wait for the neurological signs of progressive posturing and a dilated pupil to occur. Rather, results should be better if the masses are recognized, defined, and removed before severe brain compression and very major brain shift occurs.

SUMMARY

1. In severe head injury, knowledge of both the ICP and neurological examination provides strong predictive power just after admission.
2. Important aspects of the neurological examination in prognosis are motor posturing (flexor or extensor) and oculocephalic reflexes.
3. Knowledge of these three bits of information (ICP, posturing, and oculocephalic reflexes) can almost always predict outcome in broad categories.

REFERENCES

1. Fisher CM: General examination of the comatose patient. Acta Neurol Scand Suppl. 35–40, 1968–1969

2. Plum F, Posner JD: Diagnosis of Stupor and Coma (ed 2). F. A. Davis Co., 1972

George T. Tindall, M.D.
Alan S. Fleischer, M.D.

5

Intracranial Pressure (ICP) Monitoring and Prognosis in Closed Head Injury

It is generally accepted that continuous monitoring of ICP in patients with severe craniocerebral trauma facilitates their management. Elevated ICP reflects increased intracranial volume and may indicate the need for appropriate medical or surgical therapy. In addition, continuous ICP measurement monitors the effectiveness of treatment and, according to some investigators, may also provide some indication of prognosis. However, the relationship between the level of ICP and prognosis following head trauma has not been established with certainty, with some conflict present in the reported results. Troupp[1] and Vapalahti[2] have presented data which show that head injury patients with marked ICP elevations have a higher mortality than patients with normal ICP. On the other hand, Jennett's[3,4] results indicate that outcome may have no correlation with levels of ICP. Likewise, Bruce et al.[5] found that ICP does not correlate well with the severity of brain injury measured by clinical criteria except at extremely high levels. These observations have derived primarily from studying series of patients with craniocerebral trauma of various degrees associated with heterogenous intracranial pathology including intra- and extracerebral hematomas, cerebral contusions, primary brain stem injury, etc. In the present study, a group of 23 patients with severe closed head injury with no angiographic evidence of mass lesion underwent continuous ICP monitoring. The study was carried out to determine whether or not clinical presentation and ICP in this relatively homogenous group of patients could be correlated with prognosis.

PATIENTS AND METHODS

From January 1 to December 31, 1974, a total of 351 patients with severe craniocerebral trauma were admitted to Grady Memorial Hospital, Atlanta, Georgia. Clinical grading was performed shortly following admission according to the classification shown in Table 1. Cerebral

Table 1
Grades of Stupor and Coma

Grade	State of Awareness
I	Drowsy, lethargic, indifferent, uninterested and/or belligerent and uncooperative; does not lapse into sleep when left undisturbed.
II	Stuporous; will lapse into sleep when not disturbed; may be disoriented to time, place, and person.
III	Deep stupor—requires strong pain to evoke movement. May have focal neurological signs but will respond appropriately to noxious stimuli.
IV	Does not respond appropriately to any stimuli; may exhibit decerebrate or decorticate posturing; retains deep tendon reflexes. May have dilated pupil, absent corneal, or oculocephalic reflexes. Breathing spontaneously.
V	Does not respond appropriately to any stimuli; flaccid—no deep tendon reflexes. May breathe spontaneously.

Table 2

Outcome of 23 Patients with Severe Closed Head Injury Without
Angiographically Demonstrated Mass Lesion

Age	ICP	Functioning Normally in Preinjury Capacity *Coma Grade*			Vegetative *Coma Grade*			Death *Coma Grade*		
		III	IV	V	III	IV	V	III	IV	V
Below 30	High ICP	1	1						1	1
years of age	Low ICP	3	1			1				
Over 30	High ICP					1		1		
years of age	Low ICP	3				4			4	1

angiography was obtained immediately on almost all of these patients and the appropriate surgery carried out shortly thereafter on 117 patients. Of these 351 patients, 45 had continuous ICP monitoring instituted early in their hospitalization for periods ranging from 5 days to 2 weeks. All patients monitored were classified Grade III coma or worse and manifested various forms of traumatic intracranial pathology. Twenty-three of these monitored patients had no demonstrable mass lesion on angiography, had no surgery, and are the subject of this report.

ICP was monitored using an intraventricular cannula attached to a subcutaneously implanted Rickham reservoir as recently described.[6] A 23-gauge needle with a soft catheter attached (Abbott butterfly) is inserted percutaneously into the Rickham reservoir and connected to a Statham pressure transducer for pressure recording and is changed frequently to reduce the incidence of infection.

Intracranial pressure was considered elevated if it exceeded 20 mm Hg or if preplateau or plateau waves were present. Elevated ICP in this group of patients was treated with various methods, including hyperventilation, glucosteroids, osmotic diuretics (mannitol 20), and ventricular CSF aspiration.

RESULTS

The outcome in these 23 patients with relation to age, clinical presentation, and ICP is presented in Table 2. Vegetative survival and death occurred more frequently in those patients over age 30 (Table 3) and was significantly higher in patients presenting in Grade IV and V coma (Table 4). Table 5 reveals the lack of correlation between clinical presentation and ICP and the preponderance of normal ICP in all coma grades in this group of patients. In addition, there is no apparent relationship between ICP and prognosis (Table 6).

DISCUSSION

Poor prognosis following severe head injury has generally been considered related to

Table 3

Relationship of Age to Prognosis
in 23 Patients with Severe
Closed Head Injury

Age (years)	Functional Survival	Vegetative Death
Less than 30	6	3
Greater than 30	3	11

$\chi^2 = 4.8$
$p < 0.05$

Table 4

Relationship of Clinical Presentation
(Coma Grade) to Prognosis

Clinical Presentation	Functional Survival	Vegetative Death
Coma III	7	1
Coma IV and V	2	13

$\chi^2 = 18.26$
$p < 0.05$

structural alterations in the brain caused by increased ICP. Sevitt,[7] in an autopsy study, implicated transtentorial herniation of the hippocampal uncus as the cause of death in 34 percent of 250 patients dying following automobile accidents. This finding would suggest that a significant increase in ICP occurred in these patients. Adams and Graham[8] confirmed that distortion and herniation of the brain are in fact equated with increased ICP and demonstrated that pathological changes in the brain correlated with the level of ICP. In addition, some authors have emphasized the correlation between the level of ICP after injury and mortality.[1,2]

Jennett et al.[3,4] recently suggested, however, that normal ICP need not be favorable in severe head injury. When associated with signs of brain dysfunction such as decerebration, it may indicate primary brain stem injury, or severe, primary white matter damage, which is likely to lead to a persistent vegetative state if the patient survives. He emphasized that a major value of ICP monitoring in head trauma was the ability to recognize that ICP may be normal in these patients regardless of the degree of the neurological deficit following brain injury.

In our relatively homogenous series of head trauma patients with no intracranial mass lesion demonstrated angiographically, the degree of neurological impairment is clearly not related to the level of ICP. Approximately 75 percent of these patients had normal ICP, equally distributed among patients presenting with coma Grades III, IV, and V. Although all these patients were severely injured, only 25 percent manifested increased ICP. In addition to being clinically indistinguishable from those patients with normal ICP, the group with elevated ICP demonstrated no significant difference in ultimate outcome. The 6 patients with elevated ICP did no worse overall than the 17 patients with normal ICP. Conversely, although the elevated ICP in these patients was adequately treated whenever present, this afforded no advantage with regard to final outcome. This trend, although reflected in a small series of patients suggests that the level of ICP may not be a primary factor in determining outcome in this variety of head trauma. It is conceivable that elevated ICP may be superimposed in these instances where it is present on a diffuse brain injury common to all of these patients, regardless of ICP, which is the determining factor of the outcome. The only apparent reliable indicators of poor prognosis in this series of patients include advancing age and the clinical evidence of brain stem dysfunction.

While the results of the present study and those of some other investigators imply that the level of ICP does not clearly correlate with either clinical presentation or prognosis in severe head injury, the authors nevertheless believe that more clinical data are necessary before definitive conclusions in this regard can be reached. The computation of volume-pressure relationships may provide more important additional information that may enhance the value of continuous monitoring of ICP.[9]

Although there are definite risks, i.e., CNS infection associated with continuous ICP recording, they can be kept low with diligent care and attention to the technique of ICP monitoring. However, if it can be shown that elevated levels of ICP show little correlation with clinical presentation or prognosis in severe head injury, no matter how adequately the elevated ICP is treated, particularly when the presence of a mass lesion has been excluded by angiography and/or EMI scan, then the practice of ICP monitoring in head injury patients should be discontinued.

Table 5

Relationship of Clinical Presentation (Coma Grade) to ICP

Clinical Presentation	High ICP	Low ICP
Coma III	2	6
Coma IV and V	4	11

$\chi^2 < 1$

p ns

Table 6

Relationship of ICP to Prognosis

ICP	Functional Survival	Vegetative Death
Low	7	10
High	2	4

$\chi^2 = 1.94$

p ns

REFERENCES

1. Troupp H: Intraventricular pressure in patients with severe brain injuries. J Trauma 7(6):875–883, 1967
2. Vapalahti M, Troupp H: Prognosis for patients with severe brain injuries. Br Med J 3:404–407, 1971
3. Jennett B, Johnston IH: The uses of intracranial pressure monitoring in clinical management, in Brock M, Dietz H (eds): Intracranial Pressure. Berlin, Springer-Verlag, 1972, pp 353–356
4. Johnston IH, Johnston JA, Jennett B: Intracranial-pressure changes following head injury. Lancet 2:433–436, 1970
5. Bruce DA, Langfitt TW, Miller JD, et al: Regional cerebral blood flow, intracranial pressure, and brain metabolism in comatose patients. J Neurosurg, 38:131–144, 1973
6. Fleischer AS, Patton JM, Tindall GT: Intraventricular pressure monitoring using an implanted reservoir in head-injured patients—technical note. Surg Neurol 3:309–311, 1975
7. Sevitt S: Fatal road accidents. Injuries, complications and causes of death in 250 subjects. Br J Surg 55:481–505, 1968
8. Adams H, Graham DI: The relationship between ventricular fluid pressure and the neuropathology of raised intracranial pressure, in Brock M, Dietz H (eds): Intracranial Pressure. Berlin, Springer-Verlag, 1972, pp 250–253
9. Miller JD, Baribi J: Intracranial volume/pressure relationships during continuous monitoring of ventricular fluid pressure, in Brock M, Dietz H (eds): Intracranial Pressure. Berlin, Springer-Verlag, 1972, pp 270–274

William K. Hass, M.D.

6

Prognostic Value of Cerebral Oxidative Metabolism in Head Trauma

The objectives of the New York University Head Trauma Clinical Center have been to quantify major physiological parameters which are altered during head trauma; to identify those parameters which correlate closely with a poor or lethal prognosis; to develop hypotheses concerning the mechanism of development of the physiological abnormalities and to test these in experimental animal models; and to attempt in the experimental models to return the observed abnormalities toward more normal levels based on observations concerning their mode of development.

A conviction, a faith if you will, that cerebral oxidative metabolism ($CMRO_2$) was a more primary problem in head injury than cerebral blood flow (CBF) per se led us to the development of the clinical mass spectrometer which permits a continuous in vivo readout of blood gases for significant periods of time, without drawing blood, from the jugular bulb and from any systemic artery simultaneously.[1,2,3] The technique also permits concurrent measurement of a diffusable gaseous indicator in the mass range scanned, between mass 28 for nitrogen and mass 45 for carbon dioxide. Argon was found to be a highly appropriate, freely diffusable gas for this purpose and a brain-blood partition coefficient of 1.1 was established indirectly by simultaneous measurements of uptake and washout curves for nitrous oxide and argon.[4] This permitted at approximately 18-minute intervals serial determinations of CBF and oxidative metabolism since oxygen levels

could be continuously monitored at the jugular bulb and in any artery, *continuously,* along with nitrogen, argon, and carbon dioxide. The technique is thus an adaptation of Kety's classic method using the Fick principle for the safe continuous recording of changes in CBF and oxidative metabolism in head injured patients.

Forty-five patients were studied at an average period of 7 days after head injury. The patients were grouped into four definable levels of cerebral function; I—alert, II—lethargic or alert with focal neurologic symptoms, III—Stuporous or in coma without definitive signs of brain stem dysfunction, and IV—coma with clear cut brain stem signs such as decerebration, pupillary, or extra ocular muscle movement abnormality or respiratory changes typical of primary and/or secondary brain stem dysfunction.

The vast majority of patients suffered from closed head injuries which occurred in or near the New York University-Bellevue Medical Center. Only uncommonly do we see high velocity, highway accidents. Only 3 patients are included who suffered missile injuries to the brain. All patients at the time of study had received definitive surgical and/or medical therapy designed to reduce increased intracranial pressure. Indeed, subsequent studies of a group of similar patients using an epidural Numoto switch revealed that intracranial pressures in this group of patients are generally below 25 mm/Hg, usually at the level of 15 mm/Hg.

The outstanding findings were a fall of *mean* CBF values from normal in the Group I to only 2/3 of normal in Group IV. On the other hand mean values for $CMRO_2$ were never in the normal

This project was supported by Grant NSO7366 from the National Institute of Neurological Diseases and Stroke.

Table 1

N.Y.U. Primary Cerebral Blood Flow (CBF) and Cerebral Oxidative Metabolism (CMRO$_2$) Data in 45 Head Injured Patients. CMRO$_2$ differences between Group I plus Group II and Group III plus Group IV significant, p < 0.01. CMRO$_2$ differences between Group III and Group IV significant, p < 0.1. CBF differences between Group I plus II and Group III plus IV significant, p < 0.2. No significant differences in mean arterial pressure (MAP), apH, aPCO$_2$ or aPO$_2$. aPO$_2$ values include patients spontaneously respiring ambient O$_2$ or supplemental O$_2$ where necessary.

	Group I (7 Patients)	Group II (12 Patients)	Group III (13 Patients)	Group IV (13 Patients)
CBF (cc/100 g/min)	52.5	49.6	39.6	36.7
Range	(39.2–70.4)	(31.4–117)	(16.2–63.8)	(12.0–85.4)
S.D.	13.1	26.1	31.7	19.5
S.E.M.	6.6	7.5	3.8	5.4
CMRO$_2$ (ccO$_2$/100 g/min)	2.66	2.38*	1.90	1.36
Range	(12.20–3.15)	(1.61–4.8)	(0.46–3.13)	(0.12–2.12)
S.D.	0.30	0.88	0.79	0.62
S.E.M.	0.12	0.26	0.22	0.07
MAP (mm/Hg)	109	101*	96.5+	109
Range	(90–124)	(95–123)	(57–137)	(80–147)
S.D.	14	7	19.4	24
S.E.M.	5	2	5.6	7
apH	7.50	7.52	7.53	7.51
Range	(7.47–7.55)	(7.38–7.66)	(7.42–7.63)	(7.37–7.62)
S.D.	0.06	0.07	0.05	0.07
S.E.M.	0.02	0.02	0.01	0.02
aPCO$_2$ (torr)	35.4	33.5	33.4	30.6
Range	(28.4–41.0)	(27.4–44.0)	(25.4–55.0)	(22.3–42.0)
S.D.	3.6	5.7	7.1	9.2
S.E.M.	1.4	1.6	1.9	1.4
aPO$_2$ (torr)	69.6	73.1	72.0	72.2
Range	(48.5–90.0)	(31.5–100)	(34.0–175)	(42.0–145)
S.D.	11.9	17.2	34.3	26.2
S.E.M.	4.5	4.8	9.5	7.3

*Includes only 11 of 12 patients.
†Includes only 12 of 13 patients.

range, being 80 percent of normal in Group I and falling in Group IV to 40 percent of normal (Table 1).

The proportionately greater diminution of CMRO$_2$ as compared to CBF particularly in the patients in Group IV with coma and brain stem signs was striking. Further, no essential change in mean CMRO$_2$ could be demonstrated in selected Group III or Group IV patients during hyperoxia; during elevation of mean arterial blood pressure (MAP) with meteraminol bitartrate or with hypercarbia in spite of uniform, often sharp

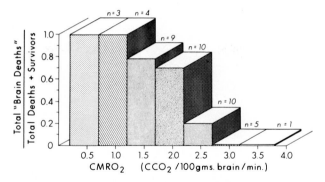

Fig. 1. Relationship of $CMRO_2$ values to deaths attributable directly to the head injury.

increases in CBF in association with increased arterial PCO_2.

Death attributable to the head injury itself, what we refer to as "brain deaths" and what others have referred to as "neurological fatalities" and define as patients who die without recovery of consciousness, claimed 100 percent of the patients when the $CMRO_2$ was below 1.2 cc/100 g/min. The brain death ratio was 75 percent if the $CMRO_2$ was 1.2–2.2. It fell to 20 percent if the $CMRO_2$ was 2.2–2.7 and to zero if the $CMRO_2$ was greater than 2.7 (Fig. 1).

The findings suggested that brain stem injury was related to the persistant supression of $CMRO_2$ and, based on the observations of Ingvar, that destruction of the reticular core *per se* decreased overall cerebral metabolism.[5,6]

Clearly, as a prognostic indicator, our findings are in agreement with those of Shalit that low $CMRO_2$ values are almost invariably poor prognostic signs.[7] This is particularly true if these values are obtained a few days after injury when intracranial pressures are known to be in the normal or near normal range and cerebral perfusion pressures appear adequate.

REFERENCES

1. Hass WK, Siew FP, Yee DJ: Progress in adaptation of mass spectrometer to study of human cerebral blood flow. Circulation 38:IV–94, 1968

2. Wald A, Hass WK, Siew FP, et al: Continuous measurements of blood gases in vivo by mass spectrography. Med Biol Eng 8:111–128, 1970

3. Wald A, Hass WK, Ransohoff J: Experience with a mass spectrometer system for blood gas analysis in humans. J Assoc Adv Med Instrum 5:325–342, 1971

4. Hass WK, Wald A, Ransohoff J, et al: Argon and nitrous oxide cerebral blood flow simultaneously monitored by mass spectrometry in patients with head injury. Eur Neurol 8:164–168, 1972

5. Ingvar DH, Haggendal E, Nilsson NS, et al: Cerebral circulation and metabolism in a comatose patient. Arch Neurol 11:13–21, 1964

6. Ingvar DH, Sorander P: Destruction of the reticular core of the brain stem; a patho-anatomical follow-up of a case of coma of three year's duration. Arch Neurol 23:1–8, 1970

7. Shalit MN, Beller AJ, Feinsod M: Clinical equivalents of cerebral oxygen consumption in coma. Neurology 22:155–160, 1972

Gleb N. Budzilovich, M.D.

7

On Pathogenesis of Primary Lesions in Blunt Head Trauma with Special Reference to the Brain Stem Injuries

The purpose of this necessarily brief communication is to describe primary traumatic injuries encountered in the brain stem of subjects dying acutely with or from craniocerebral trauma sustained mostly, but not exclusively, as a result of motor vehicle-related accidents. The illustrative material had been selected from a total of over 1000 cases of closed head trauma, personally examined by the writer in the course of the past several years. Furthermore, all findings presented and discussed below were derived from the study of material from those accident victims whose survival time was assessed as not exceeding a few minutes, at most, or whose death had been termed by witnesses as "instantaneous." Such a rapidity of fatal issue precluded further evolution of the primary lesions and development of secondary alterations; superimposition can make their exact retrospective differentiation difficult and, sometimes, impossible.

The basic lesions found in the brain stems of the victims of the acute injury were hemorrhages, which ranged from those demonstrable only with the aid of the microscope to the grossly visible ones. Failure to fully appreciate this has led to an underestimation of true incidence of the primary brain stem hemorrhages, as pointed out by Tomlinson[1] and resulted in divergence of data regarding their frequency as reported by different authors. Thus, Jellinger[2] described them in 43.5 percent of his cases, while Mayer[3] found them in 100 percent of cases comprising his series. Relative frequency of the brain stem involvement in our material was not determined.

As regards the distribution of the traumatic hemorrhages throughout the lower brain stem, the great majority of them were found in the periaqueductal gray, subjacent to the floor of the IV ventricle, in parts of the tegmentum of the midbrain deep to the lateral mesencephalic sulcus and, less often, along the ventrolateral borders of the midbrain, pons, and rarely, medulla. Most of the hemorrhages along the outer surfaces of the brain stem, as a rule, were located deep in the tissues only infrequently approaching the surface. Furthermore, majority of the periaqueductal hemorrhages were round or ovoid in shape, while those located more peripherally tended to be streaklike and their location coincided with the course of the perforating blood vessels supplying the brain stem[4] (Fig. 1).

Microscopically, many hemorrhages were clearly related to the small arteries, veins and/or capillaries, while in some others no such relationship could be ascertained in the plane of a given section (Fig. 2). While no serial or step sectioning had been utilized in the study of our material, the results of such studies by others are of interest. Thus, Krauland[5] and Mayer,[3] using serial sectioning techniques were able to identify torn arteries and veins as the source of the bleeding. Furthermore, according to Mayer,[3] the peripherally located hemorrhages are predominantly arterial, while those around the aqueduct and IV ventricle are venous in origin.

No general agreement exists regarding the pathogenesis of the primary brain stem lesions nor, to be noted in passing, of those of the ce-

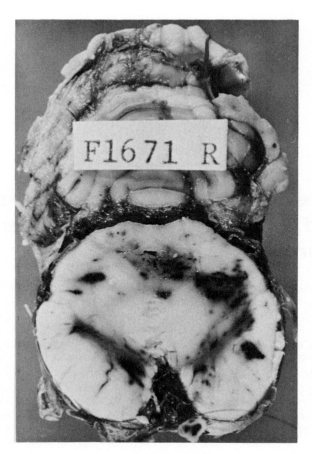

Fig. 1. Twenty-three-year-old male bicycle rider struck by auto. "Instant" death. Deep lacerations of the occipital (to the bone) and left parietal regions. Multiple fractures of the base of the skull. Dura intact. No subdural hematoma. The subarachnoid space over cerebrum and cerebellum focally filled with fresh blood clot. Viscera revealed nothing of note save for evidence of aspiration of blood. Midbrain. Fresh hemorrhages are present in the periaqueductal gray, lateral tegmentum, substantia nigra, and cerebral peduncles. (Similar hemorrhages, rapidly diminishing caudad were present in the tegmentum and basis pontis). All subsequent illustrations are from this case.

rebrum. Shearing strains were invoked by several authors,[3,4,6] some of whom, in addition, considered rotational movements of the brain stem as a significant contributory factor.[3]

On the other hand, it is a common knowledge that a caudad displacement of the mesencephalon and upper parts of the pons readily occurs under various circumstances, common to which is a sufficient rise in the intracranial pressure. Thus, it can easily be imagined that, especially in those instances of craniocerebral trauma in which an impact had caused a significant shortening of the vertical diameter of the skull, a momentary

caudad displacement, with or without a rotational component, of the brain stem can result in an avulsion and/or tearing of perforating blood vessels giving rise to hemorrhages described above. In our opinion, a caudad movement of the lower brain stem represents a major pathogenetic mechanism operating in the primary brain stem injury, the rotational component being of auxilliary significance. The role of the often invoked shearing strains appears to be unproved, since the pathological changes (presence of the axonal retraction bulbs) sometimes described in cases with prolonged survival as a proof of their effect

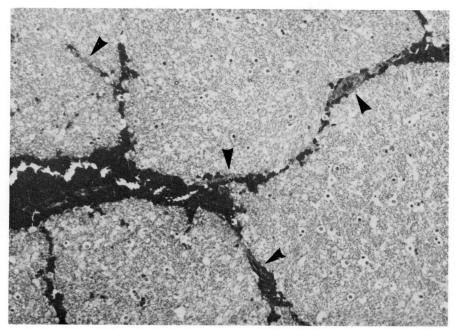

Fig. 2. Midbrain. A fresh hemorrhage along the course of branches of a short circumferential artery. Visible segments of the vessels are indicated by arrows. Azocarmine stain. (× 150.)

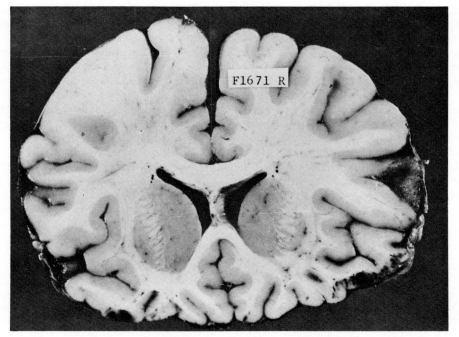

Fig. 3. Coronal section through frontal lobes. Fresh subarachnoid hemorrhage (left) and multiple intracortical hemorrhages (contusions) are seen in the subfrontal region. Note absence of grossly recognizable edema.

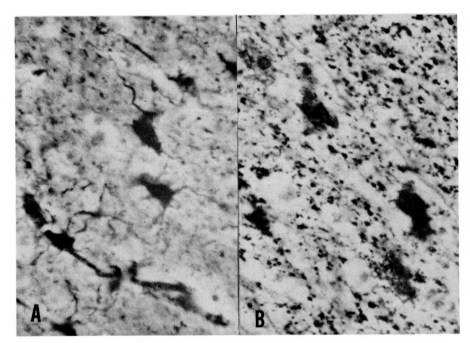

Fig. 4. Cerebral white matter. Note relatively good preservation of astrocytes in the arcuate zone (*a*) and their total disruption in the immediately subjacent deep white matter (*b*). Paraffin. Modified gold sublimate method for astrocytes. (× 400.)

may actually be due to local ischemia on the basis of vascular injury or represent Wallerian degeneration, reflecting presence of other traumatic lesions at the higher levels. It may also be added that the violence which is required to injure the relatively well-protected brain stem will practically always produce traumatic changes elsewhere in the brain (Fig. 3). Of these, diffuse cerebral edema, which, as we became aware in the course of the study of our acute cases, can be of an extremely rapid onset (minutes!), is likely to be one of the most injurious components in the complex of the trauma-induced alterations. The presence of the edema, which usually is not grossly apparent, was deduced on the basis of

characteristic degenerative changes of astroglia in the cerebral white matter as demonstrated by a modified gold sublimate technique.[7] The said changes are characterized by a relative preservation of the astrocytes in the subcortical arcuate zones and their severe degeneration in the deeper portions of the white matter, especially in the centrum ovale (Fig. 4), and are considered by some authors pathognomonic for the effects of acute cerebral edema.[8]

Although the pathogenesis of the rapidly developing diffuse cerebral edema in the acute craniocerebral trauma remains totally obscure, the clinical importance of being aware of such an early appearance cannot be overestimated.

REFERENCES

1. Tomlinson BE: Brain-stem lesions after head injury. J Clin Pathol 23, Suppl. (R Coll Pathol) 4:154–165, 1970
2. Jellinger K: Häufigkeit und Pathogenese zentraler Hirnläsionen nach stumpfer Gewalteinwirkung auf den Schädel. Wien Z Nervenheilkd 25:223–249, 1967
3. Mayer E Th: Zentrale Hirnschäden nach Einwirkung stumpfer Gewalt auf den Schädel. Arch Psychiatr Neurol 210:238–262, 1967
4. Hassler O: Arterial pattern of human brainstem. Normal appearance and deformation in expanding supratentorial conditions. Neurology 17:368–423, 1967

5. Krauland W: Über Hirnschäden durch stumpfe Gewalt. Dtsch Z Nervenheilkd 163:265–328, 1950
6. Crompton MR: Brainstem lesions due to closed head injury. Lancet 669–673, 1971
7. Naoumenko J, Feigin I: A modification for paraffin sections of the Cajal gold sublimate stain for astrocytes. J. Neuropathol Exp Neurol 20:602–604, 1961
8. Feigin I, Popoff N: Neuropathological observations on cerebral edema. Arch Neurol 6:151–160, 1962

Bryan Jennett, M.D., M.B., Ch.B.

8
Prognosis of Severe Head Injury

The prediction of outcome after severe head injury is required for two quite separate purposes. For comparing the efficacy of alternative management methods, it is adequate to know the predicted distribution of different outcomes in groups of patients identified by certain combinations of features. Statistically significant changes in the distribution of expected outcomes would indicate a treatment effect. For the clinician making management decisions, however, it is of only limited value to know that a given patient has features associated with, say, 80 percent mortality; the doctor needs to know the probability that his patient is in the 20 percent that will live, and if he does survive the probability of his making a reasonable recovery.

Plum has reported his experience with a series of patients with nontraumatic coma, in which there were certain combinations of features (absent oculovestibular reflex with motor response extensor or absent) associated with irrecoverability. Such cases were uncommon in our traumatic series, and seeking feature clusters associated exclusively with one outcome seems unlikely to solve the problem of prediction in more than a small number of extreme cases. Two alternative approaches seem to offer more promise. One is to use Bayesian probability statistics to compare the features of a newly occurring patient

with the features in a previously accumulated series of cases whose outcome is known; this allows the calculation of the probabilities that the new patient will reach each of the specified outcomes. We used this method to predict the outcome in 92 cases of traumatic coma, on the basis of data collected on 255 previous cases, using only clinical information available during the first 24 hours of coma. Outcomes were classified according to a recently described scale, already referred to by Dr. Plum.[1] All 21 patients predicted to have a bad outcome (dead or vegetative) were correctly predicted; but another 9 cases who were predicted to do better than this in fact died. This should cause no surprise, as there will always be patients with potential for good recovery, on the basis of their state in the first 24 hours, who may subsequently develop serious complications. The present system is not designed to predict such complications; it is concerned with identifying potential for recovery. The certainty of these predictions increases as more data is accumulated with the passage of time. When data from 1 to 3 days was available, the number of patients predicted with certainty ($p > 0.96$) increased from 21 to 63 percent as compared with data available in the first 24 hours. No further improvement resulted from the addition of data collected in the 4- to 7-day period.

The statistical method assumes that all items of data are independent, and it uses all the data available. By exploring and exploiting the dependence between some variables, it is likely that the amount of data required to reach predictions at a given certainty could be greatly reduced—this has been the experience of the statisticians involved with this project when they dealt with similar problems in other medical fields.[2] To de-

This study has been supported by the National Fund for Crippling Diseases and is currently supported by NIH Grant NO1-NS-4-2328.

Principal collaborators are Dr. Graham Teasdale (Department of Neurosurgery) and Dr. Robin Knill-Jones (Health Services Research Unit, Western Infirmary, Glasgow), and Dr. R. Braakman (Rotterdam), and Professor J. Minderhoud (Groningen).

termine these relationships requires a considerable computing effort, but the end result could be a simplification of the predictive scheme to a level which would make it practical for bedside use, either with a desk top computer or on the basis of a scaling system not requiring data processing.

This is of considerable practical importance because most head-injured patients are initially admitted to a community hospital; indeed in Europe only a proportion are subsequently referred to neurosurgical units. Neither computer facilities nor laboratory investigations of the kind described in the previous chapters are therefore likely to be available for many head injuries. It is for these reasons that our study is based solely on clinical data. But because of this, the study provides a yardstick by which to measure the predictive value of laboratory investigations. Their value must depend on the balance between the benefit of increased accuracy conferred by a laboratory test and the cost in terms of resources required and of possible risk to the patient.

The clinical features observed in our study were of two kinds: those related to coma per se and those that were specific to head injury. The former consisted of rating coma on the basis of a recently described practical scale[3] together with various eye signs previously mentioned (oculovestibular and oculocephalic reflexes, spontaneous eye movements, and the pupil reactions). Head injury details included, inter alia, the presence and site of skull fracture, of intracranial hematoma, of lateralizing neurological signs, and of other injuries. Only a limited list of features was observed, but the best and worst state in a number of succeeding epochs (day 1, days 2–3, days 4–7, days 7–14, etc.) were recorded, so that each feature might yield many items of predictive data.

Only severe injuries were studied—for at least 6 hours, patients had neither obeyed commands nor given any verbal response. In some, this persisting state of coma was delayed in development, following a relatively lucid interval; in that event, observations were timed from when the patient went into coma. The study began with patients from the Glasgow Institute, where cases are secondarily referred and only 50 percent were admitted to neurosurgery in the first 24 hours. More recently, we have added cases from two Netherlands units where 90 percent were under neurosurgical or neurological care within 24 hours. Apart from this, the populations proved to be remarkably similar, as indeed we had found in a previous joint study with the Netherlands. All cases were treated with the techniques and vigor which is natural in a fully equipped unit, but controlled ventilation was used only occasionally. A number of different clinicians took charge of care, but they were not asked to standardize treatment. In spite of this, the distribution of outcomes was very similar in the Glasgow and the Netherlands series.

The outcome distribution of certain characteristics was ascertained as a means of identifying which features, when considered alone or in combination with one other feature, have an influence on outcome. The following results are based on the first 350 cases from Glasgow. When age at injury was considered, a statistically significant breakpoint was found both for bad and good outcomes at age 30; 5–20 was no better than 20–29 and 40–49 and 50–59 were no worse than 30–39. Over 60 years the outlook was worse and this, like the 30-year watershed, is consistent with the findings of others.[4] More surprising was the high mortality in the small group of patients under the age of 5, because younger children are commonly believed to do well after severe injury. It seems likely that this may have been due to the inclusion in most series of pediatric head injuries of a considerable proportion of less severely affected patients, due to the natural tendency to admit younger children because of difficulty in clinical evaluation. These younger children (under the age of 5) are excluded from the remaining analyses in this presentation. The outcome distribution can be determined for groups of patients who are at different levels of coma at different intervals, by ascribing numbers to each point on the coma scale; the lowest score would be 3 and the highest 15, low score representing deep coma.

Depth and duration of coma were closely related to outcome, but there were exceptions at all levels of coma in regard to both good and bad outcomes; the coma level therefore needs to be combined with some other features in order to become a reliable predictor. Age is one other such factor; another useful one is the various eye signs which reflect brain stem function— as emphasised by Plum and Posner[5] in their study of stupor and coma, but hitherto not applied systematically to head injuries. In addition to pupil reactions, which are traditionally recorded after head injury, the oculocephalic and oculovestibular reflexes and spontaneous eye movements each correlated well with outcome. Oculocephalic reflexes were more readily disturbed than oculovestibular and were therefore a more sensitive indicator of impaired function; on the other hand, oculovestibular reflexes, if they are absent, are a more reliable sign of irrecoverable damage. Obviously care is needed in interpreting these reflexes after head trauma because of the possibility of drugs or of local injury to the pathways involved. In patients with damage to one or other cerebral hemisphere (intracranial hematoma, focal neurological signs, or epilepsy) there was no difference in the outcome between right- and left-sided lesions.

The possibility of making accurate predictions in even a proportion of severely head-injured patients implies the need to consider the practical use to which predictions might be put. Most obvious is the challenge to improve the outcome in patients currently predicted to have a bad outcome and the opportunity provided to test new management regimes for such patients. Unless some such method is available, the question may arise as to whether cases predicted as almost certain to be dead or vegetative should continue to receive full intensive care. Certainly this decision should be faced if resources for special care are limited and the choice has to made between such cases and other patients who are more likely to benefit from such treatment.[6,7]

REFERENCES

1. Jennett B, Bond M: Assessment of outcome after severe brain damage. A practical scale. Lancet I:480–484, 1957

2. Teather D, Hilder W: The analysis of diagnostic data. J R Coll Physicians Lond 9:219–225, 1975

3. Teasdale G, Jennett B: Assessment of coma and impaired consciousness. A practical scale. Lancet II:81–84, 1974

4. Overgaard J, Christensen S, Hvid-Hansen O, et al: Prognosis after head injury based on early clinical examination. Lancet II:631–635, 1973

5. Plum F, Posner J: Diagnosis of stupor and coma (ed 2). Philadelphia, Davis, 1972

6. Jennett B: Scale, scope and philosophy of the clinical problem, in Outcome of Severe CNS Damage (Ciba Found. Symp. 34), 1975 (in press)

7. Jennett B, Teasdale G, Knill-Jones R: Prognosis after severe head injury, in Outcome of Severe CNS Damage (Ciba Found. Symp. 34), 1975 (in press)

Ayub K. Ommaya, M.D., F.R.C.S.
Thomas A. Gennarelli, M.D.

9

A Physiopathologic Basis for Noninvasive Diagnosis and Prognosis of Head Injury Severity

More than in other diseases of the nervous system, neural trauma initiates a veritable avalanche of physiopathologic responses, both intracerebrally and systemically. As the mechanically induced disintegration of neural functions reverses in survivors, unique reintegrative processes develop which finally lead to recovery.[15] The varying quality of such recovery and the lack of precision in prognosis for the more severely injured are inevitable consequences of our incomplete understanding of the mechanisms of neural trauma as well as an almost total ignorance of the nature of the processes underlying cerebral reintegration after head injury. Recent advances in diagnostic methods and a clearer understanding of the mechanism of brain trauma at the *macroscopic* level now offer new hope for developing a more rational management.

At the outset, two simple but important principles must be emphasized. First, it is essential to place any diagnostic, prognostic, or even therapeutic effort squarely within some overall framework or paradigm *for the entire range of neural trauma phenomena*. This will be done by providing an explanation of our paradigm for head injury and reviewing our basic hypotheses for head injury, cerebral concussion, and the effects of intracranial masses. Second, any method to monitor the entire range of head injuries must be *noninvasive* if it is to be of any use as a practical tool and must be designed for *serial evaluation* of what is essentially a process rather than a state. Invasive methods must be reserved for the precise diagnosis of suspected states within the process, e.g., the location of clots by angiography. We thus recommend formalized neurological and neuropsychologic testing, neurophysiologic assays using skin electrodes, computerized axial tomography, and certain biochemical tests for serial use. We do not recommend the use of invasive methods for serial evaluation of neural trauma phenomena, this would include the routine use of "exploratory" angiography, invasive methods of cerebral blood flow measurement, or routine recording of intracranial pressure by implanted catheters or transducers except in very severely injured patients. The reasons for this will be made clear in what follows.

A PARADIGM FOR HEAD INJURY RESEARCH

Because we cannot control the input aspect of human head injuries it is essential to coordinate our clinical observations with careful studies in models (animal, physical, and theoretical). We assume that the loss of consciousness and traumatic amnesias of common head injuries are due to *diffuse, bilateral* damage to the brain and that

The work reported herein has been supported by Contract DOT-HS-081-1-106-1A awarded by the Bureau of Highway Safety, Department of Transportation and by the National Institute of Neurological Diseases and Stroke, National Institutes of Health. Gratitude is expressed to Mr. Larry Thibault for invaluable assistance in the experimental aspects of this research and to Mr. Arthur Hirsch for his unfailing support of our work.

no focal lesion can reproduce both of these aspects of traumatic unconsciousness. We further suggest that *focal* lesions (e.g., subdural, extradural, and intracerebral hematomas; cerebral contusions and lacerations) are key determinants for survival in the acute stage as well as for *specific* neurological deficit, particularly in the late stage; it is the diffuse set of lesions however, which are the major determinants of the quality of final outcome after the posttraumatic reintegrative processes have completed their course. Our strategy for head injury research is to conceive the experimental models as "white boxes," using the cybernetic terminology of Norbert Wiener. A "white box" is one in which both the inputs and responses can be measured and the internal mechanism of which is known to some extent. Our clinical approach is to consider the patient as a black box to which the initial traumatic input is unknown. Measurement of the responses to known inputs (noninvasive stimuli) using identical techniques (e.g., evoked response recording) to those used in measuring the responses of the white box to analogous inputs would then allow reliable inferences to be drawn concerning the mechanism of the injury process. Diagnostic and therapeutic interventions in the process carried out on this basis and using the same strategy would be more likely to yield definitive guidelines to a rational management of neural trauma.

A variety of models are available and some of these are listed in Fig. 1. After considerable experience with most available models, we believe that use of the constrained head (impact and impulse) techniques for "whole head" studies[64] and the microtrauma method for focal injury studies provide most reproducible results. The following account of our paradigm for the mechanics of head injury has been developed on this basis.

A simplified flow diagram for the most significant events occurring in head injury is shown in Fig. 2. Impairment of function and damage to neural structures can be initiated either statically (forces applied slowly, e.g., with durations > 200 msec) or dynamically (forces applied with durations < 200 msec).[31] Static loading is an uncommon cause of head injury; when brain damage does occur by such mechanism, e.g., in patients whose heads are slowly crushed, it is predominantly focal. In such cases, diffuse injuries are rarely found and loss of consciousness or amnesia for the event is unusual.[72] Dynamic loading is the common cause of head injury and this can be initiated either by direct blows to the head (impact) or by sudden movement of the head (impulse) produced by impacts elsewhere.[9] Brain injury by blast loading and penetrating wounds will not be considered here.[30] Both impact and impulse inputs can injure the brain and its adnexae by the stresses and strains of inertial loading

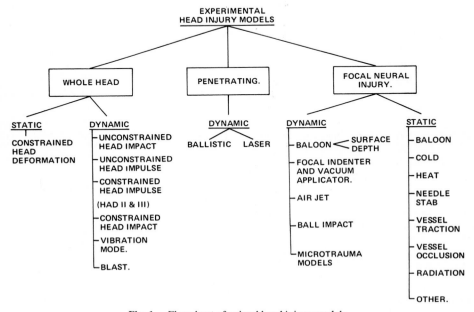

Fig. 1.   Flowchart of animal head injury models.

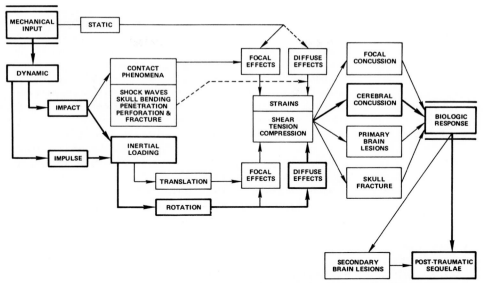

Fig. 2. A flowchart for critical factors in the mechanics of head injury. The traumatic mechanical input is shown at the top left. Heavy lines are used to indicate areas where our experimental data are adequate to begin testing of the hypothesis proposed. Lighter lines connect areas where work remains to be done and dotted lines are used to indicate predicted causal relationships which are least supported by available data.

associated with the sudden changes in motion of the head; in addition, impact adds the effects of contact phenomena, which primarily consist of skull bending, fracture, and wave propagation.[24]

The contribution of contact phenomena to *diffuse* brain damage has not yet been adequately determined. Impact to the skull will certainly produce focal effects on the brain. The extent of diffuse effects is uncertain because the duration of impact is in the order of milliseconds, i.e., one order of magnitude greater than the transit time of waves passing through brain or skull.[24] The tentative nature of such effects is therefore represented with a dotted line in Fig. 2. It should be emphasized that we are not minimizing the potentially crippling and even lethal effects of some focal lesions; we seek to emphasize however their relative simplicity of causation and their inability to explain the various manifestations of traumatic unconsciousness. Because nonimpact inertial loading can produce traumatic unconsciousness and visible brain injuries,[9,48] it is reasonable to assume that inertial loading is a major cause of brain damage in the majority of blunt head injuries. Until recently the relative significance of the two components of inertial loading, i.e., translatory and rotatory or angular movements of the head, was undecided. According to Holbourn,[31] shear strains generated by rotation should cause cerebral concussion as well as contre-coup contusions; translation was dismissed as being an insignificant cause of brain damage in head injury mechanics. Conversely, other workers produced experimental data suggesting that pressure gradients produced by translation contributed significantly to cerebral concussion as well as cerebral contusions.[28,80,81] Our recent experiments studying these components in relative isolation have shown that both points of view are only partly correct. At equivalent levels of input acceleration, rotation of the head appears to be necessary for loss of consciousness as well as productive of diffuse and focal lesions in the brain; the main damage distribution being at brain surfaces and at zones of changes in density of the intracranial tissues. Translation of the head in the horizontal plane, on the other hand, produces essentially *focal* effects only, resulting in well-circumscribed cerebral contusions and intracerebral hematomas; such focal effects do not appear adequate for the production of cerebral concussion or other evidence of diffuse effects on the brain at head acceleration levels up to 1400'g' in the squirrel monkey.[20,21,62] It is possible to conceive of a translation in the long axis of the brain stem which could result in a focal lesion: impacts at the vertex or impulsive loading in this axis, however, are not common.

Focal and diffuse stains developed within the head as a result of these inputs can thus result in a variable mixture of four operationally defined components of the biologic response to mechanical trauma (Fig. 2). *Focal concussion* is defined as the reversible or irreversible disruption of function by trauma in a restricted asymmetric zone of the brain, occurring in isolation and usually cortical in location. *Cerebral concussion* is a similar disruption of functions occurring in a diffuse symmetrical manner throughout the brain in a distribution determined primarily by certain physical rules described below. *Primary brain lesions* refer to visible structural disruptions of neural tissues. These may or may not correlate with the sites of concussion, e.g., contusions at the site of focal concussion are most likely to correlate with irreversible effects but the wide variation in such effects compared to the more steretyped nature of contusions preclude a direct causal relationship. Because of the lack of electron microscopic data, we restrict the level of such lesion visibility to that detectable by the light microscope. The fourth element, *skull fracture,* is self-explanatory. It is important to realize that the four components of the biologic response to head injury can occur in isolation of the others under specially defined conditions.[38] Correlation of primary brain lesion locations with focal and cerebral concussion is perhaps most satisfactory when concussion is of such severity that a degree of irreversibility of the functional disturbance is introduced. Here too, however, it is possible to have an essentially reversible disturbance of motor, sensory, and reflex function associated with a considerable degree of irreversible structural damage. What is emphasized, therefore, by this paradigm is the primacy of disturbance in *neural functions* while simultaneously recognizing that their structural substrates are only incompletely recognized by conventional light microscopy.

The *severity* of head injury is composed by the relative contributions of the four components in the biologic response to trauma *plus* the added deleterious effects of the secondary responses developing after the primary events outlined above. Secondary "lesions" thus produced are not only intracranial events directly related to the primary injury (e.g., ischaemic hypoxia in a zone of traumatic haemorrhage or edema)[42] but also the indirect *systemic* consequence of the impairment in neural control mechanisms precipitated by the responses to trauma (e.g., hypoxia due to airway obstruction and secondary pulmonary effects in the unconscious patient).[6] Posttraumatic sequelae will be the resultant of either the extent of primary response alone in the mild case of head injury or of the combined effects of primary and secondary responses in the more severe case.

The theoretical and experimental basis for proposing the following hypothesis is derived from the physical model experiments and theoretical analysis of head injury mechanics by Holbourn,[31] the mathematical models of Advani et al.,[1] and our own work.[50,51,54,62] The mechanics of injury to the brain in blunt head trauma revealed by such studies suggest that the distribution of damaging strains induced by inertial loading would decrease in magnitude from the surface to the center of the approximately spheroidal brain mass. Thus, at low levels of inertial loading, injurious levels of shear strain would not extend deeper than the cortex. The severity and locations of the resultant functional disconnections at the cortical and subcortical levels and the degree of associated irreversible structural damage will depend to a great extent on the material and structural properties of these tissues.[48,61] Similar disconnections at progressively deeper circumferential "layers" of the three-dimensional mass of the brain will then occur as the shear strain input magnitude increases. Paralytic coma (traumatic unconsciousness) is not developed until the magnitude of shear strain is large enough to reach the well-protected mesencephalic part of the brain stem and thus complete the disconnection of the alerting system of the brain. It must be emphasized that such circumferential disconnections are not to be conceived as an inevitable series of "onion-peel" layers with uniform neural disruption throughout that layer. As indicated above, material and structural factors will influence such disconnections. The results will be dependent in a very complex manner on the mechanical properties of the multicomponent, anisotropic, inhomogeneous brain as well as the location of bony protusions, dural partitions, vascular anatomy, and other sources of tissue interfaces with different densities. Thus, it would follow that those parts of the cortex covered by smooth surfaces (e.g., the occipital lobes) should suffer the least damage, whereas those portions covered by rough surfaces (e.g., the temporal lobes, frontal poles, and orbital cortex) would suffer the most. The contact phenomena and translatory components of inertial loading would add to such diffuse effects by contributing focal lesion effects at sites determined by the skull distortions and pressure gradients as shown experimentally by Lindgren.[40] The *site* (and area) of impact is therefore more important for the resultant *focal* effects on the brain, both via the contact phenomena and the translatory component of inertial loading. The *combination* of rotational and translational effects is possibly the reason why we have been unable to confirm experimentally the qualitative strain distribution diagrams given by Holbourn; there were significant discrepancies in our experimental results for the distribution of visible brain lesions produced by inertial loading which are not simply explicable by the difficulty in producing large strains in small animal brains.[32,57,58] It must be noted that Holbourn's data were based on two-dimensional photoelastic stress analysis in a simplified model representing only "skull" and "brain" elements and no foramen magnum or neck. These facts are also useful in explaining the distribution of cerebral contusions after head injury as elegantly described in the classic work of Lindenburg and Freytag.[39]

HYPOTHESIS FOR CEREBRAL CONCUSSION

Earlier definitions of cerebral concussion (commotio cerebri) emphasized two essentially contradictory aspects of the phenomena of traumatic unconsciousness. First, that trauma to the brain could abolish all its functions and even cause death without leaving visible pathological evidence.[69] Second, that the disturbances of consciousness thus produced could be entirely reversible. Later, the fact that traumatic unconsciousness was always associated with disturbances in memory was recognized.[14] More recently, it became evident that the traumatic amnesias exhibit a striking one-way dissociation with respect to traumatic coma; thus, although coma caused by a head injury is always associated with amnesia, varying degrees of amnesias may occur without the presence of coma or indeed any significant effect on alertness.[17] Earlier hypothesis for cerebral concussion provided no satisfactory explanation of all these diverse aspects of the problem of traumatic unconsciousness. Our experimental work has enabled us to formulate a

unifying theory for these phenomena and to provide a testable hypothesis for the mechanism of cerebral concussion.[64]

Let us define normal consciousness operationally as that state of awareness in the organism which is characterized by maximum capacity to utilize its sensory input and motor output potential in order to achieve accurate storage and retrieval of events related to contemporary time and space.[46] Our hypothesis for cerebral concussion would then be defined as *a graded set of clinical syndromes following head injury wherein increasing severity of disturbance in level and content of consciousness is caused by mechanically induced strains affecting the brain in a centripetal sequence of disruptive effect on function and structure. The effects of this sequence always begin at the surfaces of the brain in the mild cases and extend inwards to affect the diencephalic-mesencephalic core at the most severe levels of trauma.* Our proposed classification of the grades of cerebral concussion thus produced is shown in Fig. 3.

The extent of cortical and subcortical involvement in head injury is thus always significant and the probability of peripheral damage increases proportionately when the amount of strain is large enough to affect the rostral brain stem and produce the "typical" case with the paralytic coma of traumatic unconsciousness (Grade IV). Extending on either side of this level of injury severity are cases with lesser and greater damage. On the one hand may be found the less severe cases where memory disturbance occurs without loss of motor control and only partially impaired awareness (Grades I to III); in such cases, we suggest that significant strains did not reach the reticular activating system. On the other hand are the more severe cases with greater degrees of diffuse irreversible damage. When such diffuse damage reaches a critical amount and therefore not necessarily when the mesencephalon shows structural damage, the Grade V case is developed. This type of result is aptly described by the term "persistent vegetative state" as suggested by Jennett and Plum.[34]

Our hypothesis leads to three critical predictions. First, that when the level of trauma is severe enough to produce what is described as traumatic unconsciousness (shown as coma in Fig. 3), the extent of simultaneous primary injury in the brain is more severe in cortical and subcortical structures (and particularly in the critically vul-

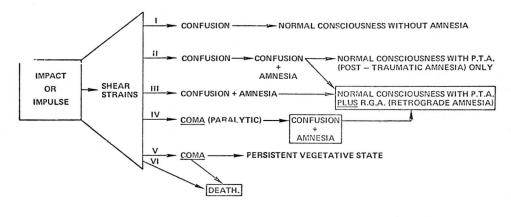

Fig. 3. Diagrammatic description of our hypothesis for the syndromes of cerebral concussion with increasing severity of primary injury causing more extensive disconnections between the cortex and the mesencephalic-diencephalic "core" of the brain. Note that Grade IV cerebral concussion is the state of traumatic unconsciousness which may be further subdivided according to duration of coma or severity of neurological sequelae.

nerable zones mentioned above) than in the rostral brain stem. Second, it follows that because the mesencephalon is the *last* to be affected by trauma, primary damage to the rostral brain stem will not occur in isolation in the vast majority of head injuries which are associated with acceleration or deceleration trauma. When a truly primary lesion of this part of the brain stem is found at postmortem, it should be found rarely and always in association with diffuse damage to the brain. If a patient with a lower grade of cerebral concussion dies from other causes, we would also predict that isolated primary rostral brain stem lesions will not be found. The third prediction from the hypothesis is that although confusion and disturbances of memory can occur without loss of consciousness the reverse should never be seen, i.e., every cause of head injury with a Grade IV cerebral concussion must have an associated period of traumatic amnesia; the mesencephalon being *less* vulnerable than the temporal lobes and limbic system. We wish to reiterate that these predictions will hold only for the commonly found head injury wherein the head is accelerated or decelerated after impact.

The validity of our hypothesis and the predictions from it will now be examined in the light of experimental, clinical and pathological observations.

EXPERIMENTAL OBSERVATIONS

In our first model for experimental head injury we discovered that wearing a cervical collar protected the brain during impact to the head.[50,51] On examination of the mechanism for this protective effect, we found that the collar did not reduce either stretching of the neck or translation of the head. Thus, by exclusion, head rotation was suggested as being the key factor in producing diffuse shear strains on the brain and that it was the reduction of the angulation of the head on the neck by the collar which minimized the shear strains in the brain during impact.[51] In further experiments aimed at testing Holbourn's hypothesis we established that inertial loading without head impact, as produced in experimental whiplash, was capable of producing experimental cerebral concussion and superficial vascular lesions in the brain but the distribution and nature of such lesions did not fit Holbourn's predicted lesion distributions precisely. We did confirm that this response was sensitive to the velocity change experienced by the head at short durations of impact (<50 msec) as predicted.[32,54,57,58] However, Holbourn's main prediction that the head rotation was the critical factor for *both* cerebral concussion and contre-coup lesions and the opposing contention that translation also played a role was not tested critically in these experiments. Measured levels of head rotations at which cerebral concussion occurred in rhesus monkeys receiving occipital head impacts were approximately half that required when the head was accelerated without direct impact in experimental whiplash.[57,58] This observation supported the idea that components other than inertial loading were significant in the genesis of cerebral concussion. In the chimpanzee however, with a brain to head mass ratio much smaller than that of 1:5 found in the rhesus and man, the levels of rotation at which concussion occurred were similar in direct and indirect impacts.[62] This was attributed to the thick scalp and skull and short muscular neck in this species; factors which would tend to minimize the contact phenomena of impact, thus making

inertial loading the prime injury mechanism. We assumed that the rotational component was critical for the diffuse effects of head injury and on the basis of these data were able to develop a tolerance curve predicting the injurious rotational acceleration threshold for man.[56–58]

In order to test this assumption and further our understanding of the mechanisms of head injury, we have recently completed experiments wherein pure inertial loading was examined more precisely and its components definitively compared. In these experiments we have also developed a quantitative and objective index of cerebral concussion to supplement clinical neurological examination; this is the somatosensory evoked response at the skull surface to median nerve stimulation at the wrist.[62] The device in

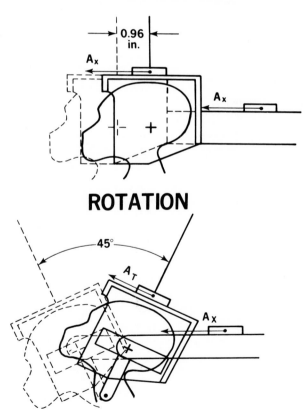

Fig. 4. Kinematics of translational and rotational modes of acceleration. The preacceleration position is depicted in solid lines and the postacceleration position by dashed lines. Note that the use of this linkage system prevents contact phenomena and that equivalent acceleration A_x (and equivalent energy input) is provided in both situations.

Table 1
Effects of Head Shaking—Rotation

Monkey Number	Peak Positive Acceleration*	Cerebral Concussion	Brain Lesions					
			SDH	SAH	CC	ICH	ICPH	BSH
SR-1	1025	+	+	+	−	−	+	−
SR-2	1025	+	+	+	+	−	+	−
SR-3	706	+	+	+	−	−	+	−
SR-4	710	+	+	+	−	−	−	−
SR-5	700	+	+	+	+	−	+	−
SR-6	961	+	+	+	−	−	−	−
SR-7	348	+	+	+	−	−	+	−
SR-8	387	+	+	+	−	−	+	−
SR-9	713	+	+	+	−	−	+	+
SR-10	488	+	+	+	+	−	+	+
SR-11	402	+	+	+	−	−	−	−
SR-12	783	+	+	+	−	−	+	−

*In "g" (resultant of the measured tangential and radial components).
+ = Lesion present.
− = Lesion absent.

SDH = Subdural hematoma,
SAH = Subarachnoid hemorrhage,
CC = Cortical contusion,
ICH = Intracerebral hematoma,
ICPH = Intracerebral petechial hemorrhages,
BSH = Brain stem hemorrhages.

Table 2
Effects of Head Shaking—Translation

Monkey Number	Peak Positive Acceleration*	Cerebral Concussion	Brain Lesions					
			SDH	SAH	CC	ICH	ICPH	BSH
SL-1	1140	−	Focal only	−	−	−	−	−
SL-2	1230	−	Focal only	−	+	−	−	−
SL-3	854	−	Focal only	−	+	+	−	−
SL-4	812	−	−	−	−	+	−	−
SL-5	830	−	−	−	+	−	−	−
SL-6	Not recorded	−	Focal only	−	−	−	−	−
SL-7	768	−	Focal only	Focal only	+	−	−	−
SL-8	802	−	−	−	−	−	−	−
SL-9	665	−	−	−	−	−	−	−
SL-10	Not recorded	−	−	−	−	−	−	−
SL-11	734	−	−	−	−	−	−	−
SL-12	1058	−	−	−	−	−	−	−

*In "g."
+ = Lesion present.
− = Lesion absent.

SDH = Subdural hematoma,
SAH = Subarachnoid hemorrhages,
CC = Cortical contusion,
ICH = Intracerebral hematoma,
ICPH = Intracerebral petechial hemorrhages,
BSH = Brain stem hemorrhages.

which we compared the two components of inertial loading directly enable the production of either pure translations or rotation of the head through 45°; in both cases the center of gravity of the head moves approximately 1 in. (Fig. 4). Identical levels of input accelerations independent of the effect of impact contact phenomena could thus be compared while varying the effect of one variable only, i.e., rotation. Serial neurological examinations of the animal before and after trauma were recorded on videotape with split-screen imaging of the simultaneous EEG and other physiological variables.[68] A PDP-12 computer enabled on-line monitoring of the somatosensory evoked responses (SER) generated by stimulation of the median nerve at the wrist. Comparison of the videotape data and SER facilitated critical on-line correlations between the neurological and electrophysiological data. All the animals in the rotated group exhibited neurological evidence of *experimental cerebral concussion* defined as the sudden onset of paralytic coma or traumatic unconsciousness. In contrast, none of the translated group showed this effect.

All animals were sacrificed after 24 hours and the location of lesions in both groups were compared. These data are shown for each animal in Tables 1 and 2; and the distribution of gross primary lesions is summarized in Fig. 5. The species used in this series of experiments was *Samiri sciureus* (squirrel monkey).

It became clear that a greater number of such lesions occurred in a more diffusely widespread symmetrical manner in the rotated group whereas only a few asymmetrically placed focal lesions developed in the translated group. Intracerebral hematomas occurred exclusively in the translated group but in only 2 out of 12 animals. These were unique lesions in one occipital lobe producing a striking separation of the gray-white interface. Conversely, petechial hemorrhage at gray-white interfaces was present in a bilaterally symmetric fashion in every member of the rotated group, but in only 2 of the translated group in a sparse asymmetrical fashion. Cortical contusions were found at approximately the same frequency in both groups, but those seen in the translated group were characteristically discrete,

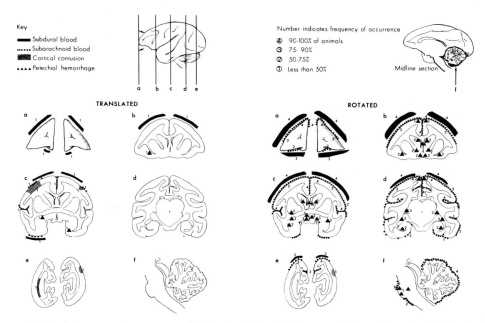

Fig. 5. Diagrammatic summary of lesion distribution in the two experimental groups. The levels of the coronal sections shown are depicted in the top left lateral view of a brain where they are alphabetically identified. The key to the types of gross primary lesions depicted is also shown here. A midline sagittal section of the brain stem and cerebellum is also shown for each group (*f*) and a numerical key to the relative *frequency* of lesion occurrence is given at the top right of the diagram. Note the bilateral symmetry and greater severity of all lesions except intracerebral hemorrhages in the rotated group as compared to the scanty, asymmetric lesion distribution in the translated group. This figure should be studied in conjunction with Tables 1 and 2.

involving only the outer cortical layers in a somewhat excavated fashion. Hemorrhages in the brain stem were remarkably scarce, occurring in only two of the rotated animals and in none of the translated animals. Both of the rotated animals in which primary brain stem hemorrhage was seen were very severely concussed with diffuse lesions throughout the brain; one dying shortly after the trauma and the other remaining in a prolonged state of depressed responsiveness to stimuli. Thus, at the levels of acceleration tested (up to 1230 "g's"), it was possible to produce cerebral concussion only when the moving head was allowed to angulate or rotate. *When rotation was prevented and the head allowed to translate only (i.e., movement in a straight line), cerebral concussion did not occur.* Conversely, evidence of *focal* primary brain damage, i.e., gross structural failure of tissue, could be produced independent of diffuse lesions or loss of consciousness under conditions of pure translation. These facts, coupled with the association of diffuse surface as well as deeper lesions with cerebral concussion only in the rotated group, support our hypothesis that cerebral concussion of a severity great enough to produce paralytic coma requires shear strains occurring in

a widespread and diffuse manner involving the cerebral cortex and deeper structures with brain stem involvement being primarily a reversible affair. In the more severe case, the diffuse damage with or without the brain stem effects are essentially irreversible; if a patient in such a category survives, it will be with varying degrees of neurological and behavioral deficits, one class of which is seen in the persistent vegetative state.

Analysis of the electrophysiologic data obtained with the somatosensory evoked response (SER) technique also supports our interpretation of the biomechanical, neurological, and pathological data.[22,23] In the squirrel monkey, the P_1 component of the SER represents conduction in primary lemniscal afferents, whereas the P_2 component represents the cortically recorded signal of sensory inputs traveling via the extralemniscal pathways (Fig. 6). Alterations in P_2 therefore provide an objective sign for adequacy of conduction through what may be considered to be the altering system in the rostral brain stem reticular formation in mesencephalic and diencephalic structures. Abolition of the P_2 wave at the cortex (recorded with extradural electrodes) was found to coincide precisely with the onset of

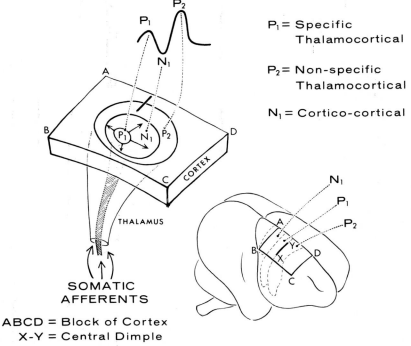

P_1 = Specific Thalamocortical

P_2 = Non-specific Thalamocortical

N_1 = Cortico-cortical

CORTEX

THALAMUS

SOMATIC AFFERENTS

ABCD = Block of Cortex
X-Y = Central Dimple

Fig. 6. Diagram (modified from Singer) of the origin and spatial distribution of cortically recorded SER in the squirrel monkey.

paralytic coma and its return with the restoration of the animals' responsiveness and motor performance (Fig. 7). In the translated animals, P_2 was always preserved and none of these animals were concussed (Fig. 8). The hypothesis that the

paralytic coma of cerebral concussion is associated with failure of activity in the mesencephalic reticular formation is thus supported.[28,82,83] We also found, however, that irrespective of such effects of trauma on the brain stem, definite and more long-lasting effects were also demonstrable at the level of the cerebral cortex. The time taken for the P_2 wave to travel from one hemisphere to the opposite side plotted as a percentage of the time taken to make the same transfer before impact is shown in Fig. 9. Note the marked slowing

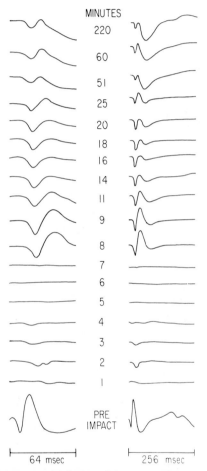

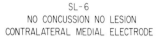
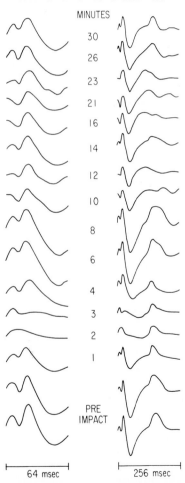

Fig. 7. Serial display of the somatosensory evoked response (SER) to median nerve stimulation in a rotated animal. Note the preimpact components which are all obliterated at impact. This animal remained unconscious for 7 minutes and the return of the second positive wave (P_2, representing conduction in the nonspecific pathways) coincided precisely with the arousal of the animal from unresponsive coma. The animal remained somnolent for over 6 hours after impact and at 220 minutes the SER component had not yet returned to normal. The SER display in this and the next two figures is shown in two time scales with the longer display on the right.

Fig. 8. The SER in a translated animal. Note that in comparison with Fig. 4, only decreases in amplitudes with no loss of the signal components are seen. This animal, like all in the translated group, showed no clinical impairment of the preimpact alert state of awareness.

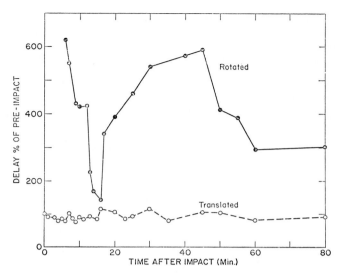

Fig. 9. Latency of contralateral to ipsilateral conduction of P_2 plotted as a function of time after impact for the two groups of animals. This reflects interhemispheric cortical functional integrity. The data clearly show the marked increase in percent delay of P_2 conduction in the rotated group as compared to the unimpaired translated group. This increased latency moreover persists far longer than either the P_2 conduction deficit noted in Fig. 4 or the duration of loss of consciousness. These data suggest that cortical injury is more significant than brain stem injury at this level of traumatic input and also that pure translation does not produce any significant diffuse effects at either brain stem or cortical levels at the levels of acceleration tested (up to 1230 "g").

of such interhemispheral cortico-cortical transfer found only in the rotated group and absent in the nonconcussed translated group; this impairment of cortical (± subcortical) function persists long after the return of P_2 indicated adequate conduction through the reticular formation. This would suggest that cortical (or telencephalic) effects of such head injury are widespread and possibly more severe than the brain stem effects. The hypothesis that cortical involvement is always significant in cerebral concussion is thus also supported.[14,33,56,61,76,82]

CLINICAL OBSERVATIONS

The complex patterns of clinical behavior after head injuries are well recognized.[33,38,82] It is possible however, to discern a general pattern of recovery in many patients after severe but relatively uncomplicated head trauma which is important to recapitulate.[33] The patient falls unconscious and remains for a while in an unresponsive, immobile coma. Emerging from this state of paralytic unconsciousness the patient successively

passes through stages of stupor, confusion with or without delirium, and finally an almost lucid phase with automatism before becoming fully alert. Stated in another way, *return of awareness to stimuli usually precedes motor and sensory recovery, which in turn recover before restoration of memory and other cognitive functions.* It is of great interest that this sequence of reintegration of normal consciousness is similar in a wide spectrum of head injuries and correlates with the severity of injury only in being much slower in cases with prolonged coma, such patients being, of course, more liable to have residual symptoms. The common element in such severe cases is that alertness always returns prior to full return of memory functions. Another feature of the "recovered" case of severe head injury is the association of a labile affect with the difficulty in learning new material.[51] These observations support the idea of a greater vulnerability of the cortex and particularly of the limbic and fronto-temporal cortices which occupy zones of great structural irregularity and variation in tissue density.

A large number of clinical observations at the less severe end of the spectrum of cerebral concussion syndromes can also be explained by our hypothesis. The lesser grades of cerebral concussion (I to III) are quite common, particularly in contact sports such as American football and boxing. The majority of such concussions do not produce paralytic coma or traumatic unconsciousness; instead, confusion and amnesia are usually seen. It is a common experience for patients who have been briefly "dazed" or confused to continue well-coordinated sensorimotor activity after a sports accident without subsequent recall of the episode.[61] Yarnell[86,87] has recently reported a group of such mildly concussed patients examined immediately after impact who were confused and disoriented in time but possessed intact recall of events immediately prior to impact; retrograde amnesia did not develop until 5 to 10 minutes *after* the impact. Yarnell also described further cases similar to that reported by Fisher[17] in which the occurrence of severe amnesia after head impact was not associated with a loss of alertness. In the latter report the author writes, "It must be concluded that a traumatic insult to the memory mechanisms can occur with complete sparing of the neural basis of alertness" and again, "In moderate to severe concussion, although both systems are usually affected together, they are not equally vulnerable, for alertness is restored first as a rule, while impaired memory almost always persists for a longer period. It might be expected therefore that amnesia would occur in the presence of retained alertness."[17]

Our hypothesis offers a reasonable explanation for the greater vulnerability of memory and the lesser vulnerability of alertness in head injury. In a recent study on memory mechanisms in humans, we presented data to support the hypothesis that it is the hippocampal gyri rather than the hippocampus per se which form the brain structures critically involved in coding experiences for retrieval from storage via the associative neocortex.[59] It would follow that if the hippocampal mesocortex and temporal neocortex bear the main brunt to the cortical damage, then the recovery of alertness should precede the return of telencephalic integrative functions controlling motor and sensory mechanisms with memory mechanisms being restored last of all. The observation by Torres and Shapiro[79] that EEG abnormalities occurring in a group of patients after nonimpact inertial loading of the head ("whiplash injury") were similar in nature and incidence to those seen after impact produced head injury is inexplicable except by invoking the common role of inertial loading with maximal effect on the cortex in both conditions.

CONTRIBUTION OF FOCAL AND DIFFUSE LESIONS TO PRIMARY AND SECONDARY EFFECTS OF CLOSED HEAD INJURIES

The primary mechanical trauma affects neural as well as vascular elements, and it is suggested that the diagnosis of head injury severity must include a clear recognition of the relative degree of localization of damage as well as the influence of each element on the other.

Recognition of focal injury is relatively easy, both by clinical and radiological methods. Besides being more easily treatable, focal lesions are also less likely to contribute to the production of a posttraumatic persistent vegetative state. Attempts to assess the state of the cerebral circulation after head injury as an index of diffuse injury have not yet provided much of value for management. Thus, Overgaard and Tweed[67] have recently confirmed earlier work by others[7] that measurement of cerebral blood flow (CBF) and functional tests of the circulation during the acute phase have limited prognostic value. They found that flows less than 22 ml/100 g/min or greater than 64 ml/100 g/min were almost equally of grave prognostic significance. Their measurements of intracranial pressure (ICP) were similarly of no great prognostic value. Thus, while very high ICP (over 25 torr) was uniformly associated with poor recovery, very low or normal ICP was no assurance of good recovery.

Our experimental data would suggest that the most significant *primary* damage for the outcome of surviving head injury patients is the extent of diffuse injury to the vascular, cortical, and subcortical structures. Damage to the brain stem is usually a secondary matter related to ischemic effects caused by the secondary responses of cerebral hyperemia, cerebral edema, metabolic acidosis, and, possibly, increased CSF volume due to impaired absorption. We would predict therefore that excluding the 10 percent of patients who have surgically treatable space occupying focal lesions (e.g., hematomas), the outcome for most head injury patients will be de-

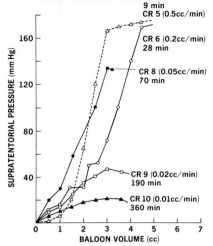

SUPRATENTORIAL PRESSURE-VOLUME RELATIONSHIPS AT VARYING RATES OF VOLUME INCREASE

Fig. 10. Pressure volume relationships are shown to differ depending on the *rate* of volume expansion. Note that classically shaped PV curves only occur in animals CR 5, 6, 8 where volume addition was rapid.

termined by the primary damage and should therefore be predictable at an early stage.

A recent report by Overgaard et al.[66] is relevant here: they found that a simple neurological examination (within 6 hours of head injury in 70 percent of patients) was reliably predictive for the final outcome with only three sets of clinical variables being recorded, i.e., the level of consciousness, motor functions, and neurophthalmological signs. Because useful recovery after head injury requires a more complete return of brain stem function compared to recovery of integrative cortical function, our hypothesis is that the critical brain damage is primary rather than secondary in recovering survivors and that the cortex is injured more than the reticular formation. The importance of early diagnosis of the degree of diffuse impairment is thus emphasized. Overgaard et al.[66] also noted that episodic systolic hypertension was significantly correlated with a poor prognosis. This suggests that the secondary factors of cerebral edema, cerebral hyperemia, and possibly increased CSF volume due to impaired absorbtion may be the prime cause of the secondary ischemic

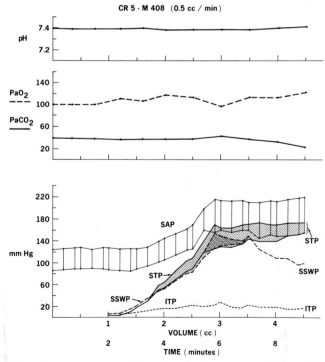

Fig. 11. Cushing response elicited in animal when rate of volume expansion was high. In Figs. 11 and 12, abbreviations are SAP-systemic arterial pressure, STP, ITP-supra and infra tentorial pressures, SSWP—sagittal sinus wedge pressure.

hypoxia and metabolic acidosis which add further brain damage to the primary insult. In coping with such intracranial volume expansion, the lack of significant correlation between prognosis and intracranial pressure or regional cerebral blood flow may well be due to the lack of correlated data on tissue pressure and the *rate* of such intracranial volumetric changes. We have shown that while relatively high rates of mass expansion in the head produces a classically exponential P/V curve, slower rates (<0.22 cc/mm in the rhesus monkey) fail to evoke a Cushing response, do not produce a marked rise in ICP but still cause brain death at the same volume of added mass as at the higher rate[44] (Figs. 10, 11, and 12). Measurement of the vascular capillaries at varying rates of mass increase has demonstrated that the crucial factor for brain death produced by added volumes is failure of capillary perfusion.[45] These data also show why the recording of ICP may not be of much diagnostic or prognostic value when taken by itself, except in the severely injured patient with a rapidly increasing mass, e.g., of cerebral

edema. We have also stressed the value of determinations of brain compliance as an index of the ability of brain tissues to survive at varying pressure gradients and in the interpretation of ICP measurements.

PATHOLOGICAL OBSERVATIONS

In spite of many detailed pathological studies, a completely adequate description of the relative three-dimensional distribution of all primary lesions throughout the brain at known intervals of time after head injury is not yet available either in humans (where it will probably never be completely obtained) or in experimental animals.[56,75,81,88] Such a study is urgently required, data being needed in cases sustaining injury at three levels of injury severity, e.g., with reversible deficits, with irreversible deficits but survival and with irreversible plus death. Review of available data, however, does enable certain aspects of the hypothesis to be examined. The observation that

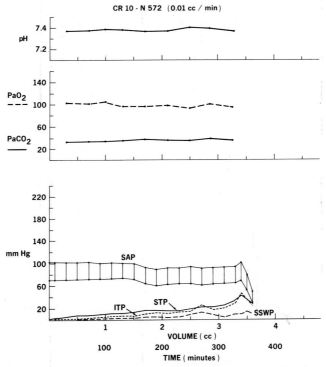

Fig. 12. Absence of Cushing response and lack of pressure rise when rate to volume expansion is low. In both Figs. 11 and 12, the end point was the same, namely death of the animal, diagnosed as an isoelectric EEG and dilated fixed pupils for 10 minutes.

the prime location of contusions is in the temporal and frontal regions *irrespective* of the site of impact has not been satisfactorily explicable by prior hypothesis.[57,58] The occurrence of subdural hematomas after falls on the buttocks and after whiplash injury alone is of course more easily attributable to the rotational components of inertial loading.[55] In a recent review of the pathology of brain damage in blunt head injuries, Strich[75] has emphasized the diffuse nature of histological changes in axons. Microglial stars around tissue tears as reported by Oppenheimer and widespread neuronal changes were found by many investigators. Grcevic and Jacob[26] have reported preliminary data on a serial-section study in fatal human head injuries showing diffuse lesions in a rostral periventricular pattern. Although cell-count data from controlled experiments in animals have been reported for a few locations, the available evidence does not enable us to decide on the relative vulnerability of cortex and subjacent white matter to mechanical trauma, nor is it yet possible to envisage the three-dimensional distribution of the diffuse lesions.[85] An important study by Mitchell and Hume Adams[43] on the incidence of primary brain stem lesions in patients dying after head injury supports the idea that such lesions probably do not occur in head injuries without severe damage elsewhere. Our hypothesis that the brain stem is the least vulnerable part of the brain for primary damage is thus not refuted.

The difficulties in interpretation of pathological data from experimental studies have been pointed out on numerous occasions.[56,75] Because of the smaller mass of brain in animals and the restriction implicit in impact techniques, it has not been possible to duplicate all the clinical and pathological observations made in man.[22,56-58,61] Critical review of the experiments claiming that primary brain stem damage and even primary rostral cervical cord damage are the substrate of acceleration concussion suggest that the data may equally well be interpreted as a consequence of the method used.[47] It is important to stress that interpretations from experimental data must provide satisfactory explanations of the clinical observations on cerebral concussion and other effects of head injury. This point was also made by Denny-Brown[13] who, in reviewing the work of Friede, pointed out the lack of immediate disturbance of consciousness and of traumatic amnesias in contusions to the medulla or upper cervical cord in man.

Our review has indicated that it is now possible to explain all the known phenomena of cerebral concussion with a unified hypothesis which is amenable to testing for validity. It is also clear that the clinicopathologic correlations required to provide the critical test of our hypothesis are still inadequate. Further pathological evidence, both in controlled animal experiments and from detailed studies in head-injured humans are urgently needed. Human data are essential for validation, but the realities of the type of available material in postmortem examination restrict our data to the most severely injured group, where the separation of primary and secondary factors in lesion genesis is difficult. Moreover, it is also clear from the discrepancy between the marked physiological disturbance and often mild pathological evidence of damage in brain trauma cases that the pathological examination will have to be extended to deeper levels of analysis, in order that more precise clinicopathologic correlations be achieved. By this we mean not only electron microscopic study of the structural details but also the application of such dynamic pathological tools as quantitative histochemical study of abnormalities in neural transmitter distribution after trauma. A more fundamental understanding of the disturbance of consciousness and memory in trauma will also require experiments aimed at providing correlations of structural change with physiologic functions at the cellular level of neural elements subjected to mechanical load.

Clinical and Neuropsychologic Testing

The recent work of Overgaard et al.[66,67] has reminded us again of the prime importance of the clinical examination. In order to develop this method in a quantitative manner, we would recommend the use of a uniform scale for the assessment of coma and impaired consciousness either by Overgaard et al.'s[66] method or as suggested by Teasdale and Jennett.[77] This latter scale is illustrated in Table 3. Following the return of consciousness and memory, the most useful clinical parameter for serial study is probably that of *motor performance*. Quantitative tests of visuomotor coordination as a measure of the sequential patterns of motor recovery could provide an index of cerebral reintegration after trauma. Such tests could include simplified versions of standardized neuropsychologic tests, e.g.,

Table 3
Chart for Recording
Assessment of Consciousness

Time	0–24 Hours
Eye opening	Spontaneous
	To speech
	To pain
	None
Best verbal response	Orientated
	Confused
	Inappropriate
	Incomprehensible
	None
Best motor response	Obeying
	Localizing
	Flexing
	Extending
	None

pointing to visual targets (as a measure of parietotemporal deficit) rotary pursuit and bimanual tracking (as measures of frontal and interhemispheric integration).

A simple but apparently sensitive test of information rate processing has recently been used by Gronwall and Wrightson.[27] This is a simple serial addition task which was given at four standard rates to patients regaining consciousness after head injury. Asymptomatic patients with uncomplicated cerebral concussion were able to develop a normal speed of performance within 35 days of the head injury. In patients with an equivalent duration of loss of consciousness but still complaining of poor concentration, fatigue, irritability, headache, and inability to work, the posttraumatic reduction of information rate processing was prolonged well beyond 35 days.

Two important variables of significance as indices of primary as well as secondary injury are the blood pressure (BP) and EKG. The deleterious effect of hypertension, probably increasing cerebral edema, has been noted above and is probably as injurious as hypotension. Electrocardiographic changes in head injury are significant but not well studied in man. Some of our data in the monkey are shown in Fig. 13. We found that persisting EKG abnormalities predicted a fatal outcome. This aspect is recommended for detailed studies in humans.[18]

Computerized Axial Tomography (CAT)

There is little doubt that this technique is a powerful new tool for head injury diagnosis. Apart from the recognition of space-occupying lesions, there is reason to suggest that the serial measurement of intracranial compartmental volumes is feasible. Figure 14 illustrates a special phantom with which the first formal tests of the EMI-Scanner device were made to determine the spatial and density resolution capability of CAT. Using the old 80×80 matrix, the spatial resolution for density differences greater than ± 1 percent was 6×6 mm. For density differences of 3 percent and greater the resolution improved to 3×3 mm.

Category	Number of Monkeys	Change in Rate	Change in Pattern	Change in Rate + Pattern	No Change	Significance
1. Concussion without fracture	22	12(55%)	10(45%)	8(36%)	10(45%)	Chi square of categories 1,2, and 3 related individually to presence or absence of electrocardiographic changes = 9.636 $P \leq .01$
2. Concussion with fracture and death	5	5(100%)	3(60%)	3(60%)	0(0%)	
3. No Concussion or fracture	11	2(18%)	1(9%)	0(0%)	9(82%)	Chi square of categories 1 + 2 compared to category 3 and related to E.C.G. change = 4.606 $P \leq .05$
Totals	38	19(50%)	14(37%)	11(29%)	19(50%)	

Fig. 13. EKG changes following free head impact in the monkey. Note the significant association of EKG rate or pattern abnormality with concussion.

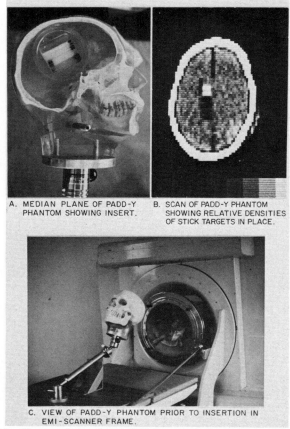

A. MEDIAN PLANE OF PADD-Y   B. SCAN OF PADD-Y PHANTOM
   PHANTOM SHOWING INSERT.   SHOWING RELATIVE DENSITIES
                                    OF STICK TARGETS IN PLACE.

C. VIEW OF PADD-Y PHANTOM PRIOR TO INSERTION IN
   EMI-SCANNER FRAME.

Fig. 14.   Phantom for use in the EMI-Scanner to determine spatial and density resolution. Impregnated stick targets of varying size and density are interchangeable and were placed in the plastic "brain" as shown photographically in (a) and in CAT scan in (b).

Density resolution was at least ±1 percent for objects 1 cm in diameter.[49,65] Recent improvements in the matrix should greatly improve this resolution, at least by a factor of 2.

Figure 15 shows the CAT scan and brain of a patient dying within 24 hours after a severe head injury. The scan was obtained within 2 hours of the injury and the lesions visible in the various views are summarized in a diagram inset in Fig. 15. Measurement of the EMI-Scan numbers related to the linear attenuation coefficients for various zones were obtained in vivo and from autopsy biopsy specimens in vitro. The absence of primary brain stem hemorrhages and the presence of severe edema plus acute hydrocephalus were diagnosed premortem. These and other preliminary data suggest that it is feasible to recognize the extent of cerebral contusions as well as measure the relative contribution of focal and diffuse lesions in vivo. This approach is currently being applied in a series of acute head injury patients, one facet of our hope to thus lay the foundations of a novel "in vivo" quantitative neuropathology.

Neurophysiologic Assay of Head Injury Severity

It is obvious that measurement of the electrical activity of the nervous system is a more direct and primary aspect of neural function as compared to such secondary aspects as cerebral blood flow or intracranial pressure. Previous investigators have documented changes of the EEG[3,4,41] or of the visual evoked response[5,16] in posttraumatic comatose patients. These studies

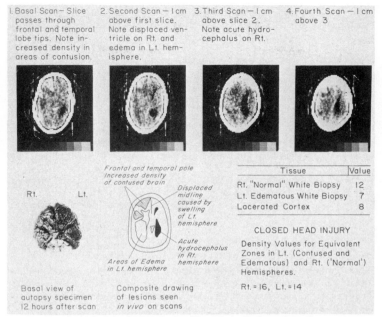

Fig. 15. Correlation of EMI-Scan with pathological specimen in acute trauma. Regional edema as well as contused areas of brain correlated well with attenuation coefficients determined premortem and autopsy data postmortem. This type of data could well form the basis for development of a quantitative in vivo neuropathology.

were aimed at documenting the nature of the change in response and did not correlate these changes for use as possible prognostic or diagnostic indices. Of the varying types of electrical activity which can be recorded (Fig. 16), we have selected a number to form a neurophysiologic assay (Fig. 17).[23]

In our experimental model, visual or computer-assisted analysis of the EEG did not provide any significant correlations between this parameter and injury severity (Figs. 18 and 19). This was in contrast to the results obtained with the somatosensory evoked response (SER) as described above (Figs. 7, 8, and 9). In addition, the

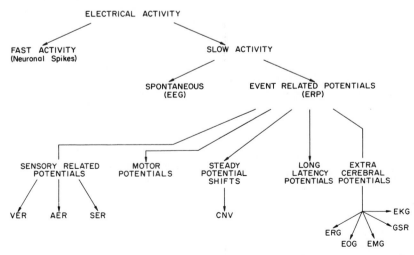

Fig. 16. Flowchart of electrical activities which may be recorded from the brain or scalp.

	MODE	SITE OF STIMULATION	SITE OF RECORDING	STIMULUS PARAMETERS
A.	EEG	NONE	10-20 ELECTRODES	NONE
B.	SER	MEDIAN NERVES BILATERAL	P_3, P_4, C_z, P_z TO Au	0.1 m sec 0.5 + 1 Hz CRC 10-200 m sec SUB TO SUPRE. MAX. TWITCH
C.	VER ERG	PHOTIC STIMULUS	MEDIAL CANTHUS Ou O_1, O_2 TO Au	1, 5, 10 Hz CRC 25-150 m sec WHITE, BLUE, RED, YELLOW 3 INTENSITIES
D.	MOTOR NCV, NAP	a) MEDIAN NERVE ELBOW b) MEDIAN NERVE WRIST	a) NAP: WRIST NCV: THENAR EMG b) NDV: THENAR EMG	SAME AS SER
E.	SENSORY NCV, NAP	a) MEDIAN NERVE WRIST b) MEDIAN NERVE ELBOW	a) NAP: ELBOW b) NCV: SER	SAME AS SER
F.	SPINAL EP	MEDIAN NERVE WRIST	NECK	SAME AS SER

HARDWARE REQUIREMENTS:
1. EEG
2. ELECTRICAL STIMULATOR
3. VISUAL STIMULATOR
4. TAPE RECORDER
5. AVERAGER

Fig. 17. The neurophysiologic assay is designed to provide data of peripheral inputs (ERG, NCV, NAP, Spinal EP) as well as central integrative processing (VER, SER). Note that the data for assessment of the peripheral systems are obtainable by the same stimulus parameters as for the central processors—the "cost" being of additional recording electrodes.

An addition should be as follows:

G. Brain stem EP—auditory click—C_2-Au—white noise @ 30 Hz 40 df above threshold.

Codes refer to:

EP, evoked potential; NCV, nerve conduction velocity; NAP, nerve action potential; AU, both ears; OU, both eyes; P_3, P_4, etc., standard electrode positions.

SER was useful in diagnosing the development of subdural hematomas as shown in Figs. 20 and 21.

In a series of head injury patients the visual evoked response was similarly useful as shown in Fig. 22. In moderately injured patients, the potentials showed a definite recovery process which paralled the clinical recovery. Figure 23 illustrates this in a case of transient posttraumatic cortical blindness which also shows concurrent restoration of normal waveforms in the electroretinogram (ERG). When the VER was evoked at a high frequency of light flash (10 Hz) it appeared that the ability of the VER to follow such higher input rates was correlated with the recovery process. This is illustrated in Fig. 24. These data have been reported[64] and allow us to draw the following tentative conclusions:

1. Patients in irreversible coma or persistent vegetative state have poorly developed, abortive evoked potentials which do not change with time. Early waves are never clearly defined. If short latency waves are absent on the first examination (hours posttrauma), such patients never recover. If such waves were present but subsequently disappeared, a progressive lesion should be suspected.

2. Moderately injured patients have mixed disorders of the waveforms. All exhibit changes as the patients recover. All became more normal. Recovery includes increase of amplitude and complexity of the waveforms with decrease of latency and interhemispheric asymmetry.

3. Symptomatic, concussed patients (posttraumatic syndrome) had mildly abnormal evoked potentials. In all, the abnormality was more manifest at higher stimulation frequencies. As symptoms cleared, the waveform inevitably normalized and the evoked response could follow higher input rates without distortion.

4. Asymptomatic concussed patients had nearly normal evoked responses which were not asymmetrical but tended to be decreased in amplitude.

The prolonged nature of posttraumatic sequelae to head injury, often of relatively minor primary severity has been a puzzle but our findings suggest a useful approach. Thus, in patients

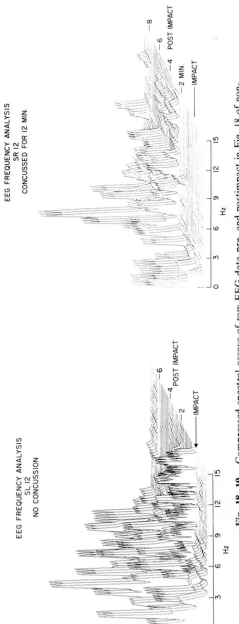

Fig. 18, 19. Compressed spectral assays of raw EEG data pre- and postimpact in Fig. 18 of non-concussed and Fig. 19 of concussed monkeys. Note the overall similarity of the pattern despite the difference in behavioral state. In Fig. 19, an apparent restoration is occurring while the animal is still unconscious.

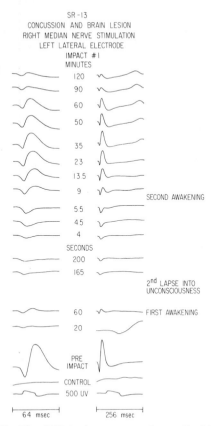

SR-13
CONCUSSION AND BRAIN LESION
RIGHT MEDIAN NERVE STIMULATION
LEFT LATERAL ELECTRODE
IMPACT #1

Fig. 20. SER is shown to correlate well with the awake or unconscious states as depicted as well as with a developing subdural hematoma (SDH). Note the progressive restoration of the waveform and amplitude form 4 to 60 minutes and then the subsequent amplitude decrease afterward (90 to 120 minutes) indicating the presence of the SDH.

recovering from cerebral concussion but with persisting complaints of the postconcussive syndrome type, the visual evoked response (VER) to light flashes at varying frequencies revealed an inability for the VER to follow an increasing rate of stimulation. As the patient recovered with time and posttraumatic symptoms improved, the VER was able to follow the higher rates of stimulation.[64] This observation may well be the neurophysiologic analog to the neuropsychologic observations of Gronwall and Wrightson,[27] who described a prolonged delay in information rate processing in patients after concussion as previously mentioned. Because the evoked response recorded at the scalp derives contributions from cortical activity and because the ability to perform cognitive tasks requires cortical integration, these

findings strongly support our contention that diffuse cortical and possibly subcortical involvement is always present when the head injury produces cerebral concussion.

Since initiating the use of this neurophysiologic assay, further definition of the auditory evoked far field potentials[35] suggests that they would be a useful addition to the assay. These potentials (also called brain stem audiometry), though recorded from the scalp, have well-defined components which have been linked to anatomic subunits of the peripheral brain stem and central auditory pathways.[19] Recent studies of comatose patients using this technique demonstrate the ability to separate these with structural anatomic lesions of the brain stem from patients comatose because of toxic, metabolic, or widespread neocortical abnormalities.[74]

Whether it will be possible to use the neurophysiologic assay as an accurate noninvasive tool to monitor and predict head injury severity remains to be shown. A correlative study of the visual, auditory, and somatosensory evoked responses with measurement of cerebral blood

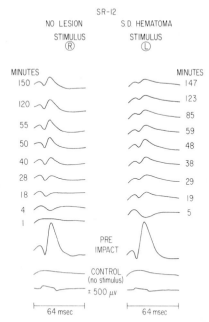

Fig. 21. Bilateral SER in a concussed monkey who subsequently developed a SDH unilaterally. The SER is absent for the 4 minutes of unconsciousness and then progressively recovers in the left hemisphere (left traces with contralateral (R) stimulus). On the right, recovery ceases at 48 minutes and subsequently the SER is diminished over the SDH.

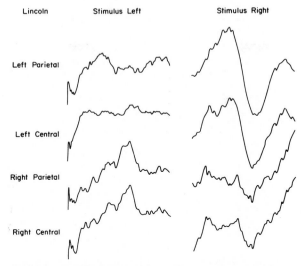

PATIENT F.L.

Right Subdural Hematoma
SER 128 MSEC

| Lincoln | Stimulus Left | Stimulus Right |

Left Parietal

Left Central

Right Parietal

Right Central

Fig. 22. SERs were obtained 4 hours after head trauma in an awake patient with no neurological deficit, who 12 hours later developed focal seizures and stupor and was shown to have an acute right subdural hematoma. Note the high amplitude SERs in the left hemisphere from right median nerve stimuli (upper right traces) and the spread of the later waves to the left side (lower right traces). Contrast these with the abnormal response over the involved hemisphere (lower left traces) and the absence of spread from right to left (upper left traces). Also compare to Fig. 21.

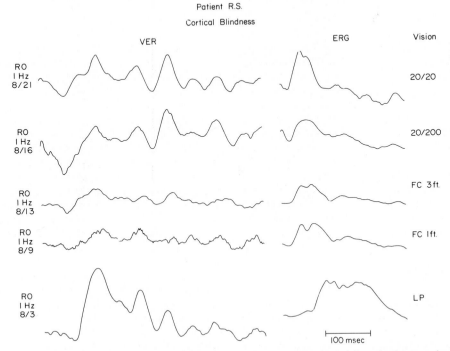

Patient R.S.

Cortical Blindness

	VER	ERG	Vision
RO 1 Hz 8/21			20/20
RO 1 Hz 8/16			20/200
RO 1 Hz 8/13			FC 3 ft.
RO 1 Hz 8/9			FC 1 ft.
RO 1 Hz 8/3			LP

100 msec

Fig. 23. Serial VER and ERG recordings in a patient who incurred a brief cerebral concussion and transient cortical blindness. Both the ERG and the VER are abnormal until visual recovery is complete. Dates are shown, the injury having occurred on 8–3.

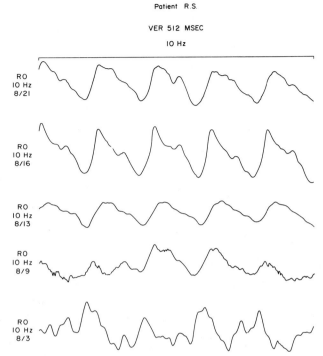

Fig. 24. Same patient as Fig. 23 showing VER in response to rapid (10 Hz) visual stimulus. Progressive restoration of amplitude and waveform correlates with restoration of visual acuity.

flow and metabolism is essential. In preliminary studies of experimental and clinical head injury we have observed that the SER does show alterations which correspond to changes in other physiological indices. As yet, these alterations have not been consistent enough to be predictive. We are currently developing an experimental study of the changes in evoked responses correlated with cerebral blood flow and O_2 metabolism using the O_{15} technique of Ter-Pogossian at different levels of head injury severity. This study should provide a more precise understanding of the interrelation between the intensity of primary damage and secondary physiopathologic responses to trauma.

Chemical Indices of Head Injury Severity

Although a number of studies on serum and CSF indices have been pursued, only two findings appear promising at this stage. First, it is now well established that the CSF acid-base balance shifts toward greater acidity and lactate is increased in the first week after trauma (metabolic acidosis).

Overgaard and Tweed[65] have noted that the period of greatest metabolic acidosis coincides with the period of cerebral hyperemia. This finding would suggest that the presence of metabolic acidosis could be an indicator of diffuse injury after head trauma, the intensity of pH shift thus reflecting the severity of primary damage.

A second aspect which holds promise is the detection of brain antigens in the serum. Thomas[78] has recently reported a preliminary study in 22 patients using antibrain rabbit serum against the patient's sera in the double diffusion method of Ouchterlony. Brain antigens were present in 71 percent of those who died and in 85 percent of those disabled for 1 month but in only 1 of 9 patients who made a good recovery. Of 4 patients dying after head injury without detectable brain antigen, 2 died of multiple trauma rather than of their relatively trivial head injury. Another was found to have no cortical contusions at autopsy. In the only patient who gave a positive antigen test with good survival there was a compound depressed fracture with cortical laceration. These important observations by Thomas suggest that the amount of primary cortical damage may well be the determining factor in releasing brain antigen. In a *nonhead-injured* group of patients with neurological disease, positive results were obtained only in 2 (of 15), both of whom had some cortical damage (temporal lobe hematoma with an aneurysm and a brain biopsy). The time course and nature of brain antigens released by trauma remain to be determined and could well provide us with an index of the extent of primary brain damage as well as a sequentially measurable index of secondarily developing progressive brain injury.

In conclusion, we wish to reiterate the extreme importance of conducting neural trauma research as a *dual* effort. Study in man must be correlated with the study of models, either aspect alone being inadequate for improved understanding of one of the most common of neurological diseases.

REFERENCES

1. Advani SH, Owings RP, Schuck LZ: Response evaluation of translational and rotational head injury models. Shock and Vibration Digest, 1972
2. Ambrose J, Hounsfield G: Computerized axial tomography. Br J Radiol 46:148–149, 1973
3. Beaussart M, Beaussart-Boulenge L: The post-concussional syndrome and the EEG, correlations in 3,100 cases. Electroenceph Clin Neurophysiol 28:649, 1970
4. Beaussart M, Beaussart-Boulenge L: EEG problems in post-concussional syndromes. Electroenceph Clin Neurophysiol 29:530, 1970
5. Bergamasco B et al: Longitudinal study of visual evoked potentials in post-traumatic coma. Schweizer Arch Neurol Neurochir Psychiatr 97:1–10, 1966
6. Brackett CE: Respiratory complications of head injury, in: Head Injuries. Proceedings of the International Symposium on Head Injuries. Baltimore, Williams and Wilkins, 225–265, 1971
7. Bruce EA, Langfitt TW, Miller JD et al: Regional cerebral blood flow, intracranial pressure, and brain metabolism in comatose patients. J Neurosurg 38:131–144, 1973
8. Bycroft GN: Mathematical model of a head subjected to angular acceleration. J Biomech 5:487–495, 1973
9. Caffey J: The whiplash shaken infant syndrome. Pediatrics 54:396–403, 1974
10. Cohen LB: Changes in neuron structure during action potential propagation and synaptic transmission. Physiol Rev 53:373–418, 1973
11. Committee to Study Head Injury Nomenclature: Report. Clin Neurosurg 12:386–387, 1966
12. Cracco RQ: Spinal evoked responses. Electroenceph Clin Neurophysiol 35:379, 1973
13. Denny-Brown D: Brain trauma and concussion. Arch Neurol 5:1–2, 1961
14. Denny-Brown D, Russel WR: Experimental cerebral concussion. Brain 64:93–164, 1941
15. Eidelberg E, Stein D: Functional recovery after lesions of the nervous system. Neurosci Res Program Bull 12:191–303, 1974
16. Feinsod M, Auerback E: Electrophysiological examinations of the visual system in the acute phase after head injury. Eur Neurol 9:56–64, 1973
17. Fisher, CM: Concussion amnesia. Neurology 16:826–830, 1966
18. Flamm ES, Ommaya AK, Fass F, et al: Cardiovascular effects of experimental head injury in the monkey. Surg Forum 27:414–416, 1966
19. Galambos R: Brain stem audiometry. Presented at the National Academy of Science Meeting, Washington DC, 1974
20. Gennarelli TA, Thibault LE, Ommaya AK: Comparison of linear and rotational acceleration in experimental cerebral concussion. Proceedings of the 15th Stapp Car Crash Conference. New York, Society of Automotive Engineers, 1971, pp 797–803
21. Gennarelli TA, Thibault LE, Ommaya AK: Pathophysiologic responses to rotational and translational accelerations of the head. Proceedings of the 16th Stapp Car Crash Conference. New York, Society of Automotive Engineers, 1972, pp 296–308
22. Gennarelli TA, Ommaya AK: Experimental head trauma. Part I. A model for inertial loading of the brain: Biomechanics and methodology. Part II. Traumatic unconsciousness. Part III. Diffuse brain lesions. The result of rotational injury. Part IV. Focal brain lesions: The result of translation injury In preparation
23. Gennarelli TA, Ommaya AK: A neurophysiological assay of head injury severity In preparation
24. Goldsmith W: Biomechanics of head injury, in Fung YC, Perrone N, Anliker M (eds): Biomechanics, Its Foundation and Objectives. Englewood Cliffs, NJ, Prentice-Hall, 1970, pp 585–634
25. Gray J, Ritchie JM: The effects of stretch on single myelinated nerve fibers. J Physiol 124:84–99, 1954
26. Grcevic N, Jacob H: Some observations on the pathology and correlative neuroanatomy of sequels of cerebral trauma, in Werner E (ed): Late Sequelae of Head Injuries. Proceedings of the 18th

International Congress of Neurology. Vienna, 1965, pp 369–374

27. Gronwall D, Wrightson P: Delayed recovery of intellectual function after minor head injury. Lancet 605-610, 1974

28. Gurdjian EG, Lissner HR, Hodgson VR, et al: Mechanisms of head injury. Clin Neurosurg 12:112–128, 1966

29. Hayashi T: Brain shear theory of head injury due to rotational impact. J Faculty Eng, University of Tokyo (B) 30: no. 4, 1970

30. Hirsch AE, Ommaya AK: Head injury caused by underwater explosion of a firecracker. J Neurosurg 37:95–99, 1972

31. Holbourn AHS: Mechanics of head injury. Lancet 2:438, 1943

32. Holbourn AHS: Personal communication to S. Strich. Quoted in Strich S: The pathology of brain damage due to blunt head injuries, in Walker AE, Caveness WF, Critchley M (eds): The Late Effects of Head Injury. Springfield, Ill: Charles C. Thomas, 1969, p 509

33. Hooper R: Patterns of Acute Head Injury. London, Edward Arnold. 1969

34. Jennett B, Plum F: Persistent vegetative state after brain damage. A syndrome in search of a name. Lancet 1:734–737, 1972

35. Jewett A: Auditory evoked far fields averaged from the scalp of humans. Brain 14:681–696, 1971

36. Joseph PD, Crisp JDC: On the evaluation of mechanical stresses in the human brain while in motion. Brain Res 26:15–35, 1972

37. Letcher F, Corrao PG, Ommaya AK: Head injury in the chimpanzee: Part II. Spontaneous and evoked epidural potentials as indices of injury severity. J Neurosurg 39:167–177, 1973

38. Lewin WS: Management of Head Injuries. Baltimore, Williams and Wilkins, 1966

39. Lindenberg R, Freytag E: The mechanism of cerebral contusion. Arch Path 69:440–469, 1960

40. Lindgren SO: Experimental studies of mechanical effects in head injury. Acta Chir Scand Suppl. 360, 1966

41. Lorenzoni E: Electroencephalographic studies before and after head injuries. Electroenceph Clin Neurophysiol 28:216, 1970

42. Meinig G, Reulen HJ, Magavly C, et al: Changes of cerebral homodynamics and energy metabolism during increased CSF pressure and brain edema, in Brock M, Dietz H (eds): Intracranial Pressure. Berlin, Springer-Verlag, 1973, pp 79–84

43. Mitchell DE, Hume Adams J: Primary focal impact damage to the brain stem in blunt head injuries: Does it exist? Lancet 215–218, 1973

44. Nakatani S, Ommaya AK: A critical rate of cerebral compression, in Brock M (ed): Intracranial Pressure. Berlin, Springer-Verlag, 1972, pp 144–148

45. Nakatani S, Ommaya AK: Pressure gradients in the cerebrovascular bed during cerebral compression at high and low rates. Proceedings of the American Association of Neurological Surgeons Annual Meeting, Miami, Florida, 1975

46. Ommaya AK: Head injuries: Aspects and problems. Med Ann DC 32:18–23, 1963

47. Ommaya AK: Trauma to the nervous system. A clinical and experimental study. Ann R Coll Surg Engl (Hunterian Lecture) 39:317–347, 1966

48. Ommaya AK: The mechanical properties of tissues of the nervous system. J Biomech 2:1–12, 1968

49. Ommaya AK: Computerized axial tomography: The EMI-Scanner, a new device for direct examination of the brain "in vivo." Surg Neurol 1:217–222, 1973

50. Ommaya AK, Rockoff SD, Baldwin M: Experimental concussion: A first report. J Neurosurg 21:249–267, 1964

51. Ommaya AK, Hirsch AE, Flamm ES, et al: Cerebral concussion in the monkey: An experimental model. Science 153:211-212, 1966

52. Ommaya AK, Hirsch AE, Martinez J: The role of "whiplash" in cerebral concussion. Proceedings of the 10th Stapp Car Crash Conference. New York, Society of Automotive Engineers, 1966, pp 197–203

53. Ommaya AK, Hirsch AE, Yarnell PR: Scaling of experimental data in cerebral concussion in subhuman primates to concussive threshold for man. Proceedings of the 11th Stapp Car Crash Conference. New York, Society of Automotive Engineers, 1967, pp 47–52

54. Ommaya AK, Faas F, Yarnell PR: Whiplash injury and brain damage: An experimental study. JAMA 204:285–289, 1968

55. Ommaya AK, Yarnell PR: Subdural haematoma after whiplash injury. Lancet 2:237–239, 1969

56. Ommaya AK, Corrao PG: Pathologic biomechanics of central nervous system injury in head impact and whiplash trauma, In Brinkhous KM (ed): Accident Pathology. Proceedings of the International Conference on Accident Pathology. Washington DC, Government Printing Office, 1970, pp 160–181

57. Ommaya AK, Grubb RL Jr., Naumann RA: Coup and contre-coupe: Observations on the mechanics of visible brain injuries in the rhesus monkey. J Neurosurg 35:503–517, 1971

58. Ommaya AK, Hirsch AE: Tolerance of cerebral concussion from head impact and whiplash in primates. J Biomech 4:13–22, 1971

59. Ommaya AK, Fedio P: The contribution of cingulum and hippocampal structures of memory mechanisms in man. Confin Neurol 34:398–411, 1972

60. Ommaya AK, Metz H, Post KE: Observations on the biomechanics of hydrocephalus, in Harbert JC

(ed): Cisternography and Hydrocephalus. Baltimore, Williams and Wilkins, 1972, pp 57–74

61. Ommaya AK, Corrao PG, Letcher F: Head injury in the chimpanzee: Part I. Biodynamics of traumatic unconsciousness. J Neurosurg 39:152–166, 1973

62. Ommaya AK, Gennarelli TA, Thibault LE: Traumatic unconsciousness: mechanisms of brain injury in violent shaking of the head, in: Proceedings of the American Association of Neurological Surgeons. Annual Meeting, Los Angeles, Paper no. 36, 1973

63. Ommaya AK, Gennarelli TA, Thibault LE: Effect of dynamic mechanical loading on frog sciatic nerve. Proceedings of the Society for Neuroscience, 4th Annual Meeting, St. Louis, Missouri, October 1974.

64. Ommaya AK, Gennarelli TA: Cerebral concussion and traumatic unconsciousness—correlation of experimental and clinical observations on blunt head injuries. Brain 97:633–654, 1974

65. Ommaya AK, Murray G, Ambrose J, Richardson A, Hounsfield G: Computerized axial tomography: estimation of spatial and density resolution capability. Brit J Radiol, in press

66. Overgaard J, Christensen S, Haase J, et al: Prognosis after head injury based on early clinical examination. Lancet 2:631–635, 1973

67. Overgaard J, Tweed WA: Cerebral circulation after head injury: Cerebral blood flow and its regulation after closed head injury with emphasis on clinical correlations. J Neurosurg, in press

68. Parsons LC, Ommaya AK: The sequelae of head injury in the rhesus monkey. Presentation at the 4th International Congress of Neurological Surgery and the 9th International Congress of Neurology, New York. Excerpta Medica 193:70–71, 1969

69. Petit JL: Oeuvres Completes de J.L. Petit. Maladie des Os, Maladies Chirurgicales. Paris, Prederic Prevost, 1944

70. Pudenz RH, Sheldon LH: The lucite calvarium:—A method for direct observation of the brain. II. Cranial trauma and brain movement. J Neurosurg 3:487–505, 1946

71. Rosenblueth A, Buylla RA, Ramos JG: The responses of axons to mechanical stimuli. J Cell Compar Physiol 3, 1957

72. Russell WR, Schiller R: Crushing injuries of the skull: Clinical and experimental observations. J Neurol Neurosurg Psychiatr 12:52–60, 1949

73. Singer P, Bignall K: Multiple somatic projections to frontal lobe of the squirrel monkey. Exp Neurol 27:438–453, 1970

74. Star A: Brain stem auditory evoked potentials in patients with coma. Presented at American Neurological Assoc. Meeting, Boston, 1974

75. Strich SJ: The pathology of brain damage due to blunt head injuries, in Walker AE, Caveness WF, Critchley M (eds): The Late Effects of Head Injury. Springfield, Ill: Charles C. Thomas, 1969, pp 501–526

76. Symonds CP: Concussion and its sequelae. Lancet 1:5, 1962

77. Teasdale G, Jennett B: Assessment of coma and impaired consciousness. A practical scale. Lancet 2:81–83, 1974

78. Thomas DGT: Brain antigen release into the peripheral blood of patients with head injuries. Paper read at Winter Meeting of Society of British Neurosurgeons, 1974

79. Torres F, Shapiro SK: Electroencephalographic abnormalities associated with whiplash injury. A comparison with the abnormalities present in closed head injuries. Arch Neurol 5:28–35, 1961

80. Unterharnschiedt F, Sellier K: Closed brain injuries: Mechanics and pathomorphology, in Caveness WF, Walker AE (eds): Head Injury Conference Proceedings. Philadelphia, J.B. Lippincott, 321–341, 1966

81. Unterharnschiedt F, Higgins LS: Neuropathologic effects of translational and rotational acceleration of the head in animal experiments, in Walker AE, Caveness WF, Critchley M (eds): The Late Effects of Head Injury. Springfield, Ill: Charles C. Thomas, 1969, pp 158–167

82. Walker AE: Mechanisms of cerebral trauma and the impairment of consciousness, in Youmans J (ed): Neurological Surgery, vol. II. Philadelphia, W.B. Saunders, 1973, pp 936–949

83. Ward AA Jr: The physiology of concussion. Clin Neurosurg 12:95–111, 1966

84. Wiener N: Cybernetics: Of control and communication in the animal and the machine. Cambridge, M.I.T. Press, 1971

85. Windle WF, Groat RA: Disappearance of nerve cells after concussion. Anat Rec 93:201–209, 1945

86. Yarnell PR: Retrograde memory immediately after concussion. Lancet 1:863–864, 1970

87. Yarnell PR, Lynch S: The "ding": Amnestic states in football trauma. Neurology 23:186–197, 1973

88. Zulch Von KJ: Pathologische anatomie physiopathologie und pathomechanismes des schadelhirntraumas. Bull Soc Sci Med Grand Duche Luxemb 106:153–211, 1969

Phanor L. Perot, Jr., M.D., Ph.D.

10

Evoked Potentials Assessment of Patients with Neural Trauma

Few days pass in the routine of the busy clinical neurosurgeon in which he does not anguish over these urgent questions: What is the extent of tissue injury in this brain- and/or spine-injured patient? What is the prognosis, the chance for recovery? Is the patient stable, improving, or deteriorating? The continuing search for answers to these questions has forced us to look for more precise techniques to supplement those of the time-honored neurological examination.

For several years, we have been interested in the application of the somatosensory evoked potential technique to the evaluation and monitoring of patients with neural trauma. We have concentrated our efforts on spinal injury and have to date used the technique in 288 studies on 116 patients. This brief summary of our work will be concerned mainly with spinal injury. A few observations will be made later concerning the use of evoked potentials in evaluating head injuries.

The mobile equipment and recording techniques have been described in detail previously.[1,2] Our standard procedure now in spinal injury cases is to record evoked potentials from appropriate areas of the scalp with stimulation of the right median nerve, right ulnar nerve, right posterior tibial nerve, left median nerve, left ulnar nerve, left posterior tibial nerve, and finally with simultaneous stimulation of both posterior tibial nerves (Fig. 1). Well-formed, consistent somatosensory evoked potentials (SEPs) can be regularly obtained from control subjects with unilateral median or ulnar nerve stimulation, but bilateral posterior tibial stimulation is definitely superior to unilateral stimulation.[3] One of our

technical problems earlier in this study was the inconsistency of SEPs from unilateral common peroneal nerve stimulation. In a recent series of 50 control subjects, definite SEPs were obtained in all cases when bilateral simultaneous posterior tibial nerve stimulation was used.

Our results in a series of 25 patients with cervical spine injury studied in the past year using the procedure outlined above show an excellent correlation of this technique with the extent of spine injury.

COMPLETE CERVICAL CORD INJURIES

These patients had no detectable motor or sensory function below the lesion on careful clinical examination. As shown in Table 1, no SEPs were recorded with stimulation of the ulnar, or unilateral or bilateral posterior tibial nerves. Three patients with low (below C5–6) lesions had responses to median nerve stimulation as might be expected. This table also points out an important technical difficulty—that of EMG contamination from cervical muscle spasm. This was much more of a problem in complete cervical injuries than in incomplete ones, and it was seen most often when the study was carried out very early (usually within several hours) in the postinjury period. Until a means can be devised to eliminate or minimize this interference, it will limit the usefulness of this method of examination in the period immediately following the injury.

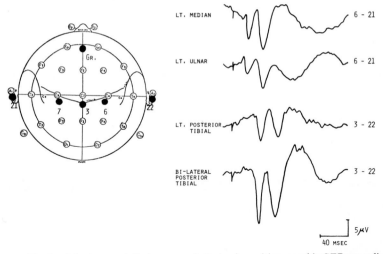

Fig. 1. Montage on left shows usual electrode positions used in SEP recording with spinal injuries. Gr., ground electrode. 21, 22, ear reference electrodes, 7, 6, electrodes for median nerve SEPs. 3, electrode for leg nerve SEPs. On right are shown normal control SEPs obtained with 128 stimulations at 1/sec. Traces redrawn from Polaroid photographs of oscilloscope. Upward deflection indicates negative potential. (This figure taken from reference 2).

Table 1
SEPs in 12 Patients with Complete
Cervical Cord Injury

Patient	Level	Med	Ulnar	PT	B-PT
G.L.	3–4	–	–	–	–
M.B.	4–5	*	*	*	*
J.J.	4–5	*	*	*	*
C.W.	4–5	–	–	–	–
P.D.	5–6	–	–	–	–
C.E.	5–6	*	*	*	*
S.C.	6–7	–	–	–	–
A.McE.	6–7	+	–	–	–
J.T.	6–7	*	–	–	–
D.W.	6–7	*	*	*	*
R.McD.	7	+	*	*	*
W.J.	7–1	+	–	–	–

Key: Level = vertebral level of injury; Med = median nerve stimulation; Ulnar = ulnar nerve stimulation; PT = posterior tibial nerve stimulation; B-PT = bilateral nerve stimulation.
+ = SEP was recorded normal or abnormal.
– = No SEP was obtained.
* = Recording was impossible due to EMG interference.

INCOMPLETE CERVICAL CORD INJURY

These patients had some preservation of motor or sensory function below the level of the lesion. In some cases, it might be extremely minimal such as preservation of deep pressure in one leg or sacral sparing. In Table 2, it can be seen that in striking contrast to the complete lesions, all patients had SEPs recorded from bilateral posterior tibial stimulation (except case J.L. where the recording was carried out on the second day after injury and EMG contamination interfered with the record). SEPs were obtained in this patient a few days later when the cervical muscle spasm had subsided. Most of the incomplete cases also had SEPs to median, ulnar, and unilateral posterior tibial stimulation as well.

These data indicate increasing accuracy in somatosensory evoked potential data as applied to spinal cord injury in the human. We are at present extending these techniques to include frequent serial studies and are actively investigating various methods of reducing EMG contamination. It would appear that the SEP technique will soon become an essential tool for the early assessment and later monitoring of spinal injuries.

EVOKED POTENTIAL STUDIES IN HEAD INJURIES

Several head injury centers are preparing at the present time to undertake comprehensive serial studies of evoked potentials in head injuries, and these will include auditory evoked potentials, visual evoked potentials, and somatosensory evoked potentials. Preliminary studies indicate that the evoked potential technique may prove extremely valuable for the assessment of head injury patients.[4,5,6] Our own observations are limited to a small series of 92 somatosensory evoked potential studies in 38 patients with head injuries of varying severity. Fourteen of the patients were in deep coma during the study. The somatosensory evoked potentials were elicited with stimulation of the median, common peroneal, or posterior tibial nerves. From these observations we have drawn a few tentative conclusions.

1. Median nerve somatosensory evoked potentials can be recorded bilaterally in severe closed head injury patients who are comatose and decerebrate. The potentials are markedly abnormal with reduction in amplitude of the early components and absence of the late components.
2. In patients with closed head injuries who are comatose and decerebrate, absent SEPs or very low voltage SEPs showing early potentials only in serial examinations over days or weeks indicates a poor prognosis for meaningful recovery. Early return of evoked potentials and particularly early return of the later components is more compatible with a good prognosis for recovery.
3. It is our preliminary impression that in deeply comatose patients, the late components of the

Table 2

SEPs in 13 Patients with Incomplete Cervical Cord Injury (Some Motor or Sensory Functions Spared)

Patient	Level	Med	Ulnar	PT	B-PT
W.Ma.	1–2	+	+	−	+
W.A.	4–5	+	+	+	+
L.C.	4–5	+	+	+	+
J.L.	4–5	*	*	*	*
F.T.	4–5	−	−	+	+
P.A.	5–6	+	+	+	+
M.J.	5–6	+	+	+	+
T.K.	5–6	+	+	+	+
W.M.	5–6	+	+	+	+
R.Ro.	5–6	+	+	+	+
S.G.	5–6	+	+	+	+
C.M.	7	+	+	+	+
N.McK.	7–1	+	+	+	+

Key: Symbols same as in Table 1.

evoked potential are more affected than the early components and that return of consciousness and improvement seem to be correlated with return of the late components of the evoked potential.

These evoked potential and other monitoring techniques have not yet reached the stage of development where they can obviate the necessity for careful clinical assessment of the patient with injury to the nervous system. However, we feel confident that the clinician will have available in the near future powerful, noninvasive, neurophysiologic techniques that will give him much more precision in the diagnosis and continuing management of these critically ill patients.

REFERENCES

1. Perot PL Jr: The clinical use of somatosensory evoked potentials in spinal cord injury, in: Clinical Neurosurgery vol. 20. Baltimore, Williams and Wilkins, 1973, p 367
2. Perot PL Jr: Somatosensory evoked potentials in the evaluation of patients with spinal cord injury, in Morley TP (ed): Controversy in Neurological Surgery. Philadelphia, W.B. Saunders (in press)
3. Vera CL, Fountain EL, Perot PL Jr: Distribution and analysis of evoked responses to unilateral and bilateral posterior tibial nerve stimulation in man (submitted to Electroenceph. Clin. Neurophysiol)
4. Numoto M, Wallman LJ, Flanagan ME, Donaghy RMP: Evoked potentials in diagnosis and prognosis in coma, particularly post-trauma. Presented at the 41st Annual Meeting of the American Association of Neurological Surgeons, Los Angeles, April 10, 1973
5. Larson SJ, Sances A, Ackmann JJ, Reigel DH: Noninvasive evaluation of head trauma patients. Surgery 74:34–40, 1973
6. Perot PL Jr: The use of somatosensory evoked potentials in the evaluation of brain and spinal cord injury. Presented at the 25th Annual Meeting of the Neurosurgical Society of America, Pebble Beach, Calif, March 22, 1972

Richard P. Greenberg, M.D.
David J. Mayer, Ph.D.
Donald P. Becker, M.D.

11

The Prognostic Value of Evoked Potentials in Human Mechanical Head Injury

Central nervous system electrical activity is a sensitive index of the functional integrity of the neuronal cell population.[1] Even mild CNS injury can be reflected in abnormal neuroelectric potentials.[2] Computer averaged evoked potentials can be used to accurately reveal the location and extent of CNS injury, can monitor the progression of the injury, and, therefore, can provide a valuable, early prognostic assessment of the magnitude of a patient's ultimate recovery or residual deficit.

We have applied evoked potentials in extensive, standardized, serial studies on severe mechanical brain injury patients in the acute phase of their hospital course in an effort to evaluate their final clinical status.

Scalp electrodes were used to symmetrically record visual, somatosensory, and auditory computer-averaged evoked potentials simultaneously from all lobes in both hemispheres. The patients were all unresponsive as a result of severe head injury and were studied after admission to the neurosurgical intensive care unit at the Medical College of Virginia Hospital. A total of 16 scalp electrodes were used for each session and placed according to the International 10-20 system. This assured intrasubject and cross-subject standardization and facilitated accurate data analysis. Both near field and far field[3] evoked potential techniques were employed to record from the cortex as well as deeper CNS areas. Electroretinograms, eighth nerve action potentials,[4] and peripheral nerve action potentials were done when indicated to verify the integrity of the respective peripheral receptor.

The evoked potential data were correlated with the clinical neurological course, acute and chronic intracranial monitoring, cerebral angiography, and the operative findings.

We have divided the multimodality evoked potential data into one of three general categories designed to help evaluate its prognostic significance: evoked potentials without electrical abnormalities; evoked potentials displaying focal electrical abnormalities; evoked potentials which seem to indicate gross topographical alteration of neuroelectric activity such as in brain stem or cerebral hemispheres.

EVOKED POTENTIAL DATA WITHOUT ELECTRICAL ABNORMALITY

Patient J.H., a 14-year-old male, victim of an automobile accident, was unresponsive to verbal command and purposeful bilaterally to painful stimulation on admission. The remainder of his neurological exam was negative. Figure 1 represents the somatosensory evoked potential data displayed with an emphasis on the anatomic location of electrical activity. Figure 2 displays his visual evoked potentials, and Fig. 3 shows a simultaneous eighth nerve action potential and auditory far field study. The patient regained consciousness and was neurologically intact on the 10th day postinjury. Acute and chronic intracranial pressure monitoring never revealed a pressure over 10 mm Hg. Cerebral angiography and skull roentgenograms were considered normal.

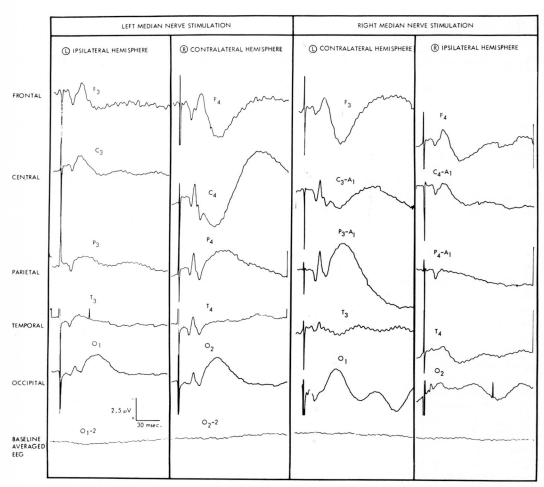

Fig. 1. J. H.; 14-year-old male normal somatosensory study.

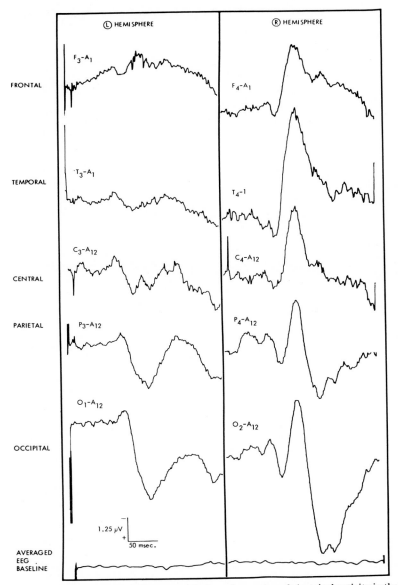

Fig. 5.   J. C.; generalized left hemisphere depression of electrical activity in the visual evoked potential study.

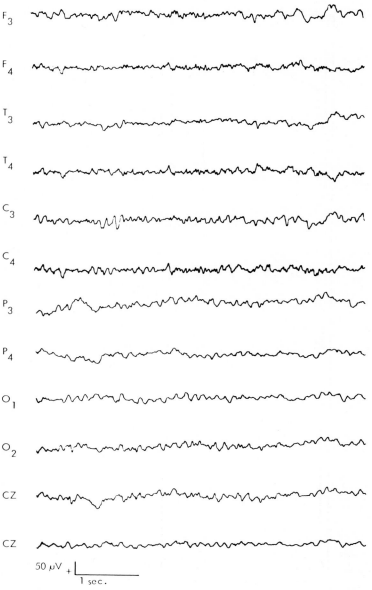

Fig. 6. J. C.; EEG appears normal even the T-3 lead overlying the left temporal lobe.

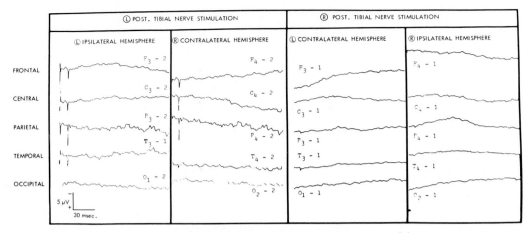

Fig. 7. R. S.; 11-year-old male absent somatosensory potentials.

EVOKED POTENTIAL DATA WITH
FOCAL ELECTRICAL ABNORMALITY

Patient J. C., a 48-year-old male, injured in a 20-foot fall, was unresponsive to verbal commands and nonpurposeful to painful stimulation on admission. Figure 4 is his somatosensory evoked potential study which localizes a left temporal lobe attenuation of electrical activity. Figure 5 displays his visual potentials, which are generally depressed in the entire left hemisphere as were his auditory potentials. Figure 6 is this patient's EEG done at the same session as the evoked potentials. These studies were done several days after he had had a 5 cm resection of a severely contused necrotic left temporal lobe tip. The patient sub-

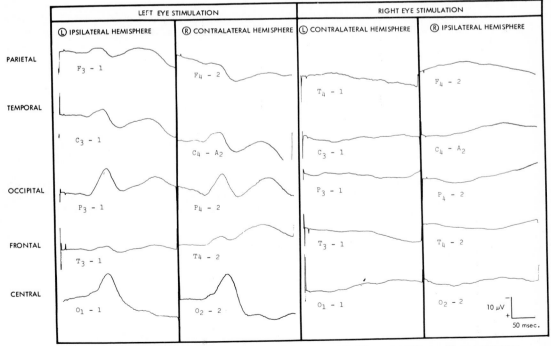

Fig. 8. R. S.; present but abnormal visual potentials as recorded from the left eye. Absent response from the right. (See Fig. 9.)

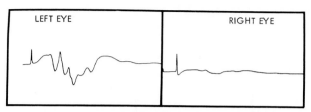

| LEFT EYE | RIGHT EYE |

Fig. 9. R. S.; absent retinal response from the right eye in the electroretinogram.

sequently became alert on the 25th hospital day after admission and surgery. Four months later he was neurologically intact except for a fluent aphasia and a visual field deficit.

EVOKED POTENTIAL DATA WITH GROSS TOPOGRAPHICAL ELECTRICAL ABNORMALITY

Patient R. S., an 11-year-old male, was decerebrate bilaterally on admission. His left pupil was fixed and dilated and the left oculocephalic reflexes were absent. His right pupil reacted sluggishly to light and a sixth cranial nerve palsy was present in this eye. The emergency ventriculogram revealed an intracranial pressure of 5 mm Hg with midposition ventricles and bloodstained CSF. Chronic intracranial pressure monitoring and four vessel cerebral angiography were normal. Figure 7 represents his somatosensory evoked potential study—no potentials could be recorded. His auditory potentials were also absent. Figure 8 represents the visual potentials which are present, although the waveform is abnormal when performed selectively on the left eye, absent when done on the right eye. The electroretinogram, Fig. 9, reveals a peripheral receptor dysfunction in the right eye explaining the right visual evoked potential absence.

These studies seem to indicate a depression of electrical activity that is greater in this patient's brain stem than in his cerebral hemispheres. Five months postinjury, this patient is essentially unchanged neurologically.

These three cases serve as examples of our preliminary observations on the value of evoked potential studies in predicting the final outcome of severe human head injury patients. Evoked potentials are a noninvasive means of evaluating CNS functional integrity and may be able to separate patients with pure brain stem injury from those with mixed supratentorial and stem damage or only supratentorial damage.

REFERENCES

1. Stohr PE, Goldring S: Origin of somatosensory evoked scalp response in man. J Neurosurg 31:117–127, 1969
2. Giblin DR: Somatosensory evoked potentials in health subjects and in patients with lesions of the nervous system. Ann NY Acad Sci 112:93–142, 1964
3. Jewett DL, Williston JS: Auditory-evoked far fields averaged from the scalp of humans. Brain 94:681–696, 1971
4. Cullen KK Jr, Ellis MS, Becker CI, Lousteau RJ: Human acoustic nerve action potential recordings from the tympanic membrane without anesthesia. Acta Otolaryng 74:15–22, 1972

Samuel A. Shelburne, Jr., M.D.
Anne N. McLaurin, M.D.
Robert L. McLaurin, M.D.

12

Effects of Graded Hypoxia on Visual Evoked Responses of Rhesus Monkeys

HYPOXIA

In recent head injury experiments on rhesus monkeys, we found a variety of changes in visual evoked responses (VERs) following controlled head injury. These changes seemed to be related to multiple factors including hypoxia, ischemia, intracranial pressure, etc. Review of the literature revealed few studies of the effect of hypoxia on the VER. The purpose of our investigations was to study the effects of graded hypoxia on visual evoked responses and the spontaneous electroencephalogram recorded by scalp electrodes.

Methods

Twelve rhesus monkeys (4.5–7 kg) were anesthetized with chloral hydrate, paralyzed with pancronium bromide, and ventilated on a Bennett model #MA-1 respirator. Nitrogen was added to room air at various concentrations to produce oxygen levels ranging down from 8 percent to 3 percent. The percent oxygen in the inspired air was kept constant throughout each separate experiment. Carbon dioxide was completely removed from the expired air and then added to the inspired air to keep the CO_2 intake constant at 6 percent. Arterial pH, pCO_2, pO_2, and hemoglobin concentrations were measured at approximately 15-minute intervals. In experiments using low

Supported by NIH Grant #NS 07253 and U.S. Public Health Service Center Grant in Mental Retardation, HD05221

oxygen concentrations (3 percent) arterial pO_2's were measured every 2 to 3 minutes. Systemic arterial pressure, EKG, and rectal temperature were measured continuously and recorded. All animals were kept normothermic with a thermal pad and arterial pH was kept within physiological limits.

For the visual evoked responses, a Grass-model 2 stroboscopic bulb was placed 10 cm in front of the monkey's face, the monkey lying prone on the operating table. One hundred flashes were presented in each group. EEG needle electrodes were inserted into the scalp over the left and right occipital areas and left and right central areas. Needle electrodes were also placed in the ears for neutral reference recordings. Four EEG channels were monitored continuously. The EEG output during visual stimulation was recorded on an Ampex model 1300 FM tape recorder. The recorded data was played back at a later date, and the VER extracted from the background activity by a computer system (Lab-8 Digital Equipment Corporation).

From the visual display, the most consistent and prominent components of the VER were the initial positive component $P_1 = 26$ msec and the initial negative wave, $N_1 = 34$ msec. For graphic analysis, the amplitudes of the P_1-N_1 complexes were calculated and the latencies of the N_1 peak were also calculated. These values were plotted separately against time of duration of hypoxia for each arterial pO_2 concentration. Statistical analysis was done using the LAB-8 system of confidence intervals. See references 1 and 2 for a complete summary of the method.

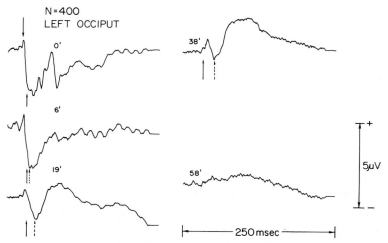

Fig. 1. Mean of 400 visual evoked responses (VERs) to stroboscopic flashes. Recording from left occiput to both ears linked. Time base is 250 msec of analysis. Positive is up. The figure in the upper left hand corner under 0′ is the mean VER in room air before the nitrogen was added. The other time intervals indicate the average time the VERs were obtained after the onset of hypoxia. The downward deflecting arrow indicates the prominent P_1 peak (latency = 28 msec) and the upward arrow the N_1 trough (latency = 38 msec). In successive figures the latency of the N_1 component at room air is shown by the solid arrow and the gradual prolongation of the N_1 latency is indicated by the dotted arrows. In addition to the increasing latency of the N_1 component the amplitude of the P_1 and N_1 complex is gradually reduced and almost disappears by 58′. Note also the upward deflection of late components. In this experiment, the mean arterial pO_2 was 121 mm Hg in room air and 24.5 ± 2.1 (1 S.D.) mm Hg after hypoxia.

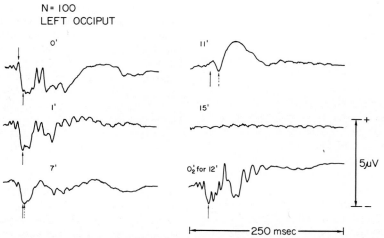

Fig. 2. Mean of 100 VERs. Recording from left occipit to linked ears. Again positive is up and the analysis time is 250 msec. The arrows indicating the P_1 and N_1 components are the same as Fig. 1. The baseline arterial pO_2 was 95 mm Hg and after the introduction of nitrogen the mean pO_2 fell to 20.5 ± 1.7 mm Hg. Note that the VER completely disappears by 15′. The last figure shows the return of the VER 12 minutes after oxygen was given to the monkey.

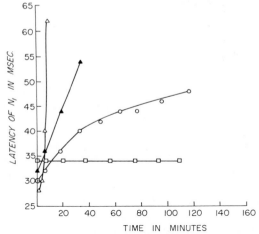

Fig. 3. Latency of N_1, in msecs, is plotted against time in minutes after hypoxia was introduced. There are three types of curves: (1) Horizontal line. Represented by the squares. The latency of N_1 remains constant throughout the experiment. Three experiments fell within this group. The mean arterial pO_2 for this group was 33.3 mm Hg and the range was from 29.7 mm Hg to 37.5 mm Hg. (2) A gradual increasing curve, similar to first order enzymatic reaction curve, represented by the circles. Five experiments fell in this group. The mean arterial pO_2 was 23.2 mm Hg and the range was 20.9–25.2 mm Hg. (3) A straight line up represented by the triangles. Four experiments fell in this group. The mean arterial pO_2 was 18.2 mm Hg and the range was 15.3–20.8 mm Hg.

Results

The following changes in the VER were seen after moderate to severe hypoxia (arterial pO_2 less than 29 mm Hg).

1. An upward (positive) shift of the late components of the VER (greater than 100 msec following the stimulus).
2. Prolongation of the latencies of the various components, particularly the first negative (N_1) component.
3. Reduction in amplitude of the VER, particularly the P_1-N_1 complex.

All of these changes are illustrated in Fig. 1. Marked changes in the visual evoked response were associated with more profound hypoxia. This is shown in Fig. 2.

Individual experiments suggested that there was a mathematical relationship between prolongation of the latency of component N_1 and the duration of hypoxia. This relationship is shown in Fig. 3. From the graph, one could accurately predict changes in the latency of the N_1 component if the initial latency (prehypoxia) and arterial pO_2 were known.

A mathematical relationship between the fall in amplitude of the P_1-N_1 complex, time and arterial pO_2 was also seen, but there was more variation in the resulting patterns. Typical examples are shown in Fig. 4. In general, there was a

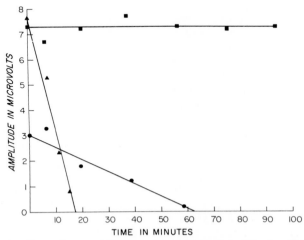

Fig. 4. Three characteristic examples of changes in amplitude with time. The amplitude in microvolts of the P_1-N_1 complex is plotted against the time in minutes after the hypoxia was introduced. There was no decrease in amplitude in the experiment represented by the squares, mean arterial pO_2 = 37.5 mm Hg. There was a gradual decrease in amplitude, the circles, with pO_2 of 24.5 mm Hg. Note the VER disappears in 62 minutes. There was a rapid decline, the triangles, with disappearance of the VER in 17' with a pO_2 of 20.5 mm Hg.

good correlation between changes in latencies and changes in amplitude, but the latency changes were more consistent, and the grouping of changes according to degree of hypoxia was more reliable.

Statistical evaluation was performed on all experiments. In such examples as Figs. 1 and 2, where the evoked response disappears, it is hardly necessary to prove a statistical difference between pre- and posthypoxic VERs. However, it is useful to show a significant difference in the experiments with milder hypoxia. All experiments showed statistical differences between the prehypoxic baseline VERs and posthypoxic VERs.

Discussion

In our review of the literature, we did not find any reports concerning the effects of graded hypoxia on the visual evoked response. There are several classical studies of the changes in visual evoked responses with anoxia. Chang and Kaada[3] stimulated the exposed optic nerves in cats and recorded the response from various areas, including the visual cortex, with an oscilloscope. After the animal was put on pure nitrogen, through the trachea, the evoked response disappeared in 96 seconds. The later components of the VER disappeared before the earlier ones. Noell and Chinn[4] found similar results using rabbits. In addition to stimulation of the optic nerve they also used photic stimulation to the retina. With the introduction of pure nitrogen, the VER disappeared completely in 88 seconds. It should be noted that both these studies used complete anoxia and implanted electrodes. Modern averaging techniques can be used to measure evoked responses through the intact scalp. Averaging techniques were used in the studies of Meldrum and Brierly,[5] although they did record from exposed cortex. They studied the decrease of somatosensory evoked responses (SERs) after ischemia in rhesus monkeys. These authors concluded that the SER is the most valuable physiological measurement of the function of the brain and, specifically, is a much better predictor of brain recovery from ischemia than the electroencephalogram or electrocorticogram.

We also found the visual evoked response to be a useful measure of brain function during hypoxia. The VER is more sensitive than the EEG. In all experiments, the EEG disappeared several minutes before the VER. When room air was started after the VER had disappeared, the VER also reappeared before the EEG.

There are several advantages to the use of the VER in this type of experiment. By using needle scalp electrodes, this method is easily applicable to clinical problems of humans and hypoxia. The rhesus monkey is close to the human and is preferable to such animals as cats, rats, and rabbits used in other experiments. Other investigations have substituted nitrous oxide for oxygen to achieve hypoxia, rather than nitrogen. Nitrous oxide is an anesthetic agent and may affect the EEG and VER. It also is important to avoid use of compounds like Phencyclidine, Nembutal, etc. These have clear effects on the EEG and VER. In our experiments we used high doses of chloral hydrate for anesthesia. This compound was selected because of its safety factor and the recognized clinical judgment that it has the least effects of sedative and anesthetic compounds on the spontaneous EEG of man. There were no previous publications found concerning effects of chloral hydrate on VERs. In five separate preliminary control experiments we compared VERs in the same rhesus monkey given pancronium bromide alone and then pancronium bromide and chloral hydrate over a 2-hour period. These animals were ventilated with room air. The chloral hydrate produced slowing of the EEG and also caused variable positive and negative deflections of the late components of the VER (125 msec). The P_1 and N_1 latencies were unchanged and the P_1 and N_1 amplitudes were essentially unchanged. We concluded that chloral hydrate had no significant effect on the components of the VER that we were studying.

Many variables can affect brain function to produce changes in VERs. As an example, ischemia can profoundly reduce the amplitude of the VER. During these experiments, vigorous efforts were made to keep all systemic factors constant during the period of hypoxia. For the group as a whole, mean arterial pressure was 119.5 ± 16.9 mm Hg in the prehypoxic baseline state and 105.6 ± 24.8 mm Hg in the hypoxic period. The fall in pressure was most likely related to the removal of blood for analysis and the effects of hypoxia. For the group as a whole, the mean control hemoglobin was $11.4 \pm .9$ g % and after hypoxia was $10.4 \pm .7$ g %. Blood loss was replaced by physiological salt solutions. In the baseline state, the average pCO_2 was 39.4 ± 4.0 mm Hg. Arterial pH was kept constant by the infusion of sodium bicarbonate. Mean arterial pH was $7.39 \pm .05$ before hypoxia and $7.37 \pm .06$ after hypoxia.

The most critical factors affecting the VER were the arterial pO_2 and the duration of hypoxia.

The critical pO_2 level for the onset of progressive reduction in amplitude of the VER and prolongation of latencies was less than 29 mm Hg. With lower pO_2's, these changes took place much more rapidly. From pO_2 levels of 29–39 mm Hg, the only change noted was an upward (+) movement of the late components of the response. There have been many recent articles[6-9] that have been concerned with the critical level of oxygen in the brain at which permanent damage will result. Many of these articles have suggested that the critical venous pO_2 is 17–19 mm Hg. In these experiments, we did not measure venous pO_2, but it is interesting that our critical level of arterial pO_2 (29 mm Hg) agrees with the calculations of Grunewald.[7] These physiological measurements seem to correlate well with biochemical results.

SUMMARY

Twelve rhesus monkeys, anesthetized with chloral hydrate and paralyzed with pancronium bromide were ventilated with oxygen concentrations ranging from 8 percent to 3 percent of the inspired air. The oxygen concentration and arterial pO_2 were kept constant in each animal throughout the experiment. EEG and visual evoked responses (VERs) were recorded continuously. Consistent changes noted after hypoxia were: upward (positive) shift of the late components (125–250 msec) of the VER, prolongation of the initial negative (N_1 = 32 msec) component, and reduction in amplitude of the early components (P_1-N_1) complex. Given the arterial pO_2, one could accurately predict subsequent changes in the latency of the N_1 component with time. Similar curves showing a mathematical relationship between reduction of amplitude of the VER, arterial pO_2, and time were also plotted. The visual evoked response appears to be a useful experimental method to study hypoxia.

REFERENCES

1. Shelburne SA Jr: Visual evoked responses to word and nonsense syllable stimuli. Electroenceph Clin Neurophysiol 32:17–25, 1972
2. Shelburne SA Jr: Visual evoked responses to language stimuli in normal children. Electroenceph Clin Neurophysiol 34:135–143, 1973
3. Chang HT, Kaada B: An analysis of primary response of visual cortex to optic nerve stimulation in cats. J Neurophysiol 13:305–318, 1950
4. Noell W, Chinn HI: Failure of the visual pathway during anoxia. Am J Physiol 161:573–590, 1950
5. Meldrum BS, Brierly JB: Brain damage in the rhesus monkey resulting from profound arterial hypotension: II Changes in spontaneous and evoked electrical activity of the neocortex. Brain Res 13:101–118, 1969
6. MacMillan V: Critical oxygen tensions in the brain. Acta Anesthesiol Scand 45:101–109, 1972
7. Grunewald W: Theoretical analysis of the oxygen supply in tissue, in Lubbers DW et al (eds): Oxygen Transport in Blood and Tissue. Stuttgart, Germany, Georg Thieme Verlag, 1968, pp 100–114
8. MacMillan V, Siesjo BK: Critical oxygen tensions in the brain. Acta Physiol Scand 82:412–414, 1971
9. Siesjo BK, Plum F: The brain in normoxia and in hypoxia. Acta Anesthesiol Scand Suppl 45:81–101, 1972

Moshe Feinsod, M.D.

13

Electrophysiological Correlates of Traumatic Visual Damage

The assessment of visual function, like any other exteroceptive sensory system, depends on verbal information from the patient in response to questions and stimuli. Consciousness and cooperation are thus imperative. There is a need, therefore, for an objective method that will enable the examination of the visual system of the head-injured patient without depending on his state of consciousness or cooperation.

In two recent papers[1,2] we reported the value of the visual evoked response (VER) in the assessment of visual function in the acute phase after head injury and in the evaluation of the posttraumatic subjective visual complaints.

After examining 75 patients suffering from visual disturbances following head injury, we wish to report some characteristics VER patterns found in the following conditions: trauma to the optic nerves; occipital lobe injury; concussion; and posttraumatic conversion reaction or malingering.

METHODS

The examinations of the VER were carried out with the patient lying, preferably in an electrically shielded cage. The pupils were dilated (Mydriaticum Roche) only when there was no danger of masking the development of neurological signs.

The VER was recorded between two 9 mm silver disc electrodes affixed to the scalp with electrode paste, at the inion and 5 cm above. The signals were amplified by AC preamplifiers (Grass PS-5) whose filters were set at 0.1 Hz and 2000 Hz. A standard calibration pulse was averaged at the beginning of each test.

One hundred 1/sec flashes at 20 cm from the patient's eyes were delivered by a Xenon discharge lamp (type 80-227) activated by a Gross photostimulator (PS-2). The responses to the flash stimuli were averaged by a computer of averaged transients (Mnemotron CAT 440b). Analysis time was 250 msec. The CAT run was triggered by the photostimulator. The averaged responses were displayed on the screen of the Tektronix CRT 502 and then photographed.

A normal VER to binocular and monocular stimulations is represented in Fig. 1. In all our recordings, positive polarity is upward. The response to binocular and monocular stimulations consists of an initial positive deflection.

RESULTS

Seventy-five patients suffering or complaining of visual disturbances were examined. Thirty-five suffered from optic nerve lesions which were unilateral in 21. Occipital lobe damage was the cause of visual deficits in 10 patients. Eighteen patients sustained cerebral concussion which caused periods of unconsciousness lasting 2 to 21 days. The other 12 patient's complaints were due to previous psychiatric disturbances, posttraumatic conversion reactions, or even to malingering.

Eight patients displaying the characteristic changes in the VER due to the above mentioned involvement of the visual pathways are presented in detail.

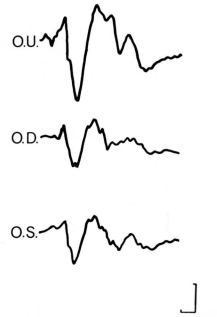

Fig. 1. A normal VER to binocular (O.U.) and monocular (O.D. and O.S.) stimulations. Calibration: 5 mv; 25 msec.

Patient One

A 20-year-old woman, involved in a road accident, was unconscious upon admission. There was a large wound in her forehead through which a fracture line could be seen. The right pupil was dilated and did not react to light. No other neurological deficits were found. Skull x-rays showed the fracture to extend into the right orbit.

The VER to stimulation of the right eye was extinct. It was normal when the left eye was stimulated (Fig. 2). After regaining consciousness the patient was found to be blind in her right eye. Vision in the left was normal.

Patient Two

A 42-year-old man fell from a truck, was hit on the head, and lost consciousness for several minutes. Later he complained of loss of vision in

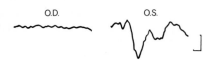

Fig. 2. Patient 1. VER to stimulation of the right (O.D.) and the left (O.S.) eyes. Note the absent VER to stimulation of the right eye. Calibration: 5 mv; 25 msec.

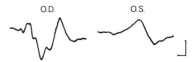

Fig. 3. Patient 2. VER to stimulation of the right (O.D.) and the left (O.S.) eyes. The latter consists of a slow wave of prolonged latency. Calibration: 5 mv; 25 msec.

the left eye. On examination, the patient could barely distinguish between light and dark in his left eye. Vision in the right eye was normal. The left pupil reacted sluggishly to light. No fracture was seen on x-ray of the skull, orbits, or optic foramina.

The VER, examined 2 days after the injury, was normal when the right eye was stimulated. Stimulation of the left eye evoked only a slow wave of prolonged latency where none of the usual VER components would be identified (Fig. 3). His visual functions did not change thereafter, and left optic atrophy was found a month later.

Patient Three

This 16-year-old boy sustained a blunt injury directed to his left temple and orbit. Vision in the left eye was lost for 3 days and later improved partially. Six weeks after the injury, his vision was 20/20 in the right eye and 20/40 in the left eye. The left pupillary reflex was slow in the left eye with Marcus Gunn sign. The left visual field was constricted and the left optic disc was pale. There was a left temporal linear fracture on skull x-ray.

The VER to stimulation of the right eye was normal. Stimulation of the left eye elicited a response of prolonged latency and lower amplitude (Fig. 4). However, the initial positive wave and the following negative deflection could be identified.

Patient Four

A 26-year-old worker was brought to the casualty room after his head was crushed between the bumpers of two cars. On admission he was

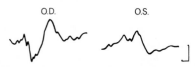

Fig. 4. Patient 3. A normal VER to stimulation of the right eye (O.D.). Stimulation of the left eye (O.S.) elicits a response of prolonged latency and reduced amplitude. Calibration: 5 mv; 25 msec.

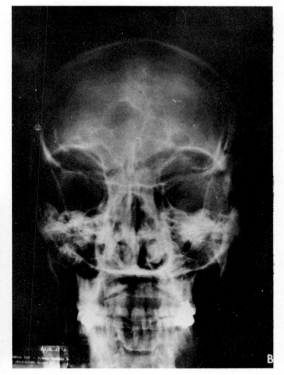

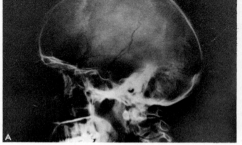

Fig. 5. (*a* and *b*) Skull x-ray of Patient 4.

semiconscious and restless. A huge hematoma extended from one temporal region to the other, causing swelling of the deformed forehead and face. The eyes were closed tightly by the swollen eyelids. On skull x-rays, many fracture lines were seen traversing the orbits and the bones of the an-terior and middle fossae (Fig. 5a, b). The patient's eyes were opened by lid retractors but any attempt to estimate his vision was futile. The pupils were moderately dilated and their reflexes to light were absent.

For the electrophysiological examination, the

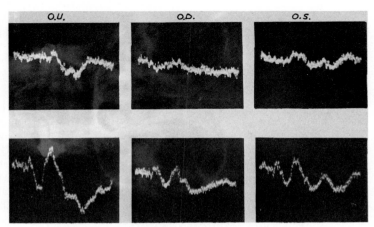

Fig. 6. Patient 4. VER to binocular (O.U.) and monocular (O.D. and O.S.) stimulation. The upper traces were recorded at the acute phase after head injury. The lower traces were recorded after recuperation.

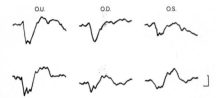

Fig. 7. Patient's VER to binocular and monocular stimulation. The upper traces were recorded shortly after the injury. The lower traces were recorded a year later. Calibration: 5 mv; 25 msec.

light source was brought close to the eyes and although much of the light was filtered by the swollen lids a long latency and low amplitude VER could be recorded from stimulation of either eye. It was, therefore, clear that the visual pathways were conducting (Fig. 6, upper traces). A week later, the eyelid hematomas were partially absorbed and consciousness regained. Visual acuity and visual fields were normal. The VER could be examined under controlled conditions and was found to be normal. (Fig. 6, lower traces).

Patient Five

This 22-year-old worker was admitted in a state of deep coma and profound shock after being injured by a falling brick. Blood and brain tissue were emerging from a large occipital wound. There was left hemiplegia and the left pupil was markedly dilated. Skull x-ray revealed a fracture

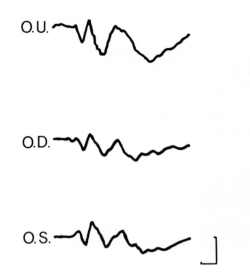

Fig. 8. Patient 6. VER in homonymous hemianopia. Note the subnormal amplitudes. Calibration: 5 mv; 25 msec.

line extending from the right parietal region to the base of the skull through the left occipital region with a large depressed bone fragment.

At operation, the superior sagittal sinus was found to be torn, there was a large laceration of the right parietal lobe, the left occipital lobe seemed completely destroyed. The torn sinus was repaired, necrotic tissues were debrided, and complete hemostasis was achieved.

The patient remained unconscious. The VER, recorded 7 days after the injury, was of normal latency, low amplitude, and somewhat distorted shape. (Fig. 7, upper traces). It was concluded that part of the visual system was spared and that there was some prognosis for vision. Ten weeks later the patient regained consciousness. He had a right homonymous hemianopia. The VER remained practically unchanged (Fig. 7, lower traces) even after a year.

Patient Six

A 20-year-old man was shot in the head. On admission he was conscious. A small amount of blood and brain tissue were coming out of a left occipital wound. Right homonymous hemianopia was suspected. No other neurological deficits were found. X-ray of the skull showed a left occipital bone defect and two intracranial metal fragments, a small one in the left occipital lobe and a larger one in the posterior region of the left temporal lobe. The left occipital region was explored; necrotic tissue was debrided and hemostasis achieved. The patient had an uneventful recovery. Right homonymous hemianopia was the only neurological sequela. The VER was of low amplitude (Fig. 8) but of normal latency and contour.

Patient Seven

A 22-year-old man was rendered unconscious for 2 days after a head injury. Skull x-rays revealed a right parietal linear fracture. He was discharged from the hospital after a week. The neurological examination did not reveal any pathological findings. At a follow-up examination 2 weeks later, the patient complained of repeated episodes of blurred vision and difficulties in reading. No objective visual symptoms were found.

The VER to stimulation of each eye was of prolonged latency and low amplitude (Fig. 9, upper traces). Three months later, the patient reported the disappearance of the visual symptoms.

The VER this time was of shorter latencies and higher amplitudes (Fig. 9, lower traces), a definite improvement.

Patient Eight

A 24-year-old soldier fell from a half-truck during combat. He immediately complained of loss of vision in one eye. Neurophthalmological examination failed, however, to disclose any objective deficit. As his complaints persisted, the VER was examined.

The VER was entirely normal (Fig. 1) in latencies and configuration.

DISCUSSION

The clinical examination of the visual system is unrivaled in accuracy. It requires, however, the cooperation of the patient and therefore depends on his state of consciousness, attention and intellect. These drawbacks are frequently encountered after head injury when consciousness may be impaired, in the acute phase, or later when conversion reaction as well as secondary gain attempts may develop.

In the present study we tried, by the use of the VER, to improve our ability for objective detection or confirmation of visual disturbances following head injury. Patients 1, 2, and 3 suffered different degrees of unilateral optic nerve injury. A satisfactory correlation was found between the severity of the clinical condition and the VER findings. Thus, stimulation of the totally blind eye of Patient 1 did not evoke any potential change (Fig. 2). Vision in the left eye of Patient 2 was reduced to light perception; the VER to stimulation of that eye was just an amplitude change at a very prolonged latency, in which none of the known VER components could be clearly identified (Fig. 3). The relatively minor damage inflicted to the optic nerve of Patient 3 was demonstrated by the mild prolongation of latencies and the reduction of the VER amplitude to about two-thirds of that evoked by stimulation of the normal eye (Fig. 4).

Patient 4 demonstrates the value of the VER in the acute phase where even a qualitative answer is of value. In spite of his state of unconsciousness and the filtering effect of the severely swollen lids which absorbed much of the stimulus energy, a VER was obtained. This was enough to demonstrate that the optic nerves were conducting, although the fractures seen (Fig. 5) seemed to make their injury likely.

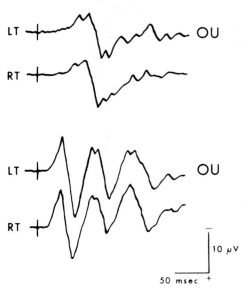

Fig. 9. Patient 7. Monopolar recordings of the VER from over the left (lt) and right (rt) occipital regions. The upper traces were recorded during a period of subjective visual complaints. The lower traces were recorded when vision cleared.

Homonymous hemianopia is best correlated in the VER by recording from over each hemisphere.[2,3,4] In the acute phase after head injury, such placement may be impossible because of scalp wounds or may be the source of artifacts because of subcutaneous hematomas etc. (Patients 5, 6). In the midline recording, the hemianopia will be correlated only by the nearly equally reduced amplitudes to stimulation of each eye. The normal latencies may exclude damage to the anterior optic pathways. Obtaining a VER from patients suffering from injuries to the occipital region may thus serve as a prognostic sign.[1] No quantitative estimation of visual functions, however, can be made on these grounds. Recording of an abnormal VER from a patient with visual complaints, though subjective, may give them an objective quality.[2,4]

In Patient 7 (Fig. 9), the latency of the initial wave indicated slowed conduction along the visual pathways. The abnormalities of the subsequent components of the VER indicated disturbances in higher levels of the visual system.[5] The fact that the patient's improvement coincided with the return to normal of his VER supported an organic basis of his subjective visual complaints.

Nonorganic nature of posttraumatic visual complaints (Patient 8) can be identified electrophysiologically by the recording of normal VER to stimulation of each eye.[1,6,7,8] A response of normal latency, amplitude, and configuration is evidence of a normally functioning visual system and effectively excludes all but trivial involvement of traumatic etiology.

SUMMARY

Examination of the visual evoked response (VER) were carried out in 75 patients suffering from visual disturbances after head injuries. The characteristic findings in optic nerve lesions, occipital lobe injuries, postconcussive visual disturbances, and posttraumatic conversion reaction or malingering are presented. The electrophysiological examination of the visual system may thus serve as an efficient tool for objective assessment of the function of the visual pathways, especially when consciousness or cooperation may be affected.

REFERENCES

1. Feinsod M, Auerbach E: Electrophysiological examinations of the visual system in the acute phase after head injury. Eur Neurol 9:56–64, 1973
2. Feinsod M, Hoyt WF, Wilson WB, Spire JP: VER in the neurologic evaluation of post-traumatic subjective visual complaints. Arch Ophthalmol (in press)
3. Vaughn HG, Katzman R. Evoked responses in visual disorders. Ann NY Acad Sci 112:305–319, 1964
4. Kooi KA: Episodic blindness as a late effect of head trauma. Neurology 20:569–573, 1970
5. Feinsod M, Hoyt WF, Wilson WB: Suprastriate hemianopia. Lancet 1:1225–1226, 1974
6. Copenhaver RM, Perry NM Jr: Factors affecting visually evoked cortical potentials such as impaired vision of varying etiology. Invest Ophthalmol 3:665–675, 1964
7. Behrman J: The visual evoked response in hysterical amblyopia. Br J Ophthalmol 53:839–845, 1969
8. Feinsod M, Rowe H, Averbach E: The diagnostic and prognostic value of electrophysiological examinations of the visual system. Harefuah 79:249–251, 1970

Edited by Z. Harry Rappaport, M.D.
and Joseph Ransohoff, M.D.

Open Discussion

The socioeconomic and ethical factors involved in arriving at therapy decisions have been stressed in the preceding presentations. Moreover, there is minimal disagreement when it comes to defining the extremes in the head injury spectrum. Certain death and very probable full recovery can be predicted on the basis of the host of clinical and technical parameters with reasonable accuracy. It is the large gray area of recovery with greater or lesser deficit that poses the problem of definition with which the presentations and discussions of this section of the 1975 Chicago Neural Trauma Conference attempted to deal. It is especially the "persistent vegetative state" as defined by Jennett and Plum,[1] and severe neurological deficit that must be avoided as an outcome, with their serious implications for family and society at large. Basic research is being carried out and has been presented at other sessions of the conference in an attempt to delineate the pathophysiology in severe head injury serving to provide a rational basis for therapy. It seems, however, reasonable to assume that in certain patients significant irreversible neural damage exists. Early in the patient's hospital course a decision concerning management of these unfortunate people is of great socioethical concern and it is the responsibility of those of us who deal with the victims of head injury to provide society with reliable criteria on which to base management decisions. Though certainty of prognostic prediction may be utopian, statistical probabilities can still be of value if they meet the standard of probability which is clearly significant.

Approaches to this problem have been outlined in the previous pages. One must at first define the deficit in the traumatized patient in order to then localize it functionally and investigate it for reversibility. As is often the case, semantics present the initial difficulty in characterizing the problem. Jennett and Plum's efforts to provide a clinical scale to describe the head injury victim assist all of us in this respect.[2,3] The parameters of best verbal and motor response, eye opening, oculocephalic and oculovestibular response, and respiratory pattern provide a practical scheme for initial evaluation of the patient and continued in-hospital monitoring. They also assist in an initial localization of neural dysfunction within the central nervous system. Jennett's outcome scale[3] is of similar import. It consists of the categories: (1) death, (2) persistent vegetative state, (3) severe disability, (4) moderate disability, and (5) good recovery. The importance of using the same terminology to clarify intercenter communication is apparent. The New York University Medical Center is currently adopting a scheme for patient evaluation based on the above scale, as are other centers around the country.

Clinical examination alone, however, leaves something to be desired regarding prognostic capability. For example, it does not take into account mode of injury and energy expended intracranially which can have great bearing on ultimate outcome. Pure translational-acceleration forces leading to localized hematomas and focal tissue destruction offer on the whole, a better prognosis than rotational-acceleration forces that produce shearing stresses with diffuse white matter and possibly vascular damage.[4,5] Patients with either type of injury, however, may have similar initial clinical presentations.

In the free discussion period of this session, Dr. Shulman (Albert Einstein College of Medicine) illustrates the prognostic significance of mode of injury in 82 patients with cerebral missile injuries. Of 39 patients who were comatose with bilateral decerebration on admission, 6 were operated upon. There were no survivors. Operation increased average survival from 1½ days to 14 days. Fifty percent of patients presenting comatose with unilateral posturing survived with severe neurological deficit. In none of the nonsurgical patients was there evidence for intracranial clots. Prognosis in these areas is extremely poor, reflecting severe irreversible tissue destruction due to the energy expenditure of the missile and direct neural disruption.

A further drawback to prognostic reliance on clinical criteria alone is that the clinical status cannot reliably differentiate between primary neural lesions of a reversible nature and those that are fixed, since initially the same functional deficit prevails. Furthermore, secondary neural dysfunction may develop as the result of increased vascular volume due to venous compression and poor respiratory function with local tissue acidosis; an increased cerebrospinal fluid volume following impaired absorption; localized and diffuse vasospasm with resultant neural dysfunction; cerebral edema, and cerebral tissue shift. Each of these factors may resolve without neurological impairment or leave a permanent deficit despite the therapy being directed toward them.

Dr. Hunt (Ohio State University) raises the possibility that the primary event post-CNS injury may be vascular-endothelial in nature with subsequent therapy being directed at secondary events. He has found a massive outpouring of Evans Blue tracer within 5 minutes of spinal cord trauma, indicating an almost immediate disruption of the endothelial vascular lining at the level of the meta-arteriole and capillary vessels.

Such considerations have led to a multifactorial analysis of the patient, adding such parameters as intracranial pressure (ICP), cerebral metabolic rate for oxygen ($CMRO_2$), cerebral blood flow (CBF), and regional cerebral blood flow (rCBF) to the clinical presentation. A correlation between $CMRO_2$ and prognosis has been presented here by Dr. Hass, but it is only in the extreme values that a high level of predictive reliability is attained. However, Bruce et al.[6] are unable to demonstrate any correlation of prognosis to $CMRO_2$, ICP, and rCBF. In Dr. Becker's presentation, an elevated ICP in association with posturing and impairment of the oculocephalic reflex was found to be associated with poor prognosis. In the reverse situation, low ICP, present oculocephalics and absence of posturing, a favorable outcome can be expected. Dr. Kurze (University of Southern California) presented data on 42 closed head injury patients in whom focal masses were excluded by echoencephalography and/or angiography. He could not correlate fatal outcomes with the level of ICP in these cases. This is in agreement with Dr. Tindall's work, presented in the previous pages. Dr. Overgaard[7] attempts to differentiate states of reversible and irreversible brain stem damage associated with cerebral dysfunction by means of

clinical parameters and rCBF. He must, however, conclude that in the majority of patients this distinction is not readily made. The numerous exceptions to general trends that are indicated in the above studies demonstrate the present inadequacy of technical parameters in defining outcome in many of the patients, even when these are evaluated in association with the clinical examination.[8,9] The basic difficulty remains: namely that initially, when the patient presents at the hospital transient neural dysfunction cannot reliably be distinguished from that which is already fixed.

The need for further localization and definition of the posttraumatic neural status has lead to the series of papers in the second part of the section. Somatosensory (SER), visual (VER), and auditory evoked potentials provide us with a noninvasive analysis of localized neural pathways. The P_2 component of the SER relates to the functional integrity of the extralemniscal transreticular brain stem pathways, while the VER and the transhemispheral relay of the SER provide information about intracerebral pathways. Evoked potential studies in cerebral trauma have been presented here by Dr. Greenberg and are planned in a number of trauma centers. They will no doubt add to our prognostic abilities as elegantly demonstrated by Dr. Feinsod in the more limited sphere of the visual system. The lability of the evoked potentials with respect to aPO_2 as outlined previously by Dr. Shelbourne and to CBF as presented in the discussion section by Dr. Crockard (University of Chicago) illustrate the limitations of the evoked potential technique. Their ultimate usefulness in reliably predicting outcome depends on the demonstration of significant correlation with the functional recovery of the pathways described.

It seems likely that further refinement in analysis of local neural dysfunction is needed before we can answer the opening question. Electromagnetometric techniques and systems for noninvasive regional cerebral metabolic analyses are as yet on the bioscientists drawing boards; such techniques will, however, eventually lead to the more precise diagnostic capabilities that are needed, both from the medical therapeutic as well as the societal point of view.

REFERENCES

1. Jennett B, Plum F: Persistent vegetative state after brain damage. Lancet 1:734–737, 1972
2. Teasdale G, Jennett B: Assessment of coma and impaired consciousness. Lancet 2:81–84, 1974
3. Jennett B, Bond M: Assessment of outcome after severe brain damage: A practical scale. Lancet 1:480–484, 1975
4. Ommaya AK, Gennarelli TA: Cerebral concussion and traumatic unconsciousness. Brain 97:633–654, 1974
5. Stritch SJ: The pathology of brain damage due to blunt injury, in Walker AE, Caveness WF, Critchley M (eds): The Late effect of Head Injury, Springfield, Ill, Thomas, 1969, pp 501–526
6. Bruce DA, Langfitt TW, Miller JD, et al: Regional cerebral blood flow, intracranial pressure, and brain metabolism in comatose patients. J Neurosurg 38:131–144, 1973
7. Overgaard J, Christensen S, Haase J, et al: Prognosis after head injury based on early clinical examination. Lancet 2:631–635, 1973
8. Jennett B, Johnston IH: The uses of intracranial pressure monitoring in clinical management, in Brock M, Dietz H (eds): Intracranial Pressure. Berlin–New York, Springer Verlag, 1972, pp 253–356
9. Fieschi C, Battescini N, Beduschi A, et al: Regional cerebral blood flow and intraventricular pressure in acute head injury. J Neurol Neurosurg Psychiatr 37:1378–1388, 1974

II

Blood-Brain Barrier

M. W. Brightman, Ph.D.
J. S. Robinson, M.D.

14

Some Attempts to Open the Blood-Brain Barrier to Protein

When a protein, such as horseradish peroxidase (HRP) (MW 40,000) or the much smaller heme-peptide, "microperoxidase" (MW 1800) are injected into the tail vein of mice, organs such as the gastrointestinal tract, skin, and muscle are infiltrated by these substances but the central nervous system is not.[4,14] This variation of old experiments made with dye-protein complexes[5] has provided a closer look at where this particular blood-brain barrier (BBB) might be situated. The reaction product of the peroxidases can be visualized with the electron microscope, and this sensitive technique has yielded convincing evidence that the barrier consists of a physical component and a kind of inactivity on the part of the endothelial cell membrane. The physical aspect is obliteration of the extracellular cleft between adjacent endothelial cells by continuous belts of tight junctions. The outer leaflets of the contiguous cell membranes are so closely apposed that the passive movement of protein on its way to the pericapillary spaces is halted (Fig. 1).[14] The second component of the barrier is the failure of the cerebral capillary to do what other blood vessels do: to ferry protein, irrespective of how much has been injected, from blood to pericapillary fluid by vesicular transport.[14]

The following summary relates our attempts to open the barrier in various ways. So far, the manipulations appear to act on the junctions while vesicular transport seems to be unaffected. In all attempts, the animal is injected first with Evans blue and HRP into a peripheral vein either before or after the barrier has been altered. Since the spread of HRP into the extracellular clefts is rapid once the barrier has been opened, short survival times of less than 2 minutes are permitted in order to distinguish primary leaks from secondary spread. The tissue, after being fixed in aldehyde is processed for peroxidatic activity[6] and examined by light and electron microscopy.

TUMORS

The increased permeability of blood vessels within brain tumors to protein is well recognized. Iodinated serum albumin injected into peripheral blood of man has been useful in locating such neoplasms because the labeled protein is able to escape from the tumor vessels and accumulate within the tumor. Our primary concern here is how the tracer is able to leave vessels that are normally impermeable. As in human malignant gliomas,[10] the route appears to be a passive extracellular one. The clefts between contiguous endothelial cells are open instead of being closed by tight junctions and permit the flow of HRP through them (Fig. 2).[3] The tumor capillary is often fenestrated, a feature associated with "leakiness."[3] This type of capillary also vascularizes choroid plexus papillomas induced by the intracerebral injection of SV_{40} virus in newborn Syrian hamsters. Fenestrae also perforate the endothelial cells of capillaries within normal areas, such as the median eminence and area postrema, that lie outside the BBB.[15] However, in vessels of normal and neoplastic tissue, each fenestra or window is covered by a thin diaphragm that may or may not be permeable to protein. Fenestrated vessels appear, nevertheless, to be one common feature of cerebral neoplasms, whether primary

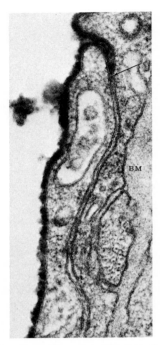

Fig. 1. Peroxidase, injected into the vascular system, moves between endothelial cells only as far as the first tight junction (arrow). The remainder of the cleft between the endothelial cells is free of protein as is the perivascular basement membrane (BM). Although this animal has been fixed 45 minutes before perfusion of the peroxidase, the distribution is the same as in animals that have received the protein before fixation.[16] (Rat × 180,000.)

or metastatic.[1,10,7] In the virally induced papilloma, the fenestrae outnumber the endothelial clefts by at least four to one and, if they are permeable, would account in part, for the extremely rapid penetration of protein from blood into tumor.

OPENING BY HYPEROSMOTIC AGENTS

When hyperosmotic solutions of polar substances are applied topically to the pial surface of the brain or infused into its vascular bed, circulating Evans blue escapes from some vessels into the surrounding brain tissue.[12] The opening of the BBB is reversible when the agents are polar, including various saccharides and urea but irreversible with nonpolar substances, such as alcohols and glycols.[11] After a thorough analysis of published data and first-hand observations, Rapoport[11] concluded that the degree of barrier opening followed expectations with osmotic cell shrinkage.

When hyperosmotic solutions (2.5 m) of urea were infused into one internal carotid artery of rabbits that had been injected intravenously with Evans blue and HRP, both the dye and the peroxidase crossed some vessels. Within 90 seconds, enough HRP crossed some segments of vessels to infiltrate the clefts around perivascular glia and neurons.[2] Most of the affected vessels appeared to

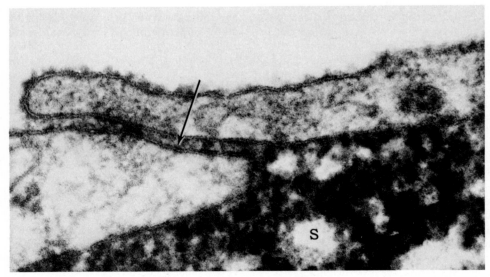

Fig. 2. The extracellular cleft (arrow) between two endothelial cells of a capillary within a choroid plexus papilloma is patent throughout its extent. No tight junctions between the cells prevented the flow of peroxidase from vessel lumen (upper third) to the pericapillary space (S). (Hamster × 100,000.)

be capillaries and in these only segments of the vessels permitted the escape of protein. The majority of arterioles, venules, and capillaries were unaffected.

The peroxidase crossed the arteriolar wall through the clefts and tight junctions between adjoined endothelial cells. The evidence that the once impermeable junctions had become opened was the accumulation of reaction product within the extracellular pockets between successive tight junctions (Fig. 3). These pockets are normally inaccessible to protein (Fig. 1). Although no actual separation of the outer leaflets at the junctions could be discerned, it is highly probable that they were separated widely enough and for sufficient time to allow the HRP to pass.

An alternative means of passage could have been by vesicular transport. These vesicles begin as invaginations of the luminal part of the endothelial cell membrane. Protein circulating in the blood enters these pits by way of their ostia which then close. The pit's membrane separates from the cell membrane and a vesicle is thus created which migrates across the thin endothelial cell to the opposite, abluminal side. At this surface, the vesicle membrane is believed to coalesce with the endothelial one to create a new ostium through which the contents of the vesicle are released into the perivascular cleft. This cleft is almost filled by basement membrane or basal lamina, which is able to bind proteins (Fig. 3).

The accumulation of HRP within the basal lamina is evidence that the protein crossed the endothelial cell in some manner. This accumulation does not, by itself, tell us how. The basement membrane appears, in some places at least, to have a limited capacity for capturing protein. Within a couple of minutes after the barrier is opened, the lamina is completely infiltrated by protein which then spills into the extracellular clefts of the neuropil. So rapid is the passive, extracellular flow of protein that, beyond the short interval of a few minutes, the walls of blood vessels unaffected by hyperosmotic urea are also surrounded by HRP reaction product. The HRP in the basal lamina around these nonshrunken vessels as well as the affected vessels then enters the abluminal pits of that portion of the endothelial cell membrane facing the lamina. Some of the protein is also able to penetrate between contiguous endothelial cells as far as the first belt of tight junctions between them.

The resulting distribution of protein which shall now be described in further detail, thus mimics vesicular transport. In a particular,

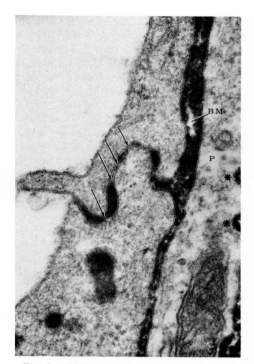

Fig. 3. While peroxidase was circulating in the blood, a solution of 2.5 m urea was infused into the carotid artery on one side and, 90 seconds later, the brain was fixed. Peroxidase has penetrated successive tight junctions (arrows) to enter interjunctional pools of extracellular space and, eventually, the perivascular basement membrane (BM). Two pits, (asterisks) made by invaginations of the cell membrane belonging to an adjacent pericyte (P), have also been penetrated by protein. The capillary lumen is at the left (Rabbit × 160,-000.)

nonaffected vessel, the luminal part of a cleft between two adjacent endothelial cells is infiltrated by protein as far as the first tight junction or perhaps a second one. In the same intercellular cleft, reaction product may also extend from basement membrane to the first or second abluminal tight junction.

The simulation is even more convincing when some of the tight junctions have been sectioned tangentially so that the cell membranes are no longer distinct but appear as a "smeared" segment that is almost as dense as HRP reaction product. To complete the false appearance of vesicular transport, many abluminal pits and a few luminal pits may also be labeled by protein.

An unequivocal sign that a blood vessel has been crossed by protein is the penetration by HRP into extracellular pools between successive tight junctions (Fig. 3). These interjunctional pools are normally inaccessible to protein (Fig. 1). If, on the other hand, the pools at the luminal and abluminal ends of endothelial clefts are filled while the intervening ones appear empty, then it is reasonable to assume that the abluminal pool was not entered by protein that had passed through these pools from the blood. It is more likely that the abluminal cleft had been filled by protein that had crossed the endothelium at some other point, to invade the basal lamina and thence the abluminal portion of endothelial clefts. In this common situation, it is unclear how and where the HRP crossed the vessel initially. In order to locate the original points at which the protein crossed the affected vessel and thereby to distinguish it from neighboring intact ones, short survival times are necessary. If only 1 or 2 minutes elapse between the infusion of hyperosmotic urea and fixation, there is not enough time for HRP to diffuse extracellularly around very many nonaffected vessels.

It is emphasized that the effects of hyperosmotic urea appear to be restricted to segments of capillaries and some muscle-coated vessels. The involved vessels are randomly distributed. We do not know why the junctions between the endothelial cells of some capillaries and arterioles are rendered more permeable to large molecules than the junctions of a far greater number of capillaries that are also exposed to hyperosmotic urea. A comparable selectivity is shown by certain vessels confronted with a sudden rise in their intraluminal pressure.

OPENING BY HYPERTENSION

The BBB to Evans blue-albumin complex is opened in some, but not all vessels during a rise in systemic arterial blood pressure.[8] When the vasopressor, aramine (metaraminol bitartrate), was injected into a peripheral vein in 10 adult rats, the arterial blood pressure, measured by a pressure transducer connected to the femoral artery, rises from an average resting level of 93

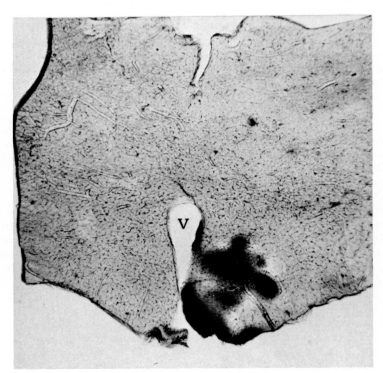

Fig. 4. After the intravenous infusion of aramine, the arterial blood pressure of this rat rose from a resting level of 115 mm Hg to 240 mm Hg, the highest increase in the aramine series. Five minutes later, the brain was fixed. During the rise in blood pressure, circulating peroxidase escaped from a few vessels to form circular exudates on both sides of the brain. Cerebrum. (Rat × 60.)

mm Hg (80 to 100 mm) to an average of 176 mm Hg (158–196 mm Hg). An estimate of the degree of barrier opening is obtained from the number and size of Evans blue spots upon the cortex and within subcortical regions of the brain. A considerably more accurate estimate, however, is gleaned when peroxidase rather than or in addition to the dye is injected into the femoral vein from 5 to 10 minutes before the infusion of aramine.

The usefulness of peroxidase as an indicator of changes in vascular permeability becomes evident when brown spots of reaction product emerge in cerebral regions free of discernible Evans-blue. What appears to be an intact area because of the absence of blue coloration actually turns out to be an altered region with several vascular leaks. Even in places where there are blue extravasations of dye, there are usually more of peroxidase (Fig. 4).

The confinement of the bulk of escaped peroxidase to the extracellular spaces can be recognized in thick sections. As in the similar globular exudates originating from vessels carrying hyperosmotic urea, the extravasated protein forms a dense reaction product that outlines individual neurons, glial cells, and cell processes (Fig. 5). Damaged cells are not as clearly differentiated from the surrounding extracellular clefts that contain protein because peroxidase becomes freely diffused within the cytoplasm of such cells.

The method of making estimates of the number of exudates is straightforward. After aldehyde fixation, the entire brain is divided into both cerebral hemispheres, diencephalon, midbrain, cerebellum and medulla. Each of these six regions is chopped at 200 μ on a Smith-Farquhar chopper and incubated in 3-3' diaminobenzidene.[6] All of the exudates in all of the sections of each region are counted. The entire brain is thus surveyed on a regional basis.

The greatest number of spots representing escaped protein occurs in the cerebrum (approximately 520). Approximately one-fifth that number (about 100) infiltrate the diencephalon and half that number (about 45), the midbrain. The cerebellum and medulla contain the least number of brown spots (about 25), approximately half that of the midbrain. The variation within each group is quite high but the differences between them are statistically significant. The consistent trend is one in which the greatest number of exudates is in the cerebrum and the least is in the medulla. This anteroposterior decrement may reflect a gradient along which hydrostatic forces may be dissipated. Another region that is often affected is the olfactory tract of either side, where at least one blue spot marks its

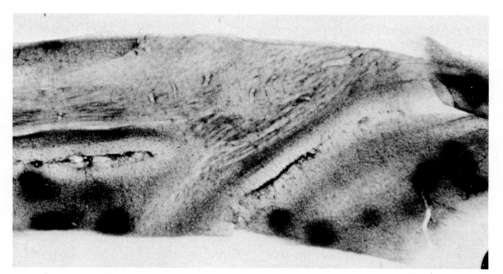

Fig. 5. An exudate of peroxidase typically appears as a dense ovoid mass surrounding neurons and glial cells in the brain of a rat whose blood pressure had been raised by Aramine administration. The neurons and glial cells appear as pale silhouettes. The affected, leaky vessel is presumably, near the middle of the exudate. The walls of some vessels, large ones, (upper right and left) contain peroxidase. (Rat × 550.)

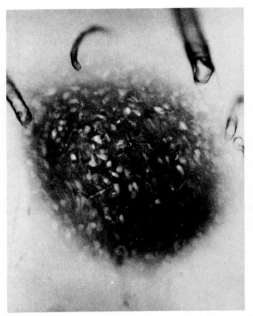

Fig. 6. A bolus of saline was infused for 10 seconds at a rate of 0.6 ml/sec into the carotid artery on one side. Ten minutes later, the brain was fixed. Peroxidase has exuded from vessels, situated to the right of the III ventricle (V) on the side that the bolus was delivered. (16) Hypothalamus. (Rat × 25.)

pial surface. This location has also been noted by Johansson.[9] Thus, a rise of somewhat less than double the resting arterial blood pressure, that is, from a mean of 93 mm Hg to an additional 83 mm Hg, is sufficient to open the barrier to protein in some vessels.

In 15 rats, peroxidase was injected from 5 minutes to 21 hours after injection of a threshold dose of aramine known to open the barrier. Four of this series were given HRP 2 hours after the aramine. Neither these rats nor 3 others given HRP at intervals longer than 2 hours had any exudates whereas those at shorter time intervals did. It would appear then, that the aramine effect is reversible after 2 hours. Beyond this period, the barrier is reestablished.

The means by which protein crosses such vessels is probably through junctions of increased permeability rather than by an increase in vesicular transport. It is, however, conceivable that aramine might, in some way, induce the formation of transferring vesicles by acting directly on the endothelium or indirectly, perhaps through a release of biogenic amines. Enhanced vesicular transport is unlikely for two reasons. First, there

is no obvious increase in the number of pits or vesicles within cerebral capillaries following aramine injections. Inasmuch as there are many more such inclusions in the endothelium of muscle-coated vessels in untreated animals, only actual counts would permit a similar conclusion to be drawn for arterioles and venules. If aramine did induce vesicle formation in these vessels, then a special responsiveness of their endothelium would have to be invoked.

The second reason for discounting vesicular transport is the results following the rapid injection of a bolus of saline into one carotid artery. When a pulse of isotonic saline is infused at the rate of 0.6 ml over a 3- to 10-second interval, Evans blue rapidly extravasates from vessels on the injected side.[13] When this type of experiment is repeated after Evans blue and peroxidase have been given intravenously, both dye and protein exude from vessels on the side receiving the bolus (Fig. 6), although a few brown spots appear in the opposite cerebral hemisphere as well.

The mean number of exudates in the affected cerebral hemisphere is 713 (78 to 2350) and is significantly greater than the mean obtained with aramine, whether the bolus infusion lasted 3 seconds or 10 seconds. As with aramine, there is an anteroposterior gradient in the rats that received the bolus. The next highest number of extravasations is in the diencephalon and midbrain with a mean of 40 to 50, less in the cerebellum with a mean of 26, and least in the medulla with a mean of 11.

These results tend to dismiss the possibility that vesicular transport accounts for the movement of protein across the affected vessels because one would have to suppose that a sudden rise in intraluminal pressure for 3 seconds would trigger a massive formation of vesicles. The vesicles would have to be numerous enough to transfer enough protein to flow for an appreciable distance beyond the affected vessel over a period of 5 minutes before fixation. One would also have to conclude that the higher the pressure, the more vesicles are formed since there is an anteroposterior gradient in the number of affected vessels. Finally, if pressure increase does trigger vesicle formation, then only certain regions of a homogenous-appearing endothelium belonging to a given vessel would be responsive. It would be simpler and more plausible to assume, instead, that the effect of the bolus pressure, as with aramine, is mechanical: the nearer to the head of pressure, the greater the number of junctions that have been made more permeable. If this effect is indeed the actual one, then it must likewise be assumed that, at a given moment, some endothelial junctions are more labile than others.

The three ways of opening the blood-brain barrier to protein that we have discussed point to the endothelial junction as the structure that is malleable. The structure of the junction can be altered, reversibly, to lower the barrier. The reversibility itself suggests that a graduated opening might be elicited. The involved vessels are only a small fraction of the total vascular bed and include both capillaries and vessels that have a tunica media. It is also suggested that this passive flow of protein through junctional channels is superimposed upon a resting vesicular transfer that occurs within the same or nearby segments of some muscle-coated vessels.[17] The combined passive and active transfer overwhelms the binding capacity of the perivascular basement membrane and appreciable protein can then flood the interstices of cerebral parenchyma. The observations to date suggest that under conditions that may physically deform tight junctions, substantial amounts of protein may rapidly cross blood vessels. The crossing is passive, extracellular, and via reversibly altered junctions rather than transcellular by means of increased numbers of transferring vesicles.

REFERENCES

1. Brightman MW, Reese TS: Types of endothelium in normal and neoplastic brain tissue. 28th Annual Proc EMSA, 1970, pp 98–99

2. Brightman MW, Hori M, Rapoport S, et al: Osmotic opening of tight junctions in cerebral endothelium. J Comp Neurol 152:317–326, 1973

3. Brightman MW, Prescott L: Blood vessels permeable to peroxidase in virally induced brain tumors (in preparation)

4. Feder N, Reese TS, Brightman MW: Microperoxidase, a new tracer of low molecular weight. A study of the interstitial compartments of the mouse brain. J Cell Biol 43:35A–36A (Abstr), 1969

5. Goldmann EE: Vital Färbung am Zentral Nervensystem. Berlin, Eimer, 1913

6. Graham RC, Karnovsky MJ: The early stages of absorption of horseradish peroxidase in the proximal tubules of the mouse kidney; ultrastructural cyclochemistry by a new technique. J Histochem Cytochem 14:291, 1966

7. Hirano A, Zimmerman HM: Fenestrated blood vessels in a metastatic renal carcinoma in the brain. Lab Invest 26:465–468, 1972

8. Johansson B, Li CL, Olsson Y, et al: The effects of acute arterial hypertension on the blood-brain barrier to protein tracers. Acta Neuropathol (Berlin) 16:117–124, 1970

9. Johansson B: Personal communication, 1975

10. Long D: Capillary ultrastructure and the blood-brain barrier in human malignant brain tumors. J Neurosurg 32:127–144, 1970

11. Rapoport SI: Effect of concentrated solutions on blood-brain barrier. Am J Physiol 219:270–274, 1970

12. Rapoport SI, Hori M, Klatzo I: Testing of a hypothesis for osmotic opening of the blood-brain barrier. Am J Physiol 223:323–331, 1972

13. Rapoport SI, Thompson HK: Opening of the blood-brain barrier (BBB) by a pulse of hydrostatic pressure. Biophys J 15:326A (Abstr), 1975

14. Reese TS, Karnovsky MJ: Fine structural localization of a blood-brain barrier for exogenous peroxidase. J Cell Biol 34:207–217, 1967

15. Reese TS, Brightman MW: Similarity in structure and permeability to peroxidase of epithelia overlying fenestrated cerebral capillaries. Anat Rec 160:414 (Abstr) 1968

16. Robinson JS, Brightman MW, Rapport, ST: Unpublished observations.

17. Westergaard E, Brightman MW: Transport of proteins across normal cerebral arterioles. J Comp Neurol 152:17–44, 1973

Stanley I. Rapoport, M.D.

15

Blood-Brain Barrier Permeability, Autoregulation of Cerebral Blood Flow and Brain Edema

The blood-brain barrier at cerebral blood vessels is due to a continuous layer of endothelial cells that are connected by tight junctions. These junctions can be deformed and made more permeable when subjected to tensile stresses. Hypertonic solutions, whether applied to the surface of the brain or injected into the carotid artery, reversibly open the barrier by shrinking endothelial cells and widening the junctions.

The barrier is opened also by a number of conditions, including cerebral concussion, hypercapnia, convulsions and acute hypertension, all of which alter autoregulation. Barrier opening follows capillary dilatation and increased pressure, and it is speculated that these changes induce widening of interendothelial tight junctions. Cerebral edema may result also from increased capillary pressure and elevated capillary permeability, caused by the loss of autoregulation.

STRUCTURAL BASIS OF BLOOD-BRAIN BARRIER

Trauma to the brain initiates a large number of changes in its function, metabolism, and ultrastructure. Cerebral blood vessels are damaged and their permeability increased, cell membranes and metabolism are modified, hemorrhage and edema often occur, hypertension may be induced, cerebral blood flow is altered, and autoregulation of flow is modified. Many of these changes progress and interact with each other, making it difficult to isolate cause from effect and therefore to modify the sequelae of trauma.

In this discussion, I shall consider the possible role of the blood-brain barrier in the posttraumatic process. I mean by the barrier the continuous layer of cerebrovascular endothelium that restricts exchange of proteins, electrolytes, and many water-soluble nonelectrolytes between brain and blood (Fig. 1).

Tight junctions (*zonulae occludentes*) connect vascular endothelial cells and limit intercellular diffusion, while transcellular macromolecular transport is restricted because of the rarity of endothelial cell pinocytosis.[1,2] These properties make cerebral blood vessels act like a continuous plasma membrane with respect to blood-brain exchange. By comparison, systemic capillaries allow for material exchange because they contain porous endothelial cells with pinocytotic vesicles.[3]

Tight junctions between epithelial cells in many cell layers are networks of fibrillar strands that can be deformed by osmotic and hydrostatic pressure stresses which increase junctional permeability.[4,5] The model which I shall employ to explain opening of the blood-brain barrier is based partially on these findings, and is illustrated in Fig. 2. Its premise is that tight junctions between cerebrovascular endothelia also can be distorted and made more permeable by mechanical stresses. Distorting stresses are produced by osmotically shrinking endothelial cells, as illustrated in Fig. 2a, or by stretching them in association with capillary dilatation and hypertension (Fig. 2b). The shrinkage mechanism is supported by physiological and electron microscopic observations,[6,7]

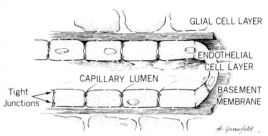

Fig. 1. Diagram of blood-brain barrier at cerebral capillary. A substance can cross the barrier either by passing through the endothelial cell membranes or through the regions of the tight junctions. Protein tracers are restricted by both routes. The tight junctions form continuous belts around the cells and are assumed to open when concentrated solutions osmotically shrink the cells.

but the dilatation mechanism requires morphological confirmation and is speculative.

OSMOTIC OPENING OF BLOOD-BRAIN BARRIER

The model for tight junctional opening in response to hypertonic solutions is based on the following observations: (1) thresholds for osmotic

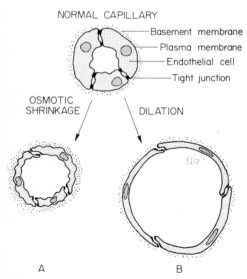

Fig. 2. Models for barrier opening by means of increased permeability of endothelial tight junctions. (a) When endothelial cells shrink in hypertonic solutions, their membranes exert tensile stresses that widen and deform tight junctions. (b) Capillary dilatation or increased intraluminal pressure stretches endothelial cells and membranes, also widening junctions and increasing their permeability.

opening of the blood-brain barrier have the same relation to solute lipid solubility as do thresholds for shrinking cells, suggesting that barrier opening is mediated by cell shrinkage; (2) osmotic opening of the barrier is reversible, showing that it is not due to destruction of cell membranes; and (3) osmotic opening is associated with observable transfer of intravascular protein *between* endothelial cells and not through them. The latter findings show that the junctions are widened and that barrier opening is not caused by increased pinocytotic transport.[6–9]

Osmotic agents like urea, lactamide, and sugars are not very lipid soluble. They open the blood-brain barrier reversibly, whether applied to the pia-arachnoid of the rabbit so as to increase the permeability of pial arterioles and venules or perfused into the internal carotid artery of the rabbit or monkey. If care is taken to avoid compromising the cerebral circulation by the perfusion procedure, the barrier can be opened over large parts of the hemisphere homolateral to perfusion without brain damage or neurological sequelae (Fig. 3).[9] Opening is reversible, and capillaries become impermeable again after 30 minutes to 4 hours.[6, 10, 11]

The absence of significant neurological effects from reversible osmotic opening shows that an impermeable barrier need not be present continuously for survival or even normal function. It is likely, however, that the barrier would be necessary if a toxic agent like an angiographic contrast medium were in the blood, or in the presence of hyperkalemia or compensated metabolic acidosis. Toxic drugs must be excluded from the brain, and the acid-base and ionic environment of neurons should be maintained within homeostatic limits.[12]

BARRIER BREAKDOWN DUE TO LOSS OF AUTOREGULATION

The evidence that capillary hypertension and dilatation open the barrier is the observed correlation between barrier breakdown and loss of autoregulation following different stresses to the brain or cerebral vasculature (Table 1). The mechanism for barrier opening, as illustrated in Fig. 2b, is suggested by finding that (1) barrier breakdown following loss of autoregulation can rapidly reverse (Table 1) indicating that vascular architecture is not disrupted; (2) tight junctions between epithelial cells of the mouse mammary gland alveolus are made more permeable and are

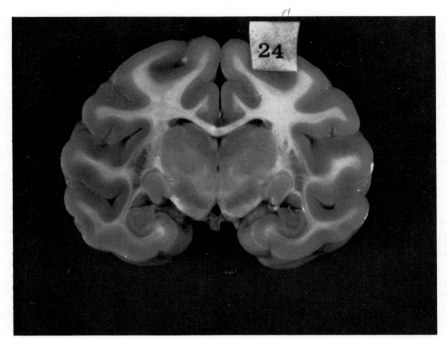

Fig. 3. Coronal section of brain of monkey sacrificed 4 days following internal carotid perfusion of 2 m urea solution. Evans blue dye (dark regions) stains the left hemisphere diffusely, indicating blood-brain barrier breakdown. The monkey was normal neurologically and had no pathological brain lesions.

Table 1

Occurrence of Blood-Brain Barrier Opening and Local Brain Edema
in Relation to Different Experimental and Clinical Conditions
which Alter Autoregulation of Cerebral Blood Flow

Conditions which Alter Autoregulation	Increased Barrier Permeability	Reversibility of Barrier Opening	Local Brain Edema	References
Acute hypertension				
Carotid perfusion	Yes	—	—	25,36
Aramine injection	Yes	3 hours	—	27, 28, 36
Hypertensive encephalopathy	Yes	—	Yes	37, 17
Convulsions	Yes	15 min	Yes	21, 22, 19
Hypercapnia (25%)	Yes	15 min	—	23, 14
Metabolic and respiratory acidosis				
with coma	—	—	Yes	38
Cerebral concussion	Yes	—	Yes	39, 34, 40, 20a
Intracranial hypertension	Yes	—	Yes	39, 26
Periphery of:				
Ischemic lesion (apoplexy)	—	—	Yes	16
Intracranial tumor	—	—	Yes	41,42

deformed by luminal hypertension,[4,13] showing that junctions are not membrane fusions and can be modified; (3) cerebral capillary junctions also are labile and can be widened by osmotic cell shrinkage (see above) and probably by hypercapnia.[14]

An alternative to junctional widening following capillary dilatation is that pinocytotic transfer is stimulated. Aramine administration appears to open the barrier on this basis,[15] but it seems doubtful to me that pinocytotic stimulation is the major factor in increased capillary permeability due to loss of autoregulation.

Loss of Autoregulation

Under normal conditions, cerebral blood flow is kept independent of systemic pressure by adjustments in the diameters and resistances of cerebral arteries and arterioles.[16] In humans, flow remains unchanged between pressures of about 60 to 150 mm Hg, and even to higher pressures in hypertensive individuals.[17] Pressures above these autoregulatory limits increase flow and dilate cerebral capillaries, while lower pressures induce cerebral ischemia.

Autoregulation of flow is lost when the pH around cerebral arterioles is reduced by cerebral lactacidosis or hypercapnia.[17,18,19] A low pH dilates the arterioles and alters their responsiveness to systemic blood pressure, so that flow follows pressure. This occurs, for example, in response to brain concussion.[20a]

Many insults to the brain or cerebral vasculature alter autoregulation by reducing periarteriorlar pH or elevating systemic pressure beyond autoregulatory limits.[16,18] Some are listed in Table 1, which also shows that brain edema and barrier opening often accompany the loss of autoregulation. When autoregulation is lost, systemic blood pressure, whether elevated or normal, is transmitted to cerebral capillaries and the capillary bed is dilated.[17] The blood-brain barrier may thereby be opened.

I shall limit my discussion to barrier opening following loss of autoregulation in concussion, convulsions, hypercapnia and acute hypertension. More extensive analyses can be found elsewhere.[16,20b]

CONCUSSION

Dr. Donald Becker[40] has informed me that concussion to the cat brain increases cerebrovascular permeability to horseradish peroxidase without tearing of cerebral capillaries. I suggest

that barrier opening in the absence of capillary damage could well reflect the loss of autoregulation of flow caused by the concussion.

HYPERCAPNIA AND CONVULSIONS

Reversible opening of the blood-brain barrier to intravascular ^{125}I-albumin or to trypan blue is caused by drug- or electrically induced convulsions, as well as by prolonged breathing of 25 percent CO_2.[21,22,23]

One report suggests that capillary tight junctions are opened by hypercapnia,[14] but some workers in the field believe that neither hypercapnia nor convulsions open the barrier by increasing cerebral blood flow.[22,23] The basis of their conclusion is that regional changes in barrier permeability do not correlate with regional increases in vascular volume.

This conclusion contradicts the model of Fig. 2*b* and is, I believe, erroneous. Local cerebral blood flow, as measured directly with a radioactive gas technique, in fact increases over all regions of the brain in which vascular permeability also is elevated.[20b,24] This means that the elevated systemic pressures that accompany hypercapnia and convulsions[19] are transmitted to cerebral capillaries.

ACUTE HYPERTENSION

Acute hypertension increases cerebrovascular permeability, whether the hypertension is produced by carotid artery perfusion or by intravenous administration of metaraminol.[20b,25-28] An elevation of systemic blood pressure within 30 to 120 seconds, furthermore, is transmitted to cerebral capillaries, because autoregulation takes this long to become established.[18,27,29]

A 10-second elevation of carotid artery pressure can be produced in the rat by perfusing isotonic saline into the common carotid artery, after ligating the external carotid.[25] The blood-brain barrier to Evans blue-albumin is opened over the cerebral hemisphere by the perfusion procedure, just as it is by osmotic barrier opening in the monkey (see Fig. 3). The threshold for barrier opening by carotid perfusion is at a carotid artery pressure of 200 mm Hg, as illustrated in Fig. 4.

Autoregulation and Brain Edema

Autoregulation might also protect the brain against edema formation by preventing transmission of excessive systemic pressures to cerebral capillaries. As shown in Table 1, brain edema often accompanies altered autoregulation.

In principle, edema of vascular origin occurs in a tissue when the rate of capillary fluid filtration exceeds the rate of fluid removal from the perivascular interstitium.[30,31] Lymphatics remove fluid from peripheral tissues, but fluid that comes from cerebral capillaries must percolate through the brain parenchyma to the CSF spaces.

Water is driven across the capillary wall by the resultant of hydrostatic and osmotic pressure differences, as modified from Starling,[30]

$$\text{Flow} = L_p[\,P^{\text{plasma}} - p^{\text{tissue}}$$
$$- \sigma(\Pi^{\text{plasma}} - \Pi^{\text{tissue}})] \quad (1)$$

In this equation, flow is in units of $\text{cm}^3\ \text{sec}^{-1}/\text{cm}^2$ of capillary wall, P and Π are mean hydrostatic and osmotic pressures in mm Hg, and L_p is the hydraulic conductivity coefficient relating flow to the net driving force.[20b,30,31]

Peripheral capillaries with porous endothelia[3] are permeable to small solutes and partially permeable to plasma proteins. For them, Π is the protein osmotic pressure and σ, a "reflection coefficient," equals 0.93.[32] (If the capillary were permeable to proteins, $\sigma = 0$.)

Cerebral capillaries with a continuous endothelium are almost impermeable to proteins, electrolytes, and most water-soluble nonelectrolytes (with the exception of glucose and other transported subtances). For them, Π is the sum of osmotic pressures of all these solutes and $\sigma = 1$.[20b]

According to Equation 1, cerebral edema could be produced by an increase in P^{plasma} when autoregulation is lost. This interpretation is consistent with findings that the rate of edema formation following brain injury is elevated by hypertension, which is transmitted to the capillary bed in the absence of autoregulation.[33,34] A similar mechanism could explain edema formation following the loss of autoregulation due to a rapidly expanding intracranial mass, as has been suggested by Symon.[42]

Edema might also be accelerated by an increase in capillary permeability. Increased permeability would increase the value of L_p and decrease the value of σ in Equation 1.[20b]

CONCLUSION

Autoregulation of cerebral blood flow, in addition to providing the brain with a constant supply of glucose and O_2, may also protect the blood-

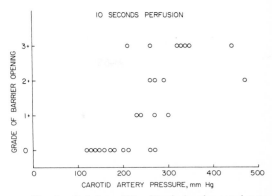

Fig. 4. Relation of blood-brain barrier opening to carotid perfusion pressure in the rat. The external carotid artery was ligated and the common was catheterized for brain perfusion. Barrier opening to intravascular Evans blue-albumin was measured after perfusing isotonic saline solution for 10 seconds, and graded from Grade 0 (no stain) to Grade 3+ (dark blue stain).

brain barrier against mechanical stress and consequent junctional widening and protect the brain against excess capillary filtration and cerebral edema. This proposition must be tested in detail. If it is correct, then the increased permeability and edema that accompany different insults and stresses to the brain could be accounted for by a common mechanism.

ADDENDUM

In the discussion following this paper, it was pointed out that measurable brain edema does not always appear when autoregulation is lost or when capillary filtration might be expected to increase. A dissociation between increased filtration and measurable edema could reflect a low tissue compliance, as illustrated by the following "back-of-the envelope" calculation.

Let intracranial volume be constant and equal to the sum of volumes of three homogeneous compartments, where csf = cerebrospinal fluid,

$$V^{\text{cranium}} = \text{Constant} = V^{\text{brain}} + V^{\text{blood}}$$
$$+ V^{\text{csf}}\ \text{cm}^3 \quad (2)$$

The net amount of fluid filtering out of brain capillaries per unit time is $F^{\text{blood}\to\text{brain}}$, and is given by Equation 1 multiplied by capillary area of the entire brain. At a steady state, this rate equals the net flow of fluid from brain to csf, $F^{\text{brain}\to\text{csf}}$, minus metabolic water production within brain, F^{brain}.

Net capillary filtration also equals flow of fluid out of csf, F^{csf}, minus metabolic water production and choroidal csf production, F^{plexus}. These equalities lead to the following expression at the steady state,

$$F^{blood \to brain} = F^{brain \to csf} - F^{metab}$$
$$= F^{csf} - F^{metab} - F^{plexus} \quad (3)$$

If capillary filtration increases because autoregulation becomes defective, the rate of change of brain volume with time equals the difference between fluid inflow to brain and outflow,

$$\frac{dV^{brain}}{dt} = F^{blood \to brain} + F^{metab} - F^{brain \to csf} \quad (4)$$

When fluid accumulates in brain, interstitial pressure (P^{brain}) and V^{brain} may increase. The ratio of the change of volume to change of pressure is defined as tissue compliance $k(P)$,

$$k(P) = \frac{dV^{brain}}{dP^{brain}} \quad (5)$$

The rate of change of brain volume with time is given by the following expression as well as that of Equation 4,

$$\frac{dV^{brain}}{dt} = \frac{dV^{brain}}{dP^{brain}} \times \frac{dP^{brain}}{dt} = k(P) \frac{dP^{brain}}{dt} \quad (6)$$

Because net volume of the cranial compartments must remain constant (Equation 2), the net volume change of the brain is the negative of the sum of sum of changes of blood and csf volumes.

Edema fluid accumulates within brain tissue when the integrals of Equations 4 and 6 exceed zero, so that the net increase in volume equals

$$\int_o^t (F^{blood \to brain} + F^{metab} - F^{brain \to csf}) \, dt$$
$$= \int_o^t k(P) \frac{dP^{brain}}{dt} \, dt > 0 \quad (7)$$

If brain compliance is negligible, measurable quantities of water may not accumulate in the brain even though capillary filtration increases (e.g., flow through a non-deformable steel pipe). If compliance is large, as in some cases of cold injury edema,[43] water accumulates easily (e.g., flow into an expansile sponge). Different compliances of white and gray matter could account for their different proclivities to develop edema. Compliance can be modified by trauma and depend on the state of hydration of brain cells.

REFERENCES

1. Reese TS, Karnovsky MJ: Fine structural localization of a blood-brain barrier to exogenous peroxidase. J Cell Biol 34:207–217, 1967
2. Brightman MW, Reese TS: Junctions between intimately apposed cell membranes in the vertebrate brain. J Cell Biol 40:648–677, 1969
3. Karnovsky MJ: The ultrastructural basis of transcapillary exchanges. J Gen Physiol 52:64s–95s, 1968
4. Pitelka DR, Hamamoto SK, Duafala JG, et al: Cell contacts in the mouse mammary gland. I. Normal gland in postnatal development and the secretory cycle. J Cell Biol 56:797–818, 1973
5. Wade JB, Revel J, DiScala VA: Effect of osmotic gradients on intercellular junctions of the toad bladder. Am J Physiol 224:407–415, 1973
6. Rapoport SI, Hori M, Klatzo, I: Testing of a hypothesis for osmotic opening of the blood-brain barrier. Am J Physiol 223:323–331, 1972
7. Brightman MW, Hori M, Rapoport, SI, et al: Osmotic opening of tight junctions in cerebral endothelium. J Comp Neurol 152:317–326, 1973
8. Rapoport SI: Effect of concentrated solutions on the blood-brain barrier. Am J Physiol 219:270–274, 1970
9. Rapoport SI, Thompson HK: Osmotic opening of the blood-brain barrier in the monkey without associated neurological deficits. Science 180:971, 1973
10. Broman T, Olsson O: The tolerance of cerebral blood vessels to a contrast medium of the diodrast group. Acta Radiol 30:326–342, 1948
11. Studer RK, Welch DM, Siegel BA: Transient alteration of the blood-brain barrier: Effect of hypertonic solutions administered via carotid artery injection. Exp Neurol 44:266–273, 1974
12. Posner JB, Plum F: Spinal-fluid pH and neurologic symptoms in systemic acidosis. N Engl J Med 277:605–613, 1967
13. Linzell JL, Peaker M: The effects of oxytocin and

milk removal on milk secretion in the goat. J Physiol (London) 216:717–734, 1971

14. Møllgard K, Sørensen SC: Changes in capillary permeability in the brain studied with alcian blue as a tracer. Acta Physiol Scand Suppl 396:12, 1973

15. Westergaard E, Brønsted HE: The effect of acute hypertension on the vesicular transport of proteins in cerebral vessels. Abstr 7th Int Congr Neuropathol Sept 1–7, Akademiai Kiado, Budapest, 1974, p 322

16. Lassen NA: Control of cerebral circulation in health and disease. Circ Res 34:749–760, 1974

17. Johansson B, Strandgaard S, Lassen NA: On the pathogenesis of hypertensive encephalopathy. The hypertensive "breakthrough" of autoregulation of cerebral blood flow with forced vasodilatation flow increase and blood-brain barrier damage. Circ Res 34 (Suppl 1):1–167 to 1–171, 1974

18. Betz E: Cerebral blood flow: Its measurement and regulation. Physiol Rev 52:595–630, 1972

19. Howse DC, Caronna JJ, Duffy TE, et al: Cerebral energy metabolism, pH and blood flow during seizures in cat. Am J Physiol 227:1444–1451, 1974

20a. Reivich M, Marshall WJS, Kassell N: Loss of autoregulation produced by cerebral trauma, in Brock M, Fieschi C, Ingvar DH, et al (eds): Cerebral Blood Flow. Clinical and Experimental Results. Berlin, Springer-Verlag, 1969, pp 205–208

20b. Rapoport SI: The Blood-Brain Barrier in Physiology and Medicine (in preparation)

21. Bjerner B, Broman T, Swensson A: Tierexperimentelle Untersuchungen über Schadigungen der Gefasse mit Permeabilitätsstorungen und Blutungen in gehirn bei Insulin-, Cardiazol- und Elektroschockbehandlung. Acta Psychiatr Neurol 19:431–452, 1944

22. Lorenzo AV, Shirahige I, Liang M, et al: Temporary alteration of cerebrovascular permeability to plasma protein during drug-induced seizures. Am J Physiol 223:268–277, 1972

23. Cutler RWP, Lorenzo AV, Barlow CF: Changes in blood brain barrier permeability during pharmacologically induced convulsions. Prog Brain Res 29:367–384, 1968

24. Freygang WH, Sokoloff L: Quantitative measurement of regional circulation in the central nervous system by the use of radioactive inert gas. Adv Biol Med Phys 6:263–279, 1958

25. Rapoport SI, Thompson HK: Opening of the blood-brain barrier (BBB) by a pulse of hydrostatic pressure. Biophys J 15 (no. 2, part 2):326a, 1975

26. Petersén I, Zwetnow N: Blood-brain barrier damage and prolonged cerebral hyperemia following changes in cerebral perfusion pressure; an experimental EEG study. Experientia 23:929–930, 1967

27. Häggendal E, Johansson B: On the pathophysiology of the increased cerebrovascular permeability in acute arterial hypertension in cats. Acta Neurol Scand 48:265–270, 1972

28. Johansson B: Regional cerebral blood flow in acute experimental hypertension. Acta Neurol Scand 50:366–372, 1974

29. Rapela CE, Green HD: Autoregulation of canine cerebral blood flow. Circ Res 15 (Suppl 1):205–212, 1964

30. Starling EH: On the absorption of fluids from the connective tissue spaces. J Physiol (London) 19:312–326, 1896

31. Landis EM, Pappenheimer JR: Exchange of substances through capillary walls, in Hamilton WF, Dow P (eds): Handbook of Physiology. Section 2: Circulation, vol. 2. Washington DC, American Physiology Society, 1963, pp 961–1034

32. Aukland KF: Autoregulation of interstitial fluid volume. Edema-preventing mechanisms. Scand J Clin Lab Invest 31:247–254, 1973

33. Klatzo I, Wísniewski H, Smith DE: Observations on penetration of serum proteins into the central nervous system. Prog Brain Res 15:73–88, 1965

34. Schutta HS, Kassell NF, Langfitt TW: Brain swelling produced by injury and aggravated by arterial hypertension. A light and electron microscopic study. Brain 91:281–294, 1968

35. Rapoport SI: Experimental modification of blood-brain barrier permeability by hypertonic solutions, convulsions, hypercapnia and acute hypertension, in Cserr H, Fencl V, Fenstermacher JD, et al (eds): Fluid Environment of the Brain. New York, Academic Press, 1975

36. Robinson JS, Brightman MW, Rapoport SI: Opening of the blood-brain barrier during aramine-induced hypertension (in preparation)

37. Byrom FB: The pathogenesis of hypertensive encephalopathy and its relation to the malignant phase of hypertension. Experimental evidence from the hypertensive rat. Lancet 2:201–211, 1954

38. Fieschi C, Agnoli A, Battistini N, et al: Cerebral vasomotor control and CSF pH in metabolic and respiratory coma, in Brock M, Fieschi C, Ingvar DH, et al (eds): Cerebral Blood Flow. Clinical and Experimental Results. Berlin, Springer-Verlag, 1969, pp 222–225

39. Langfitt TW, Weinstein JD, Sklar FH, et al: Contribution of intracranial blood volume to three forms of experimental brain swelling. Johns Hopkins Med J 122:261-270, 1968

40. Becker D: Personal communication

41. Brock M, Hadjidimos A, Schürmann K, et al: Regional cerebral blood flow in cases of brain tumor, in Brock M, Fieschi C, Ingvar DH, et al (eds): Cerebral Blood Flow. Clinical and Experimental Results. Berlin, Springer-Verlag, 1969, pp 169–171

42. Symon L: Personal communication

Patricia Tornheim, Ph.D.
Robert L. McLaurin, M.D.

16

Traumatic Cerebral Edema: An Experimental Model

One of the most serious problems associated with human head injury is that of brain edema, a phenomenon which consists of an increase in brain water content. Traumatic edema fluid seeps from injured cerebral vessels into brain tissue spaces. It accumulates preferentially in the white matter, resulting in an increased brain volume which can cause a rise in intracranial pressure that leads to brain stem compression and death.

Most experimental approaches to the study of traumatic brain edema have involved the use of models in which insults are delivered directly to brain tissue. In the present investigation, a model was developed to study cerebral edema which was initiated by a method somewhat comparable to that seen clinically—that of cranial impact. This model was tested experimentally to determine (1) the magnitude and distance of spread of edema fluid 48 hours after head injury, and (2) the reproducibility of the brain edema, in order to evaluate the suitability of the model for reliable drug testing.

TECHNIQUES

Trauma Model

A Remington Humane Stunner was used to deliver blows to the heads of anesthetized cats. This device consists essentially of a barrel containing a piston which is fitted at one end with an impacting disc (Fig. 1). An apparatus was built which holds the fixed stunner barrel and the cat

during delivery of the blow (Fig. 1). With the use of this device, accurate placement of the cat's head in relation to the impacting disc is permitted. The animal's head rests on a compressed aluminum foil support which serves to damp the unrestrained head in response to the blow.

In preliminary testing, it was found that the most consistent response to impact involved the following circumstances: (1) delivery of the blow to the dorsal surface of the exposed skull, and (2) positioning of the cat's head so that the center of the striking surface of the impacting disc was 1.6 cm above the midline area of the frontoparietal suture. With this method, approximately 70 percent of animals demonstrated the following response to impact: unilateral fracture of the frontal bone; ipsilateral contusion of the insular-temporal area of the brain (Fig. 2); subarachnoid hemorrhage; and the development of significant brain edema of the contused hemisphere by 48 hours after impact. These characteristics were considered the essential features of an impact model for study of traumatic brain edema.

Specific Gravity Determination

Quantitative analysis of brain edema is usually accomplished by direct determination of the change in brain water content from normal levels. The method used in this study for measurement of brain edema is indirect, involving the determination of tissue density or specific gravity. Nelson et al.[5] have shown that accumulation of edema fluid reduces the density of brain tissue. From specific gravity data, change in tissue volume can also be calculated.[5]

Supported in part by GRANT NS 07253.

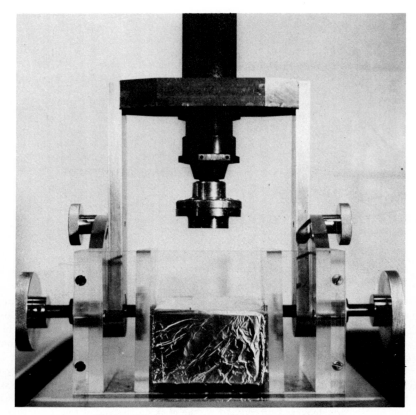

Fig. 1.   Remington Humane Stunner in its holder.

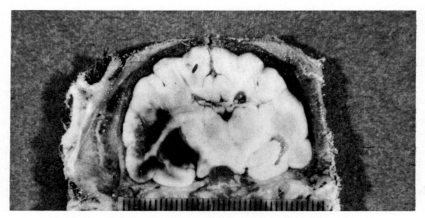

Fig. 2.   Unilateral insular-temporal contusion of cranial impact.

Table 1
Specific Gravity of Centrum Semiovale

Sectional Level	Normal Control Hemispheres (N = 6)	Contused Hemispheres			
		Gray Matter-White Matter Contusions (N = 8)		Gray Matter Contusions (N = 4)	
I (Rostral limit-caudate nucleus)	1.0494* ±.0004	1.0346 ±.0016	(P < .001)**	1.0466 ±.0016	(P < .05)
II (Lamina terminalis)	1.0491 ±.0004	1.0357 ±.0013	(P < .001)	1.0455 ±.0024	(P < .02)
III (Rostral thalamus)	1.0493 ±.0004	1.0404 ±.0019	(P < .01)	1.0484 ±.0008	(N/S)
IV (Lateral geniculate nucleus)	1.0493 ±.0004	1.0430 ±.0018	(P < .02)	1.0481 ±.0004	(N/S)
V (Occipital lobes)	1.0498 ±.0006	1.0469 ±.0022	(N/S)	1.0489 ±.0009	(N/S)

*Mean value for the group ± standard error.
**P values represent differences from normal control values at the same sectional level.

In the present study, testing was limited to uncontaminated white matter since the edema fluid seen with this model, as in human head injury, was located primarily in white matter. Specific gravity values of small (5–10 mg) samples were determined with the use of an organic density gradient column according to the procedures described by Lowry and Hunter[4] and Nelson et al.[5]

APPLICATION OF TECHNIQUES

Twenty-five adult mongrel cats, 2–3 kg in weight, were used in this study. Following anesthesia with ketamine hydrochloride and endotracheal intubation, 19 cats were subjected to cranial impact in the following manner. The scalp covering the dorsum of the skull was reflected and the animal was placed in the stunner holder. After positioning of the head as described previously, the stunner cartridge was detonated with a .22 caliber cartridge. Immediately after impact, those animals which demonstrated prolonged respiratory arrest were placed on a respirator until unassisted breathing began. Sacrifice was accom-

plished 48 hours after impact by head immersion in liquid nitrogen under ketamine anesthesia.

Normal control animals (N = 6) were not subjected to experimental intervention until the time of sacrifice. At least 1 normal control animal was sacrificed in the same manner as that used for the impacted cats on each sacrifice day.

The frozen heads of all animals were sliced with a band saw. Using the frontoparietal suture as a landmark, six coronal slices were made through the cranial vault at 5 mm intervals. The resulting five coronal sections were at the levels of the brain indicated in Table 1.

Each section, while still frozen, was immersed in kerosene to prevent evaporation and allowed to thaw. Sections were then examined under a dissecting microscope for pathology. The location, approximate size and type tissue involved in each contusion were recorded.

For each section, duplicate white matter samples (5–10 mg each) were removed from the centrum semiovale bilaterally and analyzed for specific gravity, using the organic density gradient column. In addition, for the experimental animals, specific gravity was determined for duplicate white matter samples taken at various distances

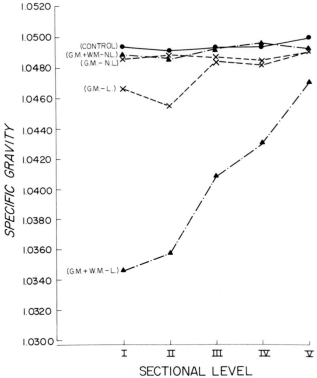

Fig. 3. Comparison of specific gravity of the centrum semiovale in normal control, GM-WM contused, GM contused, and noncontused impacted hemispheres. (CONTROL) = Mean values for normal control animals (N = 6). (GM+WM–NL) = Mean values for nonlesioned (noncontused) hemispheres of animals suffering GM-WM contusions (N = 8). (GM–NL) = Mean values for nonlesioned (noncontused) hemispheres of animals suffering GM contusions (N = 4). (GM–L) = Mean values for GM lesioned (contused) hemispheres (N = 4). (GM+WM–L) = Mean values for GM-WM lesioned (contused) hemispheres (N = 8).

from the posterior margin of each insular-temporal contusion.

RESULTS

Of the 19 animals impacted, 4 died prior to the sacrifice time of 48 hours after head injury. Twelve of the remaining 15 animals demonstrated unilateral frontal fracture with an underlying insular-temporal contusion, and these cats were selected for study.

It was found that the precise size and location of the insular-temporal contusion varied from one animal to another. All lesions, however, were found at sectional levels I and II. The type of tissue involved in contusion also varied. In 8 ani-

mals, both cortex (gray matter) and underlying white matter were contused. In 4 animals, the contusion was limited to cortex (gray matter).

Specific Gravity Data

The mean specific gravity of the centrum semiovale of control animals ranged from 1.0491 to 1.0498 at the five levels tested (Table 1). In the impacted animals, the specific gravity data from hemispheres with gray matter contusions only (GM) differed considerably from data of hemispheres with contusions involving both gray and white matter (GM-WM). GM-WM contused hemispheres demonstrated a significant decrease in density from normal values at sectional levels I through IV. The greatest density decrease was found at sectional levels I and II, the levels which had contused tissue. Proceeding caudally from section level II, the specific gravity of the centrum semiovale increased toward normal values (Table 1). For the GM contused hemisphere, significant decrease in specific gravity was seen at section levels I and II only. With these animals, both the magnitude and extent of specific gravity change was less than that seen with the GM-WM contused hemispheres (Table 1).

In Fig. 3, the mean values for specific gravity at each sectional level for the normal control, GM-WM contused, and GM contused hemispheres are compared graphically. In addition, values for the noncontused hemispheres of impacted animals have been plotted, showing an absence of significant change in density for these hemispheres.

White matter samples were taken at various distances from the posterior margins of GM-WM contusions to evaluate the change in specific gravity of white matter as a function of distance from the site of injury. In Fig. 4, the distance curves plotted for each GM-WM contused hemisphere showed a very low density close to the lesion (1 to 4 mm from the edge of contusion). For most animals, a rather sharp rise in specific gravity was seen somewhere between 6 and 10 mm posterior to the edge of contusion. In all animals, the specific gravity of white matter at the occipital pole was near normal levels.

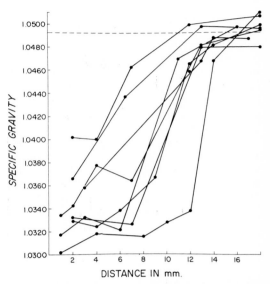

Fig. 4. Specific gravity of white matter posterior to the edge of contusion in GM–WM contused hemispheres. Each point on the graph represents the average of duplicate samples taken at a specific distance from the edge of a contusion for a single animal.

DISCUSSION

Most experimental studies of traumatic brain edema have involved the use of models in which focal insults (thermal, photic, inflammatory, mechanical) are delivered directly to brain tissue.[1,2,3,6] These models have the advantage of a rather high reproducibility of the injury and resultant edema. In addition, they permit the study of brain edema in a system uncomplicated by multifocal pathology. The main disadvantage with many of these models relates to the question of whether the resulting edema is qualitatively and quantitatively comparable to that seen in human head injury.

In the present investigation, a model was developed for study of brain edema associated with the contusion of cranial impact. The main advantage of this method relates to its similarity to clinical conditions. The primary weakness seen with this model is a lack of precise morphological reproducibility, a problem associated primarily with differences in skull characteristics from one animal to another.

Although preliminary investigations suggested an inability to reproduce consistent morphological responses with cranial impacting, it was found that with the methods described previously, approximately 70 percent of animals suffered one-sided fracture with an underlying contusion. With the use of specific gravity for quantitating edema, a method which offers excellent precision in the testing of small tissue samples, a respectable reproducibility of edema was seen in animals selected for one-sided contusion.

The quantitative aspects of the brain edema of contusion have not been described previously. The results of the present study lend support to a number of observations made with the use of other models for traumatic brain edema. In preliminary studies, it was found that density changes in gray matter were limited to the area immediately surrounding contusion. It was also seen that, 48 hours after impact, the noncontused hemispheres of impacted cats were not edematous, suggesting a failure of the spread of edema fluid to the contralateral white matter. With a comparison of specific gravity data from several levels of the brain, the greatest change in density was seen close to contusion, with a decline in edema as the distance from contusion increased. These observations suggest that with contusion, as with other local injuries to brain tissue, edema fluid spreads from the area of direct damage to distant sites. For all of the above-mentioned judgments, however, caution must be exercised because data were collected at one time period only.

Perhaps the most striking feature demonstrated in this study is the difference in specific gravity data seen in animals with GM-WM contusions versus those with contusions limited to the cortex. The great difference in data from these two groups of hemispheres suggests that direct involvement of white matter in contu-

sion represents an important factor in terms of the magnitude of resulting edema. This difference is one which certainly warrants further investigation, particularly with morphological studies.

In summary, the present study describes a method for the induction of cerebral edema associated with the contusion of cranial impact. With a selection of animals based on morphological response to impact, edema of respectable reproducibility develops. It is hoped that these methods will provide the basis for further studies concerning the pathophysiology of the edema of contusion and will permit evaluation of therapeutic measures for control of brain edema in a system somewhat comparable to that seen clinically.

REFERENCES

1. Benson VM, McLaurin RL, Foulkes EC: Traumatic cerebral edema. An experimental model with evaluation of dexamethasone. Arch Neurol 23:179–186, 1970
2. Hirani A, Becker NH, Zimmerman HM: Pathological alterations in the cerebral endothelial cell barrier to peroxidase. Arch Neurol 20:300–308, 1969
3. Klatzo I, Piraux A, Laskowski EJ: The relationship between edema, blood-brain barrier and tissue elements in a local brain injury. J Neuropath Exp Neurol 17:548–564, 1958
4. Lowry OH, Hunter TH: The determination of serum protein concentration with a gradient tube. J Biol Chem 159:465–474, 1945
5. Nelson SR, Mantz ML, Maxwell JA: Use of specific gravity in the measurement of cerebral edema. J Appl Physiol 30:268–271, 1971
6. Sperl MP Jr, Svien HJ, Goldstein NP, Kernohan JW, Grindlay JH: Experimental production of local cerebral edema by an expanding intracerebral mass. Proc Mayo Clin 32:774–749, 1957

Edited by James A. Mosso, M.D.
and Robert L. McLaurin, M.D.

Open Discussion

DR. DONALD BECKER: We have recently been looking at the blood-brain barrier status after acute traumatic injuries in animals, and have some preliminary data I would like to present. One of the major problems in using the horseradish peroxidase technique to study the blood-brain barrier in acute acceleration-deceleration injuries is that a small petechial hemorrhage, often too small to be seen by standard neuropathologic techniques, will produce leakage of the horseradish peroxidase into the extracellular space in the region of the petechial hemorrhage. It will then spread throughout the brain. In one case 4 hours after injury, there was no evidence of petechial hemorrhage but horseradish peroxidase was seen in the extracellular space adjacent to an intact tight junction. Does this occur because the tight junctions were temporarily opened, because the endothelial cells transported the peroxidase at an increased rate into the extracellular space, because trauma to the ventricular wall and bleeding into the ventricle allowed the horseradish peroxidase to enter the extracellular space, or because acute hypertension at the time of injury with injury with transient breakdown of the blood-brain barrier?

DR. ALLEN CROCKARD: We have found that immediately following missile injury to an animal brain there is a massive increase in intracranial pressure that occurs in the first few seconds (Fig. 1), and the only way we think this could happen is as a result of an acute increase in intracranial volume. The only possible source for this increased volume is the vascular compartment. This may be pertinent to Dr. Becker's question.

DR. J. D. MILLER: We have made some observations on the effects of Conray ventriculography on intracranial pressure and were surprised at the results. With an intraventricular catheter in place and a transducer taped to the side of the head so as not to record hydrostatic pressure artifact, Conray was injected with the patient in the sitting position. This produced no change in ventricular pressure. However, when the patients were tipped backward into the supine position, the pressure rose by an average of 45 mm

Hg. This rise occurred whether the pressure had been initially high or normal. The rise in pressure corresponded to the point at which the stream of Conray fell into the fourth ventricule. In a patient with aqueduct stenosis, this rise in pressure was markedly delayed. These pressure changes did not occur with intraventricular air.

In view of the comments that have been made about the barrier-opening properties of Conray, and that gap junctions exist rather than tight junctions in the ventricular ependyma, one must speculate that Conray is entering the fourth ventricular ependyma and that the acute rise in pressure must be related to a vascular dilatation. The pressure rise spontaneously subsides to baseline within about 45 minutes.

DR. EUGENE FLAMM: We have extended our interest in the effect of alcohol on spinal cord injury to that in head injury. We have found that with an 800 g/cm impact on the intact dura of the left frontal region of an animal following injection of Evans blue, only a small lesion and extravasation of dye is produced. However, following an infusion of alcohol to obtain a blood level of 350 mg %, and following this same impact, at 12 and 24 hours following injury a much more extensive extravasation of dye occurs in the animal with the high blood alcohol level.

Alcohol has been shown to produce lipid peroxidation particularly in the liver, and we have been very interested in the effects of peroxidation on lipid membranes in the nervous system. Whether this is the explanation for the alteration in blood-brain barrier, I am not sure. However, alcohol certainly produces a striking potentiation of a seemingly insignificant amount of trauma in both spinal and head injured animals.

DR. ARTHUR KOBRINE: For the last couple of years we have been measuring blood flow and autoregulation in the spinal cord, using the hydrogen clearance method. In a series of 7 or 8 animals, we measured blood flow in the white matter of the spinal cord under conditions of normocapnia, while varying the blood pressure by bleeding the animal or infusion of norepinephrine or angiotensin (Fig. 2). We found that autoregulation of

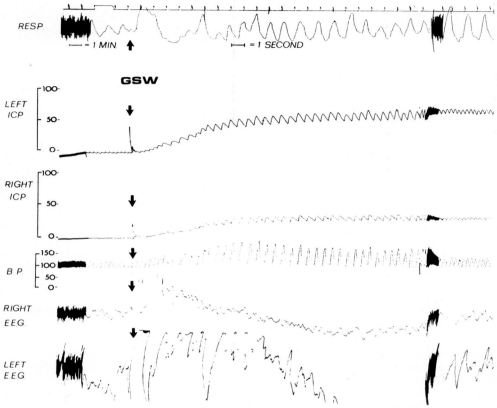

Fig. 1. The vital signs of a monkey before and immediately after a right hemispheric missile injury. Note the increase in ICP to 40 mm Hg within 4 seconds after shooting. (Right side artifactually low due to entrance wound). This sudden increase in ICP can only be due to an increase in cerebral blood volume; flow studies performed at 1 minute after injury show complete loss of autoregulation with a passive flow situation.

the spinal cord does exist between 50 to 55 mm Hg up to about 135 to 140 mm Hg, analogous to that seen in the brain. Autoregulation here also depends on changes of the resistance as the blood pressure changes. Beyond the limits of autoregulation, with a low blood pressure the vascular resistance is minimal and with a pressure above 135 mm Hg, the vessels progressively dilate and there is a marked increase in blood flow. This correlates with what has been said about the breakdown of autoregulation as the blood vessels dilate.

DR. ROSENBLUM: Dr. Rapoport has presented conditions in which edema is known to be present, and another set of conditions in which tight junction dissolution is known to be present, and yet at times these two things can be dissociated. I would like to ask him how it is that sometimes edema does not occur when tight junctions are supposedly separated?

DR. RAPOPORT: I don't mean to say that when autoregulation breaks down and the barriers open that is equivalent to opening every tight junction. I meant simply that there is evidence that intravascular material gets into the brain. I would assume that according to Starling's law, edema of vasogenic origin occurs when the rate of efflux of water from the brain (whatever the mechanism is) is less than the rate of entry of filtration into the brain.

The only instance in which I could envision tight junctional opening and edema not occurring would be under extreme hypotension, that is zero pressure.

DR. WILLIAM HUNT: There are many places in the body that do not have tight junctions and turn blue with Evan's dye, yet do not have edema.

DR. RAPOPORT: The question really should be, What is the quantitative relation between the hy-

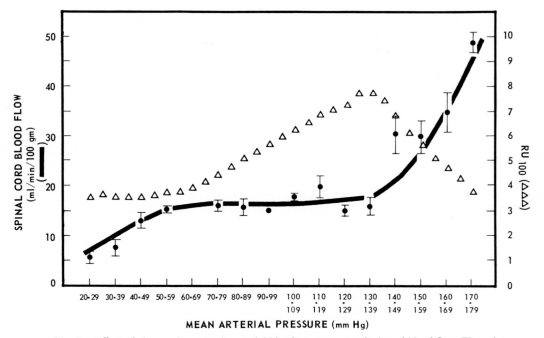

Fig. 2. Effect of changes in systemic arterial blood pressure on spinal cord blood flow. The axis on the left represents SCBF, demonstrating autoregulation between an MAP of 55–135 mm Hg. The axis on the right represents the calculated vascular resistance for each MAP value. Note the progressive *decrease* in vascular resistance, and breakthrough in autoregulation, at high MAP values, i.e., above 135 mm Hg.

draulic conductivity, which obviously increases when the tight junctions are open, and the rate of flow with the rate of edema formation? I would guess in the peripheral tissues, if there is an opening of pores, there is also a lymphatic system to rapidly clear the fluid. There is also a protective mechanism in that increased permeability or increased pressure by 10 mm Hg does not produce brain edema, because in essence the interstitial fluid is filtered and washed out, where protein-rich fluid that normally exists is replaced by protein-poor fluid. So, there are negative feedback mechanisms that protect against edema formation either by slight increase in permeability, or slight increase in hydrostatic pressure, or slight decrease in osmotic pressure. Edema does not occur until protein osmotic pressure is down to 2 mm Hg.

I suppose the real question is, What are the quantitative relations among these factors which operate, and that rate and appearance of measurable edema? I do not know. Obviously, tight junctions open up, hydraulic conductivity decreases, and one expects increased flow if pressures remain the same; and if the tight junc-

tions open up the reflection coefficients also are falling, so the driving force is also increasing. This is the sort of question that has to be addressed quantitatively.

DR. JOHN PICKARD: We did some experiments with baboons, extending Dr. Rapoport's technique in blood-brain barrier, for pharmacologic purposes. When the CO_2 was elevated, we know we were opening the blood-brain barrier for other reasons. We got no evidence of cerebral edema nor did we get it by raising blood pressure. Small molecules, such as prostaglandin, can be distributed across the blood-brain barrier if the circulatory response to cerebral autoregulation is affected. CO_2 elevation results in a far better vasodilator effect than with a breakdown of autoregulation. However, we found no evidence of increase in total brain water or increase in water content of gray or white matter after we elevated the CO_2 and after we broke the blood-brain barrier with urea. Prostaglandin did not cross the barrier under these circumstances.

DR. RAPOPORT: Nevertheless, I think the basic question is how much the permeability has to increase, how much the pressure has to be increased before edema occurs. It is a quantitative problem in principle. I can tell you that we do not get brain edema when we open up the blood-brain barrier and allow protein into the interstitial fluid, although that would produce a driving force. So there must be perhaps a threshold either with reference to the tolerance of the brain to increased water flow or threshold to the driving force.

DR. DEREK BRUCE: First of all, from the point of view of reflection coefficients, I think we have to realize that in the brain and obviously in other tissues, the reflectivity of the capillary endothelium is one coefficient only, and that there is a greater interstitial space that also has a reflection coefficient. In the brain, the makeup of the interstitial space is different from other tissues. I think the fact that we break the tight junction in one case presents only a solitary injury, whereas in trauma we are doing more than just opening a barrier.

The other thing is that in other organs, lymph flow is responsible for a very small portion of fluid clearance, and that there is a good deal of protein fluid flow along the capillary bed from the arterial end to the venous end. There is an actual pericapillary tissue flow conceivably, and the amount of lymph drainage is only what is left over.

I think it is very important that we do not equate edema with dysfunction. Cerebral edema does not uniformly lead to cerebral dysfunction. Edemas associated with an intact blood-brain barrier do not necessarily appear toxic, and patients with pseudotumor cerebri or hydrocephalus where there is extracellular edema with high pressure do not usually have neurological dysfunction.

DR. THOMAS LANGFITT: I would like to refer to some studies we did a number of years ago in the cat, in which we did craniectomies on one side of the brain and traumatized that area with a jet of nitrogen in a 500 msec blast. Prior to the nitrogen jet, we found that by elevating the blood pressure acutely, a slight increase in brain volume followed by a return to control level occurred, which was a good measure of autoregulation. Following the nitrogen jet, we observed a progressive swelling, which at times was quite massive. With injection of Evans blue, we could find no correlation between the amount of swelling and the amount of extravasation of Evans blue, and, in fact, in an occasional cat we found quite significant brain swelling and no Evans blue extravasation at all. So we concluded that we were dealing with two types of

edema, one due to conventional osmotic edema following breakdown of the blood-brain barrier in those animals in which there was an Evans blue extravasation, and a second type of edema which we termed hydrostatic edema. Here, according to Starling's hypothesis, with a perfectly intact blood-brain barrier, edema may occur purely on a physiological basis with increase in water content of the tissue.

In other words, with effective autoregulation, an elevation of blood pressure produces passive vascular dilatation, pressure is transmitted to the capillary bed, and if the osmotic pressure is the same on either side of the capillary wall, according to Starling's hypothesis, an increase in the intracapillary pressure will produce an extravasation of fluid into the brain without damage to the capillary.

DR. RAPOPORT: I think the point is, distinct from edema of cytotoxic origin, which we consider to be metabolic inhibition and accumulation of water in cells, there are many factors that could lead to transudation of fluid across capillaries. There is the hydraulic conductivity which is a function of permeability. There is the reflection coefficient which would decrease if barriers, probably serial barriers of permeability, increased. There is the interstitial osmotic pressure which would increase if lactate or material from damaged cells penetrated the interstitial tissue. If barrier permeability remained the same, then increase of hydrostatic pressure independent of a change in permeability should, by the law of Starling, lead to increased flow into the brain. At which point edema develops when flow increases, is a question. The real questions are how much pressure independent of permeability would lead to measurable brain edema, how much increase in permeability independent of pressure, and how can these things be revised.

DR. PLUM: You are talking about a physiological measurement problem. When the hydrostatic pressure changes in relation to the resistance of the tissue, there is an increase in tissue water content. You are describing a pathological threshold level.

DR. RAPOPORT: Yes. We only talk about edema that we measure, and I assume it is of the order of 2 percent change. When one says there was no observable brain edema, you really say you are not able to measure it. However, measurable edema does not occur in peripheral tissue even through pressure increases because of the feedback mechanism. The initial filtration washes out the protein, according to the Wiederheld and Aukland hypotheses.

DR. A. TAYLOR: Basically I agree with Dr. Rapoport. But I want to point out that, and this concerns peripheral tissue, tissue pressure is another factor that can increase according to swelling of the tissue. The tissue pressure-volume relationship varies for different tissues according to their compliance. Until now, we do not know what the compliance of brain tissue is, and we do not know how much volume we have to push out of the capillaries to elevate the outside pressure enough to oppose the filtration pressure.

DR. CARL DILA: It is intriguing to me that both Dr. Rapoport and Dr. Brightman demonstrated that with increases in pressure, for instance, a spike in blood pressure secondary to aramine, the tight junction might open.

I wonder if under physiological conditions, substances such as histamine may have an affect on tight junction, as they do dilate crerebral vessels. Also, plasma bradykinesia are very potent vasodilators in other organs and tissues and cause marked changes in capillary permeability. One wonders whether these substances have an effect on cerebral vessels and whether they are involved in the pathogenesis of cerebral edema.

DR. THOMAS DUCKER: Is there a significant difference in the tight junction of the capillary in gray and white matter? This is a leading question in the sense that often selectively the white matter is more edematous than the gray.

DR. BRIGHTMAN: No, we have not seen any obvious difference between the tight junction in gray or white matter, but there are some vessels described by Volt recently which he calls seamless—that is, they have no junctions at all. In cross sections, as hard as we look, we find no junctions, and it is very likely that such seamless vessels are in the heart of an edematous focus. There does appear to be a dichotomy in that, although in areas where peroxidase and Evans blue can get out if we push a bolus of saline into such a vessel, there is no appreciable edema. On the other hand, maybe the water can get across the vessel directly without having to resort to the occasional opening, the seam. So there appears to be a dichotomy between opening with respect to protein and the flood of water across the vessel wall.

With respect to Dr. Dila's question, Dr. Westgaard and I repeated the work of Broman done in the 1940s. We perfused ventricles with

maximal doses, at least 100 mcg of histamine over a period of 15 to 30 minutes and injected in the usual approach peroxidase proximally into the vessel. We found no evidence of extravasation. So histamine appears to have no effect whatever within the limits of sensitivity of these tracers.

DR. RAPOPORT: With respect to the differences between white and gray matter, I think we come back to the question of compliance again. Classen pointed out that the myelin sheaths of white matter can separate more easily under pressure, and therefore an accumulation of water may occur. I think perhaps the difference in edema between white and gray matter reflects this difference in compliance. With respect to histamine, there may be a cause for the lack of response to histamine. Dr. Carl Becker has shown that the endothelia of many peripheral capillaries apparently have actomycin-like protein within them, and do respond to histamine and shrink with an increase in permeability. Endothelia of the brain don't have this actomycin-like protein, and this may, in fact, be an explanation for the differential sensitivity of brain capillaries versus peripheral capillaries to histamine.

DR. BRUCE: In a recent paper from Roentgen's group on the effects of histamine and bradykinin on fluid concentration in the peripheral tissues of dog, they suggest that histamine and bradykinin cause an increase of capillary permeability through an increase in pinocytosis, taking up of the protein and transporting it across the cell with its release on the other side.

They base this on the fact that when they increase the venous pressure in the animals that have been treated with histamine and bradykinin, they do not get an increase in the amount of protein and dextran that comes out, suggesting this is not a hydrostatically dependent process, suggesting it is not through a fixed pore, but at least is a mixed transport. Since the transport in vesicles seems to be a relatively unimportant event in brain capillaries under normal circumstances, this may be another reason for lack of effect of these substances on the brain.

DR. ALVIN WALD: We have been working with Dr. Hochwald measuring cerebrospinal fluid formation by the technique of ventriculo-cisternal perfusion in cats and altering at the same time the serum osmolality by intravenously infusing sucrose solutions of different osmolalities. If we change serum osmolality, either increase or decrease, by up to 10 percent we find no change in either gray or white matter content, but we do find a linear relationship to CSF formation. In other words, we can increase CSF formation by two- to threefold by decreasing serum osmolality and conversely completely inhibit CSF formation by increasing serum osmolarity. This suggests to us that CSF is acting as a sink of water during this vasogenic water intoxication and in some ways is replacing lymphatic system.

DR. RAPOPORT: An alternative mechanism relates to the high rate of blood flow through the choroid plexus.

III

Respiratory Pathophysiology

Gerald Moss, Ph.D., M.D.

17

Respiratory Distress Syndrome as a Manifestation of Primary CNS Disturbance

The focus of the medical profession has turned toward the "respiratory distress syndrome" (RDS) as it has become recognized as the major cause of death of patients under intensive hospital care. The etiology in most cases is still not clear, but attention had been directed toward the CNS as the primary "trigger" site.

Classical studies in the past have shown that CNS disturbance can lead to the pathological lung changes of this complex (congestion, edema, atelectasis, and hemorrhage). Stereotaxic preoptic hypothalamic lesions or focal deposition of stimulant caused these changes.[1,2] Increasing intracranial pressure leads to the picture.[3] Instillation of fibrin or endotoxin into the CSF bathing the brain will result in the complication.[4] The past explanation for this "neurogenic pulmonary edema" will require reexamination. The accepted theory was a generalized sympathetic response with massive peripheral vasoconstriction, and left heart failure as the ultimate result, leading to the pulmonary complication. Indeed, increased pulmonary capillary pressure with resultant congestion, transudation of protein-rich fluid into the interstitium and alveoli, etc. will lead to this gross and microscopic pathology. However, in many cases of RDS, as follows various types of shock, left ventricular dynamics, both clinically and experimentally, have been measured to be normal. We still postulate increased capillary pressure as the underlying hemodynamic alteration, but this would require the interposition of a high resistance to vascular flow between the capillary and the pulmonary veins, the site of the "venule" or "postcapillary sphincter." We believe that direct autonomically mediated constriction at

this site, as demonstrated by Webb's group after canine hemorrhage,[5] provides a plausible explanation. We feel that the initiating insult (hypoxia, hemorrhagic or septic shock, etc.) causes a disturbance directly in the hypothalamus, leading to this pulmonary "tourniquet" effect.

In our research, we subjected the arterially isolated brain of several species of experimental animals to hypoxemia.[6,7] Systemic blood pressure and volume remained in the normal ranges, as did the pO_2, pCO_2, and pH of the systemic arterial blood. Our perfusate was the subject's own mixed venous blood, whose major difference from its arterial blood was a pO_2 of only 35 mm Hg. After exposure to this hypoxemic blood in lieu of normal cerebral arterial flow for 2 hours, all subjects developed progressive, fatal pulmonary failure and the anatomic features of RDS.[8,9]

We perfected a technique for denervation of the left canine lung that required only 10 minutes of ischemia time[10] so that we could prepare large numbers of these subjects with minimal mechanical and metabolic trauma to the reimplanted lung. When these dogs were subjected to isolated cerebral hypoxemia, they did not succumb. The pulmonary lesions developed in the normally innervated right lung, but the denervated left lung remained anatomically and functionally normal.[11] Similarly, the changes developed in the right but not left lungs when the dogs were subjected to hemorrhagic shock or to 100 percent O_2 ("oxygen toxicity").[12]

Many workers have sought the site of "irreversibility" in shock. It was found that a level of canine hemorrhage that proved uniformly fatal (removal of 50 ml/kg, with mean arterial pressure at 25 mm Hg for 4 hours) could result in 50 percent survival if a constricting clamp was placed around the thoracic aorta. The decreased cardiac output was artificially redistributed, so that the upper half of the body received an augmented flow, at the expense of the lower half.[13] These workers speculated as to the possible sites of irreversibility: heart, brain, or lungs.

More recently, Hardy's group at Mississippi showed that the heart was not the critical site.[14] Dogs subjected to "irreversible shock" then were donors of their hearts, transplanted orthotopically into equal-sized recipients. These hearts were then able to recover from their metabolic derangements, which had occurred, to provide the pumping function for the recipients, until rejection difficulties, many days later, became the limitations to survival. The heart had not been irreversibly damaged by the hemorrhagic shock.

In a similar vein, Dr. Baue's group in St. Louis examined energy metabolism in liver and lung, as well as the cell's ability to maintain its cation "pumping" activity. Liver slices from rats subjected to hemorrhagic shock had decreased levels of ATP. Further, when chilled to 0.5°C in a Krebs Ringer's solution, the liver slices were unable to restore the normal internal Na^+ and K^+ after rewarming to 37°C. By contrast, lung slices from rats in shock were virtually unchanged in these functions from control lung slices from normal rats. Pulmonary cellular integrity and energy production were apparently unimpaired by hemorrhagic shock.[15] The focus seems to sharpen on the CNS.

We obtained additional evidence that the CNS was the "trigger" for RDS when we showed that diphenylhydantoin protected dogs and rats from development of the pulmonary lesions after hemorrhagic shock.[16] We are uncertain of the exact actions by which diphenylhydantoin maintains cerebral cellular function and integrity under conditions of oxygen deprivation, but this has been observed empirically in rats subjected to respiratory hypoxia.[17]

It formerly was thought that the CNS was "spared" during shock. In the "wisdom of the body," a disproportionately larger share of the reduced cardiac output flowed to the brain, virtually maintaining its normal support. This view is no longer tenable. The brain soon shares the full brunt of the total reduced cardiac output under conditions of severe shock, within minutes.[18] CSF and cerebral cortical pO_2 levels fall precipitously.[19] Anerobic metabolism supervenes, with rapid accumulation of lactic acid in the brain.[20] Cellular integrity and function are jeopardized, as K^+ and pseudocholinesterase "leak" into the CSF.[21] With more severe shock, lethal neuronal changes are demonstrable.[22] In hemorrhage studies upon trained, awake dogs, Shoemaker's group used sequential "tagged" microspheres to follow the pattern of cerebral blood flow in shock.[23] As taught classically, the percentage of cardiac output going to the brain rose initially, almost offsetting the effect of decreased cardiac output. Then, even the fraction of the reduced flow going to the brain fell below basal levels. The deficit was found to be uniformly distributed throughout the brain, with the same proportionate fall in white and gray matter, in brain stem, hypothalamus, cerebellum, etc.

Our laboratory has not yet addressed itself to the subject of neural trauma and the subsequent pulmonary changes. Yet this is of great clinical significance. Of the servicemen dying in Vietnam of brain injury, fully 85 percent had the lung complex at autopsy.[24] Some died too soon to have been the "victims" of overenthusiastic resuscitation. There is grave doubt as to whether any of those dying with the pulmonary lesions had been transfused "too much." A prospective study showed that none of those developing the syndrome ("Da Nang lung") had reached a measured blood volume that would have been normal for those youngsters, let alone exceeded it.[25] Indeed, the greatest blood volume deficits were found in those given the largest volumes of blood and fluid. This parallels our civilian OR experience, where we usually underestimate the extent of blood loss; the greater the hemorrhage, the further we "fall behind." Why did the CNS injured GIs die with or of their pulmonary complication? Why does it develop among our civilian patients? Further work is indicated to explore the interconnections between CNS and respiratory function, and the autonomic control of the pulmonary vasculature would appear to be a likely subject for closer scrutiny.

REFERENCES

1. Gamble JE, Patton HD: Pulmonary edema and hemorrhage from preoptic lesions in rats. Am J Physiol 172:623, 1953

2. Wood CD, Seager LD, Ferrell G: Influence of autonomic blockade on aconitine induced pulmonary edema. Proc Soc Exp Biol Med 116:809, 1964

3. Ducker TB: Increased intracranial pressure and pulmonary edema. I Clinical study of 11 patients. J Neurosurg 28:112, 1968

4. Simmons RL, Ducker TB, Martin AM, Anderson RW, Noyes HE: The role of the central nervous system in septic shock: Pathological changes following intraventricular and intracisternal endotoxin in the dog. Ann Surg 167:145, 1968

5. Sugg WL, Craver WD, Webb WR, Ecker RR: Pressure changes in the dog lung secondary to hemorrhagic shock: Protective effect of pulmonary reimplantation. Ann Surg 169:592, 1969

6. Moss G: Cerebral arterial isolation: The effects of differential pressure perfusion. J Surg Res 4:170, 1964

7. Moss G: Total cerebral perfusion: Applicability of technique to several species of experimental animals. Surgery 61:265, 1967

8. Moss G, Staunton C, Stein AA: Cerebral etiology of the shock lung syndrome. J Trauma 12:885, 1972

9. Moss G, The role of the central nervous system in shock: The centroneurogenic etiology of the respiratory distress syndrome. Crit Care Med 2:181, 1974

10. Moss G: Simplified experimental unilateral pulmonary autotransplantation. J Thorac Cardiovasc Surg 65:899, 1973

11. Staunton C, Stein AA, Moss G: Cerebral etiology of the respiratory distress syndrome: Universal response with prevention by unilateral pulmonary denervation. Surg Forum 24:229, 1973

12. Dworkin P, Moss G, Cerebral etiology of the pulmonary lesions of oxygen toxicity. Surg Forum 24:211, 1973

13. Golden PF, Jane JA: Survival following profound hypovolemia: Role of heart, lung, and brain. J Trauma 9:784, 1969

14. Culpepper RD, Kondo Y, Hardy JD: Successful orthotopic allotransplantation of hearts from dogs in irreversible shock. Surgery 77:126, 1975

15. Sayeed MM, Chaudry IH, Baue AE: Na^+-K^+ Transport and adenosine nucleotides in the lung in hemorrhagic shock. Surgery 77:395, 1975

16. Moss G, Stein AA: Cerebral etiology of the acute respiratory distress syndrome: Diphenylhydantoin prophylaxis. J Trauma 15: May, 1975 (in press); Surg Forum 24:433, 1973

17. Naiman JG, Williams HL: Effects of diphenylhydantoin on the duration of respiratory activity during anoxia. J Pharm Exp Ther 145:34, 1964

18. Rutherford RB, Kaihara S, Schwentker EP, Wagner NH Jr: Regional blood flow in hemorrhagic shock by the distribution of labeled microspheres. Surg Forum 19: 14, 1968

19. Vranova Z, Keszler H, Vrana M: Oxygen tension in the cerebral cortex of dogs in hemorrhagic shock and its changes after oxygen therapy. Acta Anesth Scand 12:171, 1968

20. Yashon D, Locke GE, Paulson G, Miller CA: Brain, CSF, and blood lactate levels during hemorrhagic shock. Surg Forum 22:23, 1971

21. Simeone FA, Witoszaka MM: The central nervous system in experimental hemorrhagic shock. Am J Surg 119:427, 1970

22. Tamura H, Simeone FA: The nervous system in experimental hemorrhagic shock. J Trauma 12:869, 1972

23. Slater G, Vladek BC, Bassin R, Brown RS, Shoemaker WC: Sequential changes in cerebral blood flow and distribution of flow within the brain during hemorrhagic shock. Ann Surg 181:1, 1975

24. Shoemaker WC, Bryan-Brown CW, Quigley L, Stahr L, Elwyn DH, Kark AE: Body fluid shifts in depletion and poststress states and their correction with adequate nutrition. Surg Gynecol Obstet 136:371, 1973

25. Simmons RL, Heisterkamp CA III, Moseley RV: Postresuscitative blood volumes in combat casualties. Surg Gynecol Obstet 128:1193, 1969

J. Hoff, M.D.
M. Nishimura, A.B.
L. Pitts, M.D.

18

A Quantitative Method of Neurogenic Pulmonary Edema in Cats

Hemorrhagic pulmonary edema occurs commonly in patients with fatal head injury.[1] Similar pulmonary changes have been observed after brain injury in experimental animals.[2-5] Presumably the brain insult initiates a neurogenically mediated hemodynamic storm.[3,6] The insult, whether generalized[6,7] or localized,[4,8] evokes sympathetic discharge, effecting peripheral vasoconstriction. As systemic arterial pressure then rises, the left ventricle may fail as hypertension becomes severe. Left heart failure, manifested by left atrial and pulmonary venous hypertension, develops, ultimately causing hemorrhagic pulmonary edema.

Whether this sequence of events is essential to the production of neurogenic pulmonary edema or whether the pulmonary changes are caused by the brain insult without a systemic vasomotor crisis remains unresolved. Efforts to study the pathophysiology of neurogenic pulmonary edema further have been frustrated by little human data[9,10,11] and inconsistent animal observations.[6,7,12,13]

We have developed an animal model in which hemorrhagic pulmonary edema may be produced consistently by raised intracranial pressure. The model may allow quantitative as well as qualitative measurement of neurogenic pulmonary edema.

Supported in part by NIH Grants NS 5593, GM 18470, and NS 11539. Dr. Hoff is recipient of Teacher-Investigator Award NS 11051

METHOD

Adult cats (2–4 kg) were anesthetized (pentobarbital 30 mg/kg IP), paralyzed (gallamine 20 mg IV), and ventilated by a Harvard respirator. The animals were fixed prone in a stereotaxic frame with the chest free. Anesthesia was supplemented half-hourly with pentobarbital, 5 mg/cc IV. Systemic arterial pressure (SAP), central venous pressure (CVP), intracranial pressure (ICP), and end tidal CO_2 (P_{ET} CO_2) were measured continuously. Body temperature was controlled (36–38°) and arterial PCO_2, PO_2, pH, and hematocrit were determined periodically.

ICP was raised (1 mm Hg/sec) by the intraventricular infusion of mock CSF (pH 7.22–7.25) to 100 mm Hg (5 animals), 150 mm Hg (5 animals), and 200 mm Hg (5 animals) and maintained there for 30 minutes or until cerebral perfusion pressure (CPP) was zero (CPP = SAP−ICP). CSF infusion was then stopped and ICP allowed to return to baseline. CSF volumes were recorded for each group of animals with raised ICP (100 mm Hg: 20 ± 4 cc/kg; 150 mm Hg: 35 ± 11 cc/kg; 200 mm Hg: 41 ± 11 cc/kg). After a 30-minute recovery period, the animals were heparinized and killed by an overdose of barbiturate. Elapsed anesthesia time was 3 hours for each experiment. The brains were removed and examined grossly. The lungs were removed, drained of blood for 1 minute, and weighed. A representative section of lung from a few animals was studied microscopically.

Lung weight, total lung water, and lung blood

$$\text{Blood Wt. (BW)} = \frac{\text{Hb (supernatant)}}{\text{Hb (whole blood)}} \times \frac{\% H_2O \text{ (homogenate)}}{\% H_2O \text{ (supernatant)}} \times \text{Wt. homogenate}$$

$$\text{Blood } H_2O = \% H_2O \text{ (blood)} \times BW$$

$$\text{Total lung } H_2O \text{ (TLW)} = \% H_2O \text{ (homogenate)} \times \text{Wt. homogenate} - \text{added } H_2O$$

$$\text{Extravascular lung water (EVLW)} = TLW - \text{Blood } H_2O$$

$$\text{Extravascular dry weight (EVDW)} = \text{Lung weight (LW)} - \text{(BW)} - \text{(EVLW)}$$

Fig. 1. Lung water formulas according to Holcroft's modification of Pearce's method for measurement of pulmonary edema.

weight were calculated by Holcroft's modification of the Pearce method.[14,15] Formulas used for the lung water analyses are shown in Fig. 1.

Control animals (5) with no CSF infusion and control animals (5) with mock CSF infused intravenously (50 cc/kg in 30 min) were studied similarly.

RESULTS

Animals with raised ICP developed hemorrhagic pulmonary edema, while control animals did not. The severity of hemorrhage evident grossly was greater in animals with higher ICP. Hemorrhage was uniformly distributed

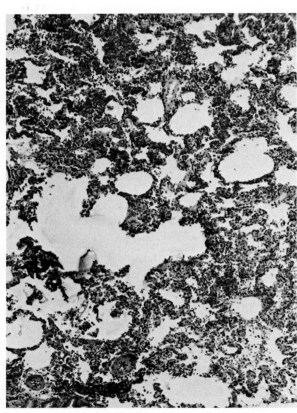

Fig. 2. Microscopic section of cat lung with ICP raised to 150 mm Hg for 30 minutes (H & E stain, 100 ×). Hemorrhage and edema are seen within the alveoli and the interstitial spaces.

Table 1

	Lung Weight (% Body Wt.)	TLW (% Lung Wt.)	EVLW (ml/g EVDW)	Blood Weight (g/g EVDW)
Control without infusion	0.6 ± 0.1	74 ± 10	3.5 ± 0.4	0.6 ± 0.2
Control with CSF infusion	0.7 ± 0.2	77 ± 10	3.7 ± 0.1	0.8 ± 0.3
ICP = 100 mm Hg	0.7 ± 0.1	81 ± 0.4	3.6 ± 0.8	3.1 ± 1.8*
ICP = 150 mm Hg	1.2 ± 0.4*	83 ± 1.0	$4.6 \pm 0.3^+$	6.2 ± 3.9**
ICP = 200 mm Hg	1.0 ± 0.2*	77 ± 10	$5.5 \pm 0.8^+$	$2.8 \pm 1.1^+$

Note: Animals with raised ICP were compared to control animals with CSF infusion
*$P < .05$.
**$P < .01$.
$^+P < .005$.

throughout the lungs, being most obvious in interstitial tissue (Fig. 2). Edema fluid was found commonly in alveoli, bronchioles, and bronchi. The lungs of test animals were heavy (lung weight), congested (blood weight), and edematous (extravascular lung water). Comparative values for the experimental and control groups are shown in Table 1.

The lungs of control animals were grossly normal except for segmental atelectasis in 2 animals without CSF infusion and in 1 with CSF infused intravenously. The brains of all animals were grossly normal.

Throughout each experiment with raised ICP arterial oxygenation remained adequate (> 70 mm Hg) despite the development of hemorrhagic pulmonary edema (Table 2). Usually PaO_2 fell modestly while $PaCo_2$ rose during the recovery period.[16] Similarly, CVP rose during ICP elevation

(14cm H_2O, maximum), to fall toward normal during recovery. CVP changed little in control animals with or without an intravenous infusion of mock CSF.

SAP rose during ICP elevation in all animals when ICP was 150 mm Hg or greater. SAP failed to rise in 3 of the 5 animals with ICP raised to 100 mm Hg, yet CPP was still maintained above 50 mm Hg in all 5. Cerebral perfusion pressure remained greater than 50 mm Hg in all animals with ICP raised to 150 mm Hg, in each instance effected by a rise of SAP. When ICP reached 200 mm Hg, CPP fell below 50 mm Hg in all, remaining above 20 mm Hg in 3, but approaching zero in 2.

Hematocrit fell during CSF infusion, whether fluid was given intraventricularly or intravenously, then rose toward baseline during the recovery period.

Table 2

	$PaCO_2$ (mm Hg)	pHa	PaO_2 (mm Hg)	Hct
Control	37.6 ± 1.4	$7.34 \pm .03$	92 ± 8	41 ± 4
100 mm Hg	39.4 ± 2.9	$7.34 \pm .06$	90 ± 7	33 ± 5
Recovery	38.2 ± 2.6	$7.35 \pm .04$	91 ± 7	35 ± 8
Control	37.7 ± 3.0	$7.31 \pm .06$	91 ± 12	35 ± 7
150 mm Hg	41.3 ± 2.4	$7.29 \pm .04$	88 ± 8	37 ± 8
Recovery	37.8 ± 2.1	$7.32 \pm .03$	94 ± 6	31 ± 8
Control	36.3 ± 3.9	$7.33 \pm .07$	104 ± 15	41 ± 4
200 mm Hg	42.3 ± 2.1	$7.24 \pm .04$	91 ± 12	37 ± 7
Recovery	41.4 ± 4.9	$7.23 \pm .08$	99 ± 17	37 ± 6

DISCUSSION

The hemodynamic events that precede hemorrhagic pulmonary edema caused by intracranial hypertension have been documented experimentally.[3,6,13] Typically, pulmonary arterial and wedge pressure rise in animals that develop neurogenic pulmonary edema, accompanied by systemic arterial hypertension. These pressure responses of the pulmonary vasculature have not been observed consistently, however.[12]

Patients with clinical and pathological evidence of neurogenic pulmonary edema have not shown consistent pressure changes either. Of 4 patients with neurogenic pulmonary edema studied soon after head injury by us, only 1 developed pulmonary artery (36/20 mm Hg) and pulmonary wedge pressure (18 mm Hg) elevations. In that 1 patient, SAP failed to rise, despite pulmonary pressure changes; he ultimately recovered without neurological or pulmonary sequelae.

That pulmonary changes occur abruptly, soon after injury, without fluid overload, was documented by Simmons et al. in combat casualties who had severe head injuries.[11] During a recent 2-year period, we found similar necropsy data in civilian patients with fatal gunshot wounds of the brain who died within minutes to hours of injury. In spite of normal physical examinations of the chest, normal chest roentgenograms, and often normal blood gases, 60 percent of the patients had wet, heavy, and sometimes hemorrhagic lungs at autopsy.

Whether hemorrhagic, edematous lungs are the final result of sympathetically mediated stress upon the entire vascular system or simply the result of massive autonomic discharge directly from the brain to the lungs remains unresolved. Moss and colleagues provide evidence that pressure changes of the systemic vasculature are not prerequisites of neurogenic pulmonary edema.[7] Rather, they suggest a specific cerebral (hypothalamic) insult may cause increased pulmonary vascular resistance and subsequent pulmonary edema without a systemic pressor response. On the other hand, Szidon and Fishman have documented decreased resistance in pulmonary vessels when sympathetic nerves of the lungs were stimulated.[17]

Hemorrhagic pulmonary edema of neural origin is probably one end of a spectrum of pulmonary lesions commonly seen in patients with brain injury. Other parts of the same spectrum may include arteriovenous shunting, ventilation/perfusion maldistribution, and subclinical pulmonary edema with vascular congestion.[10] The animal model described here, by allowing quantitation of pulmonary pathology, will enable more detailed study of the lung lesions associated with brain injury and may provide a means for evaluating therapy.

REFERENCES

1. Weisman SJ: Edema and congestion of the lungs resulting from intracranial hemorrhage. Surg 6:772–729, 1939
2. Campbell GS et al: Circulatory changes and pulmonary lesions in dogs following increased ICP. Am J Physiol 158:96–102, 1949
3. Sarnoff SJ, Sarnoff LC: Neurohemodynamics of pulmonary edema. II. The role of sympathetic pathways. Circ 6:51–62, 1952
4. Gamble JE et al: Pulmonary edema and hemorrhage from preoptic lesions in rats. Am J Physiol 172:623–631, 1953
5. Bean JW, Beckman DL: Centrogenic pulmonary pathology in mechanical head injury. J Appl Physiol 27:807–812, 1969
6. Ducker TB et al: Increased intracranial pressure and pulmonary edema, Part II. JNS 28:118–123, 1968

7. Moss G et al: Cerebral etiology of the 'shock lung syndrome'. J Trauma 12:885–890, 1972
8. Reynolds R: Pulmonary edema as a consequence of hypothalamic lesions in rats. Science 141:930–932, 1963
9. Ducker TB et al: Increased intracranial pressure and pulmonary edema, Part I. Clinical study of 11 patients. JNS 28:112–117, 1968
10. Brackett CE: Respiratory complications of head injury, in Gillingham, Obrador (eds): Head Injuries. Baltimore, Williams & Wilkins, 1971, pp 255–265
11. Simmons RL et al: Respiratory insufficiency in combat casualties: II. Pulmonary edema following head injury. Ann Surg 170:39–44, 1969
12. Pitts LH et al: The role of increased ICP in the production of neurogenic pulmonary edema, in

Proc 2nd Int Symp on ICP. Berlin-New York, Springer-Verlag, 1975

13. Brashear RE, Ross JC: Hemodynamic effects of elevated CSF pressure: Alterations with adrenergic blockade. J Clin Invest 49:1324–1333, 1970

14. Holcroft JW, Trunkey DD: Extravascular lung water following hemorrhagic shock in the baboon. Ann Surg 180:408–417, 1974

15. Pearce ML et al: Measurement of pulmonary edema. Circ Res 16:482–488, 1965

16. Jennett S, Hoff J: Arterial blood gases during raised intracranial pressure in anesthetized cats. Br J Anesth (in press)

17. Szidon JP, Fishman AP: Participation of pulmonary circulation in the defense reaction. Am J Physiol 220:364–370, 1971

Allan M. Parham, M.D.
Thomas B. Ducker, M.D.
Joseph S. Redding, M.D.

19

Lung Dysfunction in the Presence of Central Nervous System Disease

Pulmonary complications are common in patients who have injury to the central nervous system. Patients with only minor CNS injuries rarely have pulmonary complications; however, in patients who die as a result of CNS injury, autopsy studies show that over 85 percent have significant lung pathology. The lung disease usually is a complex mixture of atelectasis, infection, and edema due to multiple pathological processes.

Lung pathology following CNS trauma may be subdivided into three major categories: (1) mechanical insufficiency, (2) acute pulmonary edema, and (3) subacute respiratory distress syndrome. The mechanical insufficiency disorders are caused by obtunded airway reflexes, obstruction of the small bronchioles, muscle paralysis, and monotonous respiratory patterns with associated microatelectasis. Acute pulmonary edema is a dramatic event most commonly associated with sudden severe increased intracranial pressure and its associated cardiovascular events. The "subacute" respiratory distress syndrome is indistinguishable from the "shock" lung disorder in general trauma—now termed the respiratory distress syndrome of the adult—and is a general term which includes many types of interstitial pulmonary congestion that occur hours to days after injury and are not due to heart failure.

MECHANICAL INSUFFICIENCY

Mechanical insufficiency is by far the most common problem following central nervous system injury, and obtunded airway reflexes are the most common type of mechanical problem.

Complete airway obstruction must be corrected immediately. The hazards of partial airway obstruction—that is, heavy snoring—are often overlooked. Partial airway obstruction is frequently accompanied by copious saliva production. When these secretions stimulate the vocal cords of an obtunded patient, severe laryngospasm may result. Moderately severe partial obstruction may lead to air swallowing, gastric distention, and explosive vomiting. If the obstruction is so severe that the patient must labor forcefully during inspiration to pull in air, he may generate enough negative airway pressure to pull capillary and interstitial fluid into his alveoli and thus precipitate pulmonary edema.

Even if the patient is capable of maintaining an unobstructed airway, his reflexes may still be inadequate to protect him from aspiration of gastric contents in the event that he vomits or passively regurgitates. The consequences of such aspiration vary greatly and depend on the volume, acidity, and size of food particles contained in the aspirate. Sudden cardiac arrest may immediately follow aspiration, apparently by reflex action, even before systemic hypoxia has developed. Shortly following aspiration, many small bronchioles may be obstructed and bronchospasm may occur, further limiting the size of the small airways. Hypoxemia is severe, and it may be difficult to ventilate the patient even with a mechanical ventilator. A more common result of aspiration is a chemical pneumonia, which is often clinically indistinguishable from a bacterial pneumonia. The presence of inadequate airway reflexes may be the only indication that aspiration has occurred.

Severe airway obstruction is most reliably

recognized by placing the hand over the nose and mouth and feeling absent or diminished air flow. Partial airway obstruction is recognized by hearing a "snore" on inspiration or palpating it immediately above the larynx. If a patient is too obtunded to respond to command, he may aspirate if he regurgitates as long as that clinical state persists. Not infrequently, a patient will respond to command when stimulated but lapse into a deeper state of unconsciousness when he is left alone. Not only the physicians but also the intensive care nurses should check the patient's "lash" reflex by stroking his eyelash and observing for a winking response. If this reflex remains present in the unstimulated patient whose eyes are closed, he will not aspirate even if he regurgitates while asleep. If it is absent, he should have a cuffed endotracheal tube placed to prevent aspiration.

The immediate treatment of inadequate airway reflexes is placement of a cuffed endotracheal tube. This should be followed by tracheostomy if long-term management is anticipated. Irritation of the posterior pharynx may precipitate gagging and vomiting. Therefore, an oral or nasal airway should be used for a brief time only until an endotracheal tube is placed, and nasogastric intubation should be deferred until after the endotracheal tube is placed. The endotracheal tube cuff should be inflated until there is only a slight leak when the patient is sighed with an Ambu bag. This minimal leak technique should be used continously until airway reflexes are intact. Humidification and warming of inspired gases, frequent aseptic suctioning of the trachea, and frequent change of the patient's position will decrease the incidence of superimposed infection. If aspiration has occurred prior to intubation, methylprednisolone is administered in a dose of 250 mg immediately and then maintained for at least 2 days to reduce the inflammatory response. When wheezing is present, an intravenous aminophylline drip is started. If the chest roentgenogram shows segmental or lobar atelectasis, bronchoscopy may be necessary to remove solid material that is obstructing the bronchus.

Another type of mechanical insufficiency is that seen with muscle paralysis from trauma to the spinal cord or the phrenic nerve. Although the patient is usually left with adequate muscle strength to breathe and maintain normal blood gases initially, he may not have enough muscle strength to sigh, take deep breaths, and cough effectively. A monotonous respiratory pattern,

unbroken by the occasional sigh or deep breath, will lead to diffuse microatelectasis of the lungs. The chest roentgenogram is frequently normal in such instances, and the only manifestation is hypoxia. If the patient cannot cough effectively, secretions will accumulate and obstruct small bronchioles; the unventilated areas of lung will subsequently develop atelectasis and later pneumonia. These conditions may be predicted and prevented by measuring the patient's vital capacity upon admission. The vital capacity is an index of the ability to cough effectively. Awake patients can take their deepest breath and blow into the spirometer; obtunded patients should be intubated and the volume of a forceful cough determined. If the patient's vital capacity is less than 25 percent of their predicted normal, a tracheostomy should be performed and a mechanical ventilator needs to be utilized. Even if there is no neurological improvement, the vital capacity and respiratory function will improve in 1 week to 10 days. Initially, the thorax will sink inward as the diaphragm descends during inspiration. As intercostal muscle tone increases, this effect will decrease, and the patient will be able to take deeper breaths and cough more effectively.

A very similar type of problem is seen in patients who have the muscular ability to sigh and cough effectively but who simply fail to do so. Commonly, this is seen in patients during protracted recovery from frontal lobe injuries and cerebrovascular accidents. Occasionally, this abnormal pattern is seen in trauma patients with very subtle changes in intracranial pressure. While these patients may be responsive to command, they are frequently totally disinterested in their surroundings. The respiratory pattern is marked by a monotonously constant rate and depth of respiration, uninterrupted by sighing, deep breathing, or coughing. The result is diffuse microatelectasis and hypoxemia. Reduction of the intracranial pressure on occasion will reverse the abnormal respiratory pattern in certain trauma patients. Frequent intermittent positive pressure breathing will help others. In the more severe cases, mechanical ventilation for 24 hours followed by intermittent mandatory ventilation at a rate of two breaths per minute is more effective.

ACUTE PULMONARY EDEMA

In recent years, the occurrence of pulmonary edema in association with central nervous system and multisystem trauma has received much attention. Clinically, at least one variant of this syndrome is clearly neurogenic in origin: the acute fulminating type of pulmonary edema which may follow within minutes after a sudden rise of intracranial pressure. The occurrence of this syndrome is the absence of cardiovascular disease, right heart failure, blood loss, fluid therapy, fractures, shock, or sepsis is well documented. In the experimental animal, an increase in intracranial pressure is followed by a Cushing reflex with an increase in blood pressure and slowing of pulse. Cardiac output initially increased, but decreased later in those rare animals which developed pulmonary edema. Right ventricular failure did not occur in either experimental animals or in our series of patients. While it is possible that cerebral ischemia caused pulmonary changes, the most probable explanation is that left ventricular failure and pulmonary edema occurred due to the extremely high peripheral resistance. Regardless of the vascular mechanism, it was clear that head injury in association with acute pulmonary edema may be secondary to increased intracranial pressure. The patient should be intubated, ventilated with 100 percent O_2, and given maximum cardiopulmonary support. If intracranial pressure is elevated, further treatment of the pulmonary edema should be continued during an immediate decompressive procedure. If pulmonary edema persists postoperatively, positive end expiratory pressure must be applied sparingly to minimize its effect on increasing intracranial pressure.

(SUBACUTE) RESPIRATORY DISTRESS SYNDROME

In addition to the acute form of pulmonary edema mentioned above, there is a more subacute variation which is generally referred to as the "respiratory distress syndrome of the adult." This appears to follow a variety of multisystem traumatic injuries, particularly after hemorrhagic or septic shock has occurred. The etiology remains uncertain, but it has generally been considered a result of various direct influences on the pulmonary capillary endothelium. More recently, an attractive unifying theory has been proposed which blames central nervous system hypoxemia as the initial event. Once the central nervous system has been injured, the sympathetic nervous system reacts with constriction of small pulmonary venules as well as peripheral vaso-

constriction. When the pulmonary venular constriction persists, interstitial pulmonary edema is created. Subsequently, there is loss of albumin into the interstitial space, pulmonary capillary damage, closure of small airways, loss of pulmonary compliance, and hypoxemia. A vicious cycle is set in motion which leads to progressive pulmonary edema and respiratory failure. The edematous lung appears more susceptible to infection, and a superimposed pneumonia may obscure the diagnosis as well as adding further pulmonary damage.

The diagnosis is made primarily on the basis of history, severe hypoxemia, and usually the presence of interstitial edema on the chest film. Treatment is primarily supportive at this time. Mechanical ventilation with positive end expiratory pressure (PEEP) helps to prevent small airway closure and permits adequate oxygenation with nontoxic oxygen concentrations. An adequate level of PEEP appears to prevent further deterioration and may actually reduce the amount of edema present. Fluid restriction, mild diuresis, and the osmotic activity of albumin help prevent the accumulation of interstitial pulmonary edema. Maintenance of a hemoglobin concentration greater than 12 g% is essential and helps assure adequate oxygen delivery to the brain and other vital tissues.

CONCLUSION

The classification system we have reported is notable in that it does not include infection as a primary source of lung pathology. The relationship of bacteria in the bronchial tree is similar to that of bacteria in a decubitus ulcer; antibiotic therapy may be necessary for resolution of the infection, but antibiotics alone will be unsuccessful unless the underlying mechanism is recognized and treated. Endotracheal tubes and tracheostomies have been recognized as predisposing to infection, but too little attention has been paid to the other mechanical factors causing infections in patients who require this type of airway.

Our purpose has been to elucidate mechanisms whereby primary central nervous system injury may lead to pulmonary damage. With proper attention to these mechanisms, with adequate supplemental oxygen and blood gas monitoring, pulmonary damage should rarely be the cause of further central nervous system injury.

Alan Crockard, F.R.C.S.

20

Controlled Ventilation in Curarized Patients with Severe Head Injuries

There are few centers now where ventilation or respiratory assistance of some variety would not be used for some head injuries. The actual method employed, the duration of treatment, the selection of cases, and the analysis of the results are still a matter of considerable debate. There are those who quite rightly point out that our knowledge of the "natural history of severe head injuries" is poor, and thus our ability to predict the outcome in many cases is questionable.[15] On the other hand, it is a common experience of those dealing with neurosurgical emergencies that a short period of manual hyperventilation may result in unresponsive dilated pupils becoming reactive again. A further difficulty is the wide variety of trauma and the presence of various combinations of other injuries complicating the evaluation of data; thus, it is difficult for even a major accident center to acquire a large series of head injuries without involvement of other systems.

The way in which mechanical ventilation alters the pathophysiology is also in dispute. The vasoconstrictive effect of hyperventilation by reduction of blood carbon dioxide levels induces a reduction in brain volume and intracranial pressure.[18] A reversal of "intracerebral steals" and consequent improved nutrition of damaged areas is also postulated[1] but not so easily proven in head injury. Opponents of hyperventilation point out that most of the deceleration-induced head injuries are already tachypnoeic with low blood CO_2 levels. Controlled volume ventilation of such

Supported by the Royal Victoria Hospital, Belfast, and United States Public Health Service fellowship (1-F05 TW-02144-01).

patients reduces unnecessary work,[4] improves lung function, raises blood oxygen levels,[5] and may reduce ICP.

This communication emphasizes two facets of the problem; first, the use of controlled ventilation in the immediate postinjury period of gunshot would of the head, an injury in which the effect of the therapy can be directly assessed. The second aspect deals with the intracranial effects of variations in the method of ventilation. Only if the maximum effect of ventilation is achieved can there be a rational assessment of further therapeutic adjuvants; (differing methods of ventilation may account for divergent results in the evaluation of barbiturate therapy in train trauma). While controlled ventilation can be used with sedation alone, it is the author's opinion that muscle paralysis with curare-like drugs affords optimum conditions for brain and lungs.

BULLET INJURIES

The hospital at which this work was carried out is situated in an area of Belfast, Northern Ireland, where some of the most violent disturbances have occurred; gunfire frequently occurred close to the hospital. This, coupled with an excellent ambulance service, resulted in a record evacuation time of casualties directly into a major hospital containing the Neurosurgical Unit for the Province. Seventy-five percent of approximately 140 patients with gunshot wound of the brain were seen within 30 minutes of wounding, and along with resuscitative measures, it was possible to monitor vital signs and intracranial pressure. An AKERS AE830 vented subdural transducer was

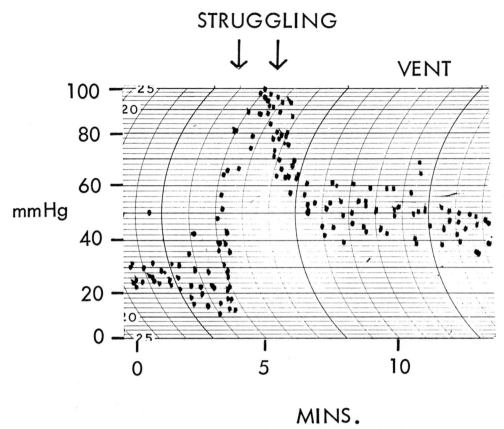

Fig. 1. The ICP record of a patient with an occipital high velocity wound, 20 minutes after injury. Drowsy on admission, he lapsed into coma after struggling. Despite controlled ventilation, ICP never returned to original values, an example of the extreme lability of such patients in the early postinjury period. Only by curarization and controlled ventilation can this be prevented. (Reprinted by permission. Ann R Coll Surg (Engl) 55:111.)

inserted directly through the missile wound when possible and the head bandaged routinely. In some of the high velocity injuries, there were large skull and skin deficits, and while this obviously affected the pressure recorded, it was considered that although the absolute level of pressure might be questioned, the sudden rise or falls could not be dismissed. Unlike the deceleration type of head injury which renders the victim unconscious from the time of impact, many patients with bullet injuries seen at this early stage were drowsy, irritable, struggling, coughing, or vomiting, and with each exertion, blood and brain extruded from the wound. It was not uncommon to examine an obtunded patient some minutes after injury only to see him lapse into coma some hours later. An example of this liability is illustrated in Fig. 1. This

patient received an occipital tangential injury with a high velocity missile and on admission, 15 minutes later, was only slightly obtunded, irritable, with no gross neurological deficit. ICP transducer inserted into the wound registered a pressure of 20 mm Hg. During treatment, he began to struggle and at the height of this his pupils became dilated. An endotracheal tube was inserted, he was given Suxamethonium, 50 mg intravenously, and mechanically ventilated. During the struggling, his ICP rose to at least 100 mm Hg and following the muscle relaxants it fell but never to the original level. At emergency operation, a small tear in transverse sinus was repaired and a large hematoma removed along with necrotic brain and bone fragments. Postoperatively, he was ventilated for 6 days until ICP remained

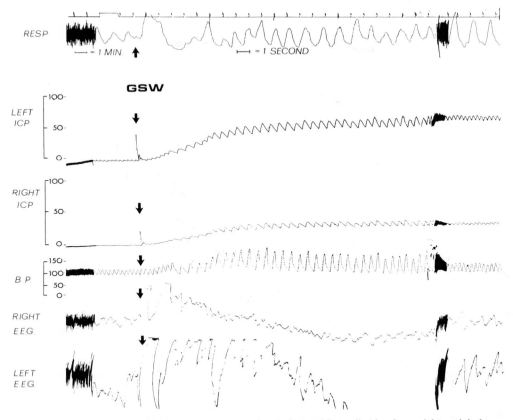

RESP

—— = 1 MIN. ↑   ⊢—⊣ = 1 SECOND

GSW

LEFT ICP

RIGHT ICP

B.P.

RIGHT EEG

LEFT EEG

Fig. 2. Recording of vital signs in a rhesus monkey before and immediately after a right occipital to frontal BB missile injury (GSW). Note the rise in ICP within a few seconds of impact indicating a sudden increase in intracranial blood volume. No hematoma was found at autopsy, excluding bleeding as a cause for this ICP rise.

low. He survived and was discharged from the hospital with a monoparesis and hemianopia.[10,11]

It was experiences like these which convinced us in Belfast that the best method of managing bullet injuries with any alteration in conscious level was immediate, controlled ventilation using muscle relaxants, before, during, and after surgery.[6] While it is known that the deceleration type of injury will eventually "settle" on controlled ventilation with large doses of sedation,[3] it is obvious from our experience that every cough and struggle will produce irrevocable rises in ICP. The most likely mechanism is increasing intracranial blood volume, and in the damaged brain some fluid is bound to leak from the vascular compartment. While there is less gross trauma in the conventional road accident head injury, there are numerous microscopic areas where this leakage might occur.[23] In an experimental animal model, it

has been shown that following a cerebral hemispheric bullet injury, ICP rises within a few seconds (Fig. 2), an indication of increasing blood volume, and cerebral blood flow passively follows blood pressure.[12] In such a situation, the brain can pass very rapidly from a compliant to a completely noncompliant state.

So, such patients were intubated with a low pressure cuffed endotracheal and kept relaxed with hourly pancuronium bromide 2–4 mg as necessary. No volatile anesthetic gases were given during operation, intravenous agents being used instead.

Hypovolemia or hypotension from whatever cause was rigorously treated by plasma expanders and blood transfusion; saline was avoided. There were problems with transfusion; in some cases while the blood volume was being restored, there was massive cerebral swelling, perhaps due to vasoparalysis and leakage of fluid from the capillaries (vasogenic oedema).[16] An unexpected bonus from controlled ventilation in cerebral bullet injuries was the marked reduction in bleeding from the damaged area during surgery. Initially, it had been our practice to take these patients immediately to the operating room and found great difficulty in controlling hemorrhage. Later, if there were no signs of deterioration, we delayed the surgery for 1 to 2 hours, while the patient was ventilated and found that hemorrhage was less of a problem.[8] If the patient was injured in a rural area, it was our advice that he be intubated and ventilated prior to and during transportation to the region's neurosurgery unit in Belfast, accompanied by a medical practitioner.

Obviously, not all patients were ventilated; those who were fully conscious were carefully observed prior to surgery, but any deterioration in clinical condition resulted in immediate endotracheal intubation and mechanical ventilation. Patients admitted comatose following bullet injury were inevitably fatal and were excluded from these measures.

Postoperatively, the bullet injuries were treated similarly to the serious road traffic head injuries, with regular doses of muscle relaxant and ventilated at a tidal volume of 10–15 ml/kg, 12 to 14 times per minute. Blood gases throughout the period of ventilation were carefully maintained (CO_2 30 ± 5 mm Hg, O_2 100 – 150 mm Hg). Every 24 to 48 hours, the patients were decurarized and assessed clinically. Pancuronium bromide, a curare-like drug was routinely used. It has fewer of the ganglion-blocking effects of curate. Pupillary reponses are intact. Dilated pupils and rising ICP in the absence of a mass lesion were taken as signs of lack of response and the ventilation discontinued. Tracheostomy was performed at 48 hours if ventilation was continued. In successful cases, ventilation is discontinued as soon as the ICP remained low during spontaneous respiration. In general terms, relatively short periods of controlled ventilation were used, rarely longer than 7 to 10 days.[9] Our most depressing results of vegetative survival have been in patients ventilated for 6 to 8 weeks.

Intracranial pressure should be measured during controlled ventilation, especially in those who have had devastating cranial injuries. Several patients requiring 10–12 l of blood and plasma expander before and during surgery had mild transfusion coagulopathies and required evacuation of clot from the wound cavity. An early postoperative rise in ICP warned of this complication.

METHODS AND ASSESSMENT OF VENTILATION

As already mentioned, we used a muscle relaxant with a moderate volume zero to positive pressure cycle. This has been satisfactory in long-term control of ICP. Pupil reactions can still be assessed and neurological examination can be performed with reversal of the muscle relaxant drugs. While it is possible to maintain controlled ventilation with high doses of sedative,[2] it has been our experience that this does not abolish motor activity and any movement of endotracheal tube, general nursing duties, etc., may rouse the patient, increase intrathoracic pressure, which is directly mediated to a "tight" brain, and produce a rise in ICP. While many such disturbances are transitory, the experience with the bullet injuries has made us wary of unnecessary rises in ICP.

Currently, compliance is being assessed by the volume pressure response (VPR), i.e., the change in pressure with unit change in volume[20] before, during, and after controlled ventilation. In some survivors of conventional deceleration injuries with moderate ICP rises (25–35 mm Hg), we have found a reduction in VPR within a few hours of ventilation before any marked reduction in ICP (Fig. 3). In other cases, the results have not been clear-cut, with wide variations in VPR over a period of hours. This may be due to inconstant ventilation conditions but may also be associated with fluctuations in cerebral blood volume, depending on changes in perfusion pressure in a passive flow situation as seen in our experimental gunshot model. Further work will be needed to evaluate this parameter. Leech and Miller[17] showed in the baboon that hyperventilation reduced ICP but not compliance as judged by VPR, but none of their animals had an injury comparable to human brain trauma, and no estimations were made during spontaneous and controlled ventilation. It is this type of experimental data which would be useful in the assessment of the role of controlled ventilation or hyperventilation in head injuries.

The effects of various methods of ventilation on ICP in head injuries have also been examined.[14] Positive End Expiratory Pressure, (PEEP) has been used to reexpand atelectasis or improve ventilation perfusion in the lung and has been invaluable with blast lung injuries in Belfast.[19]

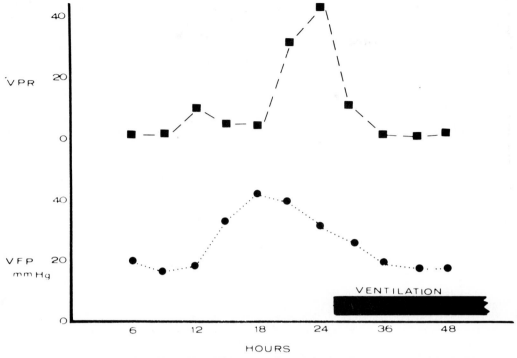

Fig. 3. Ventricular fluid pressure (VFP) and volume pressure response (VPR) of a patient with a deceleration injury. For the first few hours, mannitol and dexamethasone did not control the pressure, and following mechanical ventilation, though the VFP decreased marginally, there was a marked reduction in the VPR, indicating that the brain had become much more compliant.

Powers et al.[21] have studied the systemic effects of PEEP in trauma patients and concluded that one-third of their patients deteriorated with PEEP, for although the arterial PO_2 increased, the decrease in cardiac output offset the improved pulmonary ventilation-perfusion.

In head injuries, we have had at best slight increases in ICP when the end expiratory pressure increased above 5 cm water, but in a "tight" brain situation with loss of autoregulation, the effects have been more dramatic with stepwise ICP changes in line with fluctuations in systemic blood pressure and diminution in perfusion pressure, with ICP occasionally exceeding mean blood pressure. Our experience with negative end expiratory pressure in head injuries has not been encouraging. We found a rise in ICP as soon as the negative phase was applied which in compliant brain situations gradually reduced back to but never less that is original level. Pressure-triggered ventilation (assisted ventilation) using a Bird or Bennett ventilator has also raised the ICP in head

injuries; in fact, it has not been unusual to find the ICP higher during this type of respiratory assistance than during spontaneous respiration. Others have investigated the relative merits of increased volume hyperventilation (IVH) and constant volume hyperventilation[22] and have found in the normal and brain-damaged experimental animal that IVH reduced cardiac output and decreased cerebral blood flow and cerebral metabolic rate for oxygen. These changes were only noted at arterial PCO_2 less than 30 mm Hg. There was little difference at normal levels.

There is a degree of cerebral vasoconstriction with the moderate hypocapnic levels employed, but its contribution is considered to be small in the overall reduction of ICP in head injuries. Profound hypocapnea (PCO_2 15 or less) had been advocated by some[13] as means of further reducing ICP some 12 to 18 percent; they also noted a tissue lactic acidosis. In several of our cases inadvertently ventilated to a PCO_2 20 mm Hg, there was a rise in CSF lactate, indicating cerebral anaerobic glycolysis, and this fell only after the hyperventilation was discontinued. No such CSF acidosis was noted during controlled ventilation.[7]

CONCLUSION

To summarize, it can be said that the observations on gunshot wounds in the early post-injury period have convinced the author of the importance of controlled ventilation using muscle relaxants to prevent irrevocable rises in ICP and reduce the incidence of intracerebral hematoma. The same treatment has been applied to deceleration injuries.

In our experience, the best form of ventilation is a moderate volume zero to positive cycle; positive or negative end expiratory pressures may raise ICP in injured patients and should only be used for pulmonary complications.

REFERENCES

1. Alexander RSC, Lassen NA: Cerebral circulatory response to acute brain disease: Implications for anesthetic practice. Anaesthesiology 32:60, 1970
2. Becker DP, Vries JK, Young HF, et al: Controlled cerebral perfusion pressure and ventilation in human mechanical brain injury, in Ponten U (ed): Second International Symposium on ICP, Lund. Munich, Springer-Verlag, 1974
3. Becker DP: Controlled ventilation in head injury treatment. Second Chicago Conference on Neural Trauma. New York, Grune & Stratton, 1976
4. Bendixen HH, Ebgert LD, Hedley-White J, et al: Respiratory Care. St. Louis, Mosby, 1965, p 123
5. Brackett C: (untitled) Second Chicago Conference on Neural Trauma. New York, Grune & Stratton, 1976
6. Byrnes, DP, Crockard HA, Gordon DS, et al: Penetrating craniocerebral missile injuries in civil disturbances in Northern Ireland. Br J Surg 61:169, 1974
7. Crockard HA, Taylor, AR: Serial CSF lactate-pyruvate values as a guide to prognosis in head injury coma. Eur Neurol 8:151, 1972
8. Crockard HA: Gunshot wounds of the brain, in Taylor S (ed): Recent Advances in Surgery, no. 8. London, Churchill-Livingstone, 1973, p 213
9. Crockard HA, Coppel DL, Morrow WFK: Evaluation of hyperventilation in severe head injuries. Br Med J 4:634, 1973
10. Crockard HA: Bullet injuries of the brain. Ann R Coll Surg (Engl) 55:111, 1974
11. Crockard HA: Early ICP studies in gunshot wounds of the brain. J Trauma 15(3):182, 1975
12. Crockard HA, Brown FD, Mullan SF: Pathophysiological changes in experimental cerebral bullet injury in primates (in prep)
13. Czernicki, A, Jurkiewicz J, Kunicki A: Effect of hypocapnia on normal and increased ICP in cats and rabbits, in Ponten U (ed): Second International Symposium on ICP, Lund. Munich, Springer-Verlag, 1974
14. Gamble J, Coppel DL, Crockard HA: End expiratory pressure and ICP in head injuries (in prep)
15. Jennett WB: (discussion) Fiesci C (ed): Cerebral blood flow and intracranial pressure, Symposium Rome. Basel, Karger, 1972, p 235
16. Klatzo I: Oedema following experimental brain trauma, in Gillingham FS (ed): Head Injury Conference Procedings. Edinburgh, Churchill-Livingstone, 1972
17. Leech P, Miller JD: Intracranial volume pressure relationships during experimental brain compression in primates. J Neurol Neurosurg Psychiatr 37:1093, 1974
18. Lundberg N, Kjallquist A, Bien C: Reduction of increased intracranial pressure by hyperventilation. Acta Psychiat Scand 34:4–64, 1959
19. McCaughey E, Coppel DL, Dundee JW: Blast injuries to lungs. Anaesthesia 28:2, 1972
20. Miller JD, Leech P: Intracranial volume pressure relationships. J Neurosurg 42(3):274, 1975
21. Powers SR, Mannal R, Neclerio M: Physiologic consequences of positive end-expiratory pressure (PEEP). Ann Surg 178:265, 1973
22. Stoyka WA, Schultz H: Effects of increased volume hyperventilation (IVH) and controlled volume ventilation on cerebral metabolism in normal and brain injured dogs. Can Anaesth Soc J 21(2):265, 1974
23. Stritch SJ: Shearing of nerve fibres as a cause of brain damage due to head injury. Lancet 2:443, 1961

D. P. Becker, M.D., H. G. Sullivan, M.D.,
W. E. Adams, M.D., R. Greenberg, M.D.,
M. Rosner, M.D.

21

Controlled Hyperventilation in Severe Mechanical Brain Injury

Controlled hyperventilation in severe mechanical brain injury has been vigorously proposed.[1,2] However, its usefulness has often been denied and despite its advocates, it has been little applied. This dichotomy exists for two reasons. First, since we lack adequate strong prognostic criteria in head-injured humans, it has not been possible to statistically demonstrate improvement in morbidity or mortality with controlled ventilation. Second, it requires a major new commitment to patient management. Patients must be more intensely cared for, observed, and studied. Frequent blood gas analyses must be obtained. Depressant drugs or paralyzing agents must be used to phase the patient into the ventilator. Thus, increased use of ICP monitoring and computerized axial tomography or angiography is necessary. Finally, without close attention of skilled nurses, pulmonary therapy experts or anesthesiologists, new complications from this therapy, such as sudden mechanical respirator failure, pneumothorax, etc., may occur.

Our own experience in this area began when we observed a distressing incidence of pulmonary insufficiency causing secondary hypoxic brain insults in our patients with severe brain injury. This was occurring despite intensive care unit management and resulted from various problems such as progressive hypoxia and acute airway obstruction. To obviate this problem, we initially instituted respirator-assisted ventilation. In this situation, patients often resisted the ventilator or still received inadequate ventilation. We then moved to controlled ventilation. We subsequently observed that secondary hypoxic brain insults and progressive pulmonary insufficiency were no longer a serious problem. We also noted a decreased incidence of delayed elevated ICP. However, because overall therapy of our patients has simultaneously been altered and intensified, we have been unable to define whether controlled ventilation per se reduces overall morbidity and mortality in severe brain injury.

METHODS

Only patients with severe mechanical brain injury are managed with controlled ventilation. These patients are defined as those who are unable to obey more than one-stage commands because of a disordered level of consciousness. This includes patients with brain stem posturing and patients with inappropriate or incoherent verbal responses to painful stimulation.

The overall management is outlined in Fig. 1. After establishment of the airway, initial management is determined by an immediate twist drill ICP measurement and ventriculogram (see flow sheet). Controlled ventilation is then instituted (Fig. 2). A volume respirator is utilized and in adults is initially set at a rate of 12 per minute with a tidal volume varying between 700 and 1000 cc (15 cc/kg body weight). In order to "phase" the patient into the ventilator, adults receive 25 mg of chlorpromazine intramuscularly every 6 hours. This is often sufficient, but occasional patients still resist the ventilator. Should this occur, intravenous morphine at a dose of 1 to 3 mg is administered as required to achieve total control.

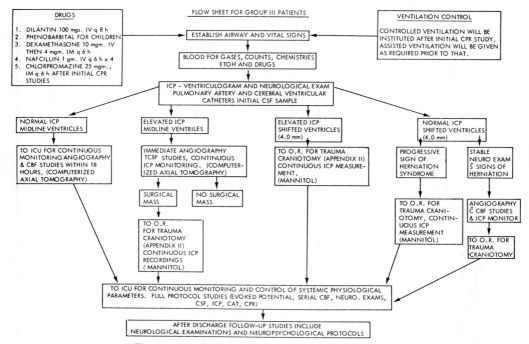

Fig. 1. Flow sheet of management of severe head injury.

We prefer these agents over drugs that cause motor paralysis because satisfactory neurological examinations of the patient's motor status, oculocephalic reflexes, and response to noxious stimuli can still be obtained. PaO_2 is maintained above 70 mm Hg and $PaCO_2$ in a range of 25–30 mm Hg. Ventilatory control is continued until the patient becomes awake and alert enough to follow more than one-stage commands or until he is stable with a normal ICP for several days. The total time period rarely exceeds 1 week. In addition to ventilatory control, ICP is measured continuously, temperature maintained at normothermia, and electrolytes kept in a normal range (Fig. 3).

RESULTS

The intracranial pressure on admission in 100 consecutive patients treated with this protocol is shown in Table 1. All but 18 patients had elevated ICP in the emergency room. Patients with acute subdural and epidural hematomas usually had very high ICPs, varying from 30 to over 50 mm Hg.

Despite the very high ICP levels on admission, with rapid removal of intracranial masses, use of controlled ventilation, and management by the protocol, ICP usually returns to a normal or only slightly elevated level (less than 15

Volume Respirator

Rate 12 per minute

Tidal Volume 700-1000 cc.

    (15 cc/kg body weight)

Chlorpromazine IM $PaO_2 > 70$ mm Hg

    (25 mgm q6h)

Morphine IV $PaCO_2$ 25-30 mm Hg

    (1-3 mgm PRN)

Fig. 2. Controlled ventilation.

1. Intracranial Pressure

2. Cerebral Perfusion Pressure

3. PaO_2

4. $PaCO_2$

5. Temperature

6. Hematocrit

7. Electrolytes and glucose

Fig. 3. Parameters monitored in severe brain injury.

Table 1
Severe Mechanical Brain Injury

	ICP (mm Hg) at Admission				
	0–10	11–29	30–50	>50	Total
Acute subdural hematoma		2	6	9	17
Acute epidural hematoma			5	1	6
Acute major intracerebral mass		10		3	13
Diffuse cerebral injury	18	35	9	2	64
Total					100

mm Hg). Progressively elevating ICP associated with neurological deterioration leading to death appears to have been reduced.

The overall mortality rate in these 100 patients was 27 percent (Table 2). However, death from progressively elevating ICP leading to inadequate perfusion pressures accounted for only 12 percent of the total deaths. The remaining deaths occurred from systemic medical complications usually resulting from withdrawal of intensive medical therapy weeks after the injury when it was apparent that useful recovery was impossible.

DISCUSSION

Firm conclusions based on statistical analysis regarding the efficacy of controlled ventilation cannot be made. This is so because a control group is not available, and each patient cannot serve as his own control. Our observations suggest, however, that early institution of controlled ventilation helps reduce ICP from pressure levels recorded on hospital admission (Fig. 4). Perhaps the most important contribution of this tool is the reduction in incidence of secondary hypoxic brain damage occurring from unexpected apnea, respiratory obstruction, or respiratory insufficiency. It also appears to reduce the incidence of progressive pulmonary insufficiency. Whereas

Table 2
Severe Mechanical Brain Injury

	Cause of death & Mortality Rate		
	Death Preceded by ICP & C.P.P.	Death from Systemic Medical Complication	Total— Dead (Mortality Rate)
Acute subdural hematoma N = 17	4	5	9 (53%)
Acute epidural hematoma N = 6	1	0	1 (17%)
Acute major intracerebral mass N = 13	1	2	3 (23%)
Diffuse cerebral injury N = 64	6	8	14 (22%)
Total N = 100	12	15	27 (27%)

1. Reduces ICP from admission ICP level.

2. Reduces incidence of secondary hypoxic brain insults.

3. Reduces incidence of progressive pulmonary insufficiency.

4. Probably reduces mortality rate.

5. Possibly reduces morbidity.

Fig. 4. Results of controlled ventilation in severe brain injury.

we had previously observed the respiratory distress syndrome, none of the 100 consecutive patients in this series developed this complication.

As a result of these three factors, controlled ventilation probably contributes to a lowered mortality rate. Similarly, if secondary hypoxic brain insults are obviated, and the incidence of progressively elevating ICP is reduced, morbidity may be expected to decrease.

REFERENCES

1. Gordon E: Controlled respiration in the management of patients with traumatic brain injuries. Acta Anaesth Scand 15:193–208, 1971

2. Rossanda M, Bozza-Marrubini M, Beduschi A: Clinical results of respirator treatment in the unconscious patients with brain lesions, in Brock M, Frieschi C, Ingvar DH, Lassen NA, Shürmann K (eds): Cerebral Blood Flow. Berlin-New York, Springer-Verlag, 1969

Robert G. Loudon, M.B., Ch.B., F.R.C.P.E.
Martin W. Brueggemann, M.D.
Robert L. McLaurin, M.D.

22

Respiratory Patterns and Compliance Changes after Experimental Head Injury

The importance of respiratory complications following head injury is well established. The mechanism of their production is less clear. Clinical and experimental observations by several investigators present at this conference suggest that the damaged brain may directly influence the lungs, damaging them in their turn. Beckman and Bean have shown changes in the static compliance of lungs removed from animals receiving immediately lethal head trauma; these changes were not seen in animals pretreated with dibenzyline.

We have recently been studying respiratory changes in monkeys subjected to head injury in an effort to develop an experimental approach which would more closely simulate the type of situation encountered clinically and use the type of measurement which could be applied clinically. Young adult rhesus monkeys were premedicated with phencyclidine and intubated with a cuffed oral endotracheal tube. An esophageal balloon, venous and arterial lines, and a spinal needle were inserted. The positions of the orotracheal tube and the esophageal balloon were checked by x-ray. The animal was then positioned prone (Fig. 1) and connected to a recorder so that continuous measurements could be made of air flow at the mouth (by pneumotachygraph); intrathoracic pressure (by esophageal balloon); venous, arterial, and CSF pressures; electrocardiogram; and expired carbon dioxide concentration. Intermittent arterial blood gas measurements were made. Additional phencyclidine was added as required to maintain the animals in a quiet state. After a 2-

hour control period of observation, the monkey was subjected to a blow on the head, using a Remington Humane Stunner. Measurements were continued as before for 2 further hours, or until the death of the animal if this occurred earlier. Eighteen monkeys were studied in this way. Two animals died immediately after trauma, and 2 died during the 2-hour period of observation. Tape recording of the physiological measurements allowed more detailed subsequent analysis than would otherwise have been possible.

Minute ventilation was measured and mean values were calculated for each animal at 30-minute intervals. There was no consistent change in minute ventilation after head trauma, as shown in Fig. 2 for a representative selection of animals.

Pulmonary dynamic compliance was measured at 30-minute intervals, plotting volume change against pressure change on an X-Y plotter for a series of 10 to 20 successive breaths (Fig. 3), and measuring the angle of the loop. Figure 4 shows the mean dynamic compliance for the 14 monkeys which survived for 2 hours after trauma, together with the standard error of the mean for each set of measurements. There was no consistent difference in dynamic compliance after trauma in these animals. Pulmonary dynamic compliance is affectd by volume history of the lungs. Sighs were noted to occur before and after trauma, and Table 1 shows compliance values measured for five breaths preceding and five breaths after a sigh. The variability of this measurement should be noted, and the fact that the dynamic compliance for these monkeys was in the range of 20–30 ml/cm of water pressure. Measurements made just before death and after

This work was supported by NIH Grant NS07253 and NIH Grant HD05221.

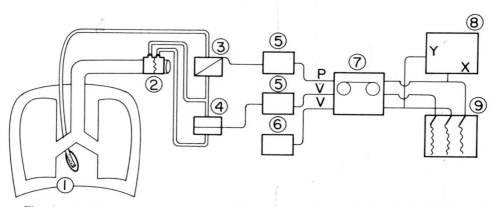

Fig. 1. Apparatus used to measure pulmonary compliance. 1. Esophageal balloon. 2. Pneumotachygraph. 3. Transducer measuring transpulmonary pressure. 4. Transducer measuring air flow. 5. Preamplifiers for pressure and flow. 6. Respirator integrator for measuring volume. 7. F.M. tape recorder. 8. X-Y recorder. 9. Strip-chart recorder.

Table 1
Cdyn Before and After Sighs
(1/cm H₂O)

	Before Trauma		After Trauma	
	Before Sighs	After Sighs	Before Sighs	After Sighs
	0.0103	0.0200	0.0238	0.0284
	0.0305	0.0272	0.0305	0.0219
	0.0122	0.0174	0.0197	0.0164
	0.0162	0.0291	0.0228	0.0289
	0.0146	0.0147	0.0343	0.0502
	0.0511	0.0362	0.0273	0.0301
Mean	0.0225	0.0241	0.0264	0.0293

Table 2
Cdyn Before and After Death
(1/cm H₂O)

	Before Death	After Death
Monkey 6		0.0079
Monkey 7	0.0048	0.0031
Monkey 10	0.0095	0.0095
Monkey 13		0.0036
Mean	0.0072	0.0060

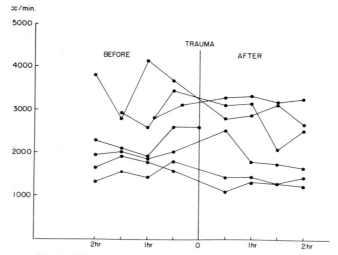

Fig. 2. Minute ventilation before and after head trauma.

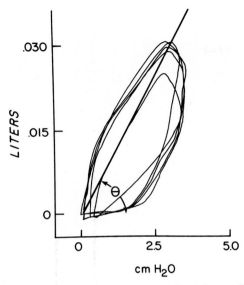

Fig. 3. Loop used to measure pulmonary dynamic compliance.

cessation of spontaneous breathing, while the heart was still beating, show marked reduction in compliance (Table 2). The measurements after death were made by using an Ambu bag to imitate the flow rates and volumes of that animal prior to death. They were all made before the animal's heart rate began to slow or become irregular.

In the four monkeys that died, respirations became irregular for 10 or 15 minutes prior to cessation of spontaneous respiration. The animals were all breathing spontaneously throughout the study, breathing room air. Figure 5 shows the air flow and minute ventilation in 1 animal that died 108 minutes after trauma. It was during this period of about 15 minutes that sizable compliance changes were first noted in the animals that died.

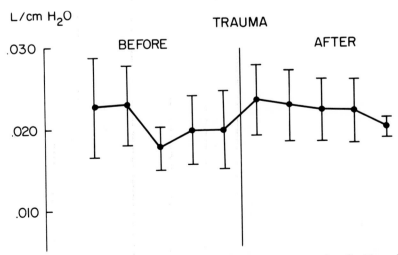

Fig. 4. Pulmonary dynamic compliance before and after trauma: mean values for 14 monkeys which survived for two hours after trauma.

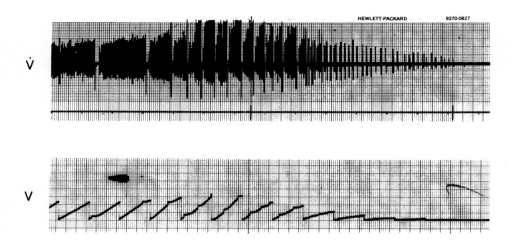

Fig. 5.   Respiratory pattern at time of death in monkey which died 108 minutes after trauma. Upper trace: air flow. Lower trace: minute ventilation.

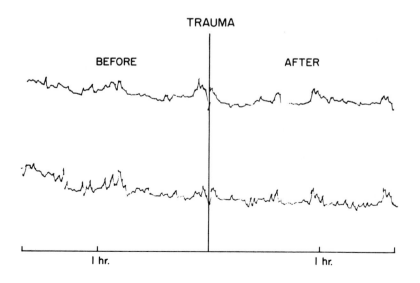

Fig. 6.   Minute ventilation (upper trace) and work of breathing (lower trace): same monkey as Fig. 5.

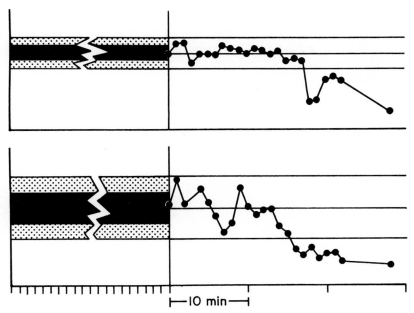

Fig. 7. Volume of air moved per unit work of breathing: upper trace—tidal volume/tidal work, mean for each minute; lower trace—minute volume/minute work. Bands to left of figure show range of values prior to last 30 minutes. Same monkey as Fig. 5.

Minute ventilation and work of breathing minute by minute are shown in Fig. 6 for this same monkey whose last gasps are shown in Fig. 5. Ventilation and work of breathing did not change to any extent during the 2 hours before and after trauma. But changes occurred in the work of breathing, as in the compliance, in the 10 minutes preceding its death. In Fig. 7, the upper trace shows the tidal volume/tidal work ratio minute by minute as it falls below the previous range during the last few minutes. The last point to the right represents the postmortem ratio obtained during Ambu bag breathing. The lower trace shows a similar ratio, minute ventilation divided by minute work of breathing.

These ratios would be expected to give quite a sensitive indication of deterioration in the mechanical characteristics of the lung. In this experimental situation, it appears that these changes in pulmonary mechanics occurred only very shortly before death of the animal.

Edited by Javad Hekmatpanah, M.D.
and John Mullan, M.D.

Open Discussion

DR. PLUM: I have a sense that perhaps the neurosurgical fraternity is suffering from looking at people who get desperately ill very, very quickly, and my reasons for saying that are that if I go onto the general medical floors and look at the people who are sick, I can find what was talked about this morning on any medical floor in the hospital, whether or not the patient has an injury to the brain.

Dr. Moss, I think, brought out a number of pieces of extremely interesting information to suggest that perhaps hypoxia is responsible through a neurogenic mechanism for inducing some of these changes in the brain. But it must be said that a great many children with congenital heart disease tolerate very low PO₂s for long periods of time without any pulmonary complication. I have had a disquieting number of friends with whom I have gone mountain climbing in the Pacific Northwest, in a rather modest way, and have done a number of laboratory experiments with PO₂s of less than 55 or 50, without any of us having developed pulmonary changes. That was unfortunately what we were looking for, so we never could write the paper.

I believe Dr. Brackett's and Dr. Hoff's and Dr. Ducker's emphasis that pulmonary edema really is rare with head injury is a correct statement. I think [Dr. Hoff] correctly identified the only neurogenic basis I know for direct pulmonary changes secondary to central nervous system disease, and that is via the beta adrenergic pathway which is invoked as part of the Cushing response with essentially dumping of volume into the lung so that one gets fluid in the interstitial compartment, where two things may happen. One is that intrapulmonary stretch receptors are stimulated, producing tachypnea, which has its own limiting influence including the push of expiration, and the other is that that fluid then begins to diffuse out because resistances in those tissues are very, very low.

Cecil Drinker, as you may remember, was able to identify fluid within the pulmonary capillary at a PO₂—he wasn't doing PO₂s in those days; it was before the days of PO₂s—but an oxygen saturation of 85 percent. Lymphatic flow from the lung increased to a substantial degree,

and by the time it was down to 80 percent, it had very materially increased to the lung, and one could get heavy lungs without any evidence of central nervous system disease. Those of us who were so heavily involved with the poliomyelitis problem, where one did have autonomic disease because of central infiltration of the virus, were very much concerned with this.

So, at the moment, one of the things which has really struck me—and I thought Dr. Ducker made one of the really most important observations about pulmonary damage in severe illness, in those extraordinary observations made on the battlefield in Korea a decade ago, in which he illustrated that proportional to the degree of injury, and in many instances including injury, patients progressively developed pulmonary insufficiency, suggesting that something went along with the very severe ill state, and possibly the traumatized state, which led to injury of the lung.

This is readily demonstrated, of course, in fracture, where it is often attributed to fat embolization even when one can't find the fat emboli, and one does wonder whether a great deal of what has been talked about here isn't secondary to problems which are intravascular in their origin. I would hope that perhaps we will come back to it in terms of microcirculatory issues in neurological injury, because I think they probably account for some of the cerebral dysfunction that all of us are used to seeing in patients with severe illness.

So, it isn't with any sense of deprecation but a sense of having been terribly disappointed in my own experimental work of not being able to be specifically able to relate the changes in the lung and in pulmonary ventilation to central problems, that I make these comments. . . .

It is awfully difficult to contradict Dr. Loudon, who just plain does not observe changes in compliance. Compliance is a very sensitive instrument for assessing modifications in the mechanical structure of the chest lung tissue, and his observation that these changes come about only in the presence of terminal conditions strikes me as a matter of the greatest importance. That they don't come about in the lung which has been separated from its parent structures and then put back in, I find to be a matter of the greatest interest. I wouldn't be able to note, though, just to conclude that that was because the nerve supply had been interrupted in that particular tissue.

Maybe I can just very briefly comment about pulmonary reflexes and lung reflexes. You will remember that pulmonary ventilation essentially serves two functions, one of which is behavioral and the other of which is metabolic, and these have to be sort of linked together. By and large, structures which lie rostral to the middle third of the pons regulate the behavioral aspects of breathing, sighing, sobbing, laughing, speaking, the modulations which essentially have made sapien primates communicate effectively with each other, while structures which lie caudal to the middle third of the pons and the reticular formation of the dorsomedial pons and the medulla down to the cervical-medullary junction regulate what can be considered the metabolic functions of breathing, namely, the control of the hydrogen ion concentration of the body and the supplying of the oxidants.

So, essentially one has a ponto-medullary reticulum sensitive somewhere in there to a hydrogen ion receptor, the main one of which lies either subarachnoid or interstitial in the brain stem, and the secondary one of which lies in the chemoreceptor of the carotid body. It is possible that even the oxygen sensitivity of the carotid body is a hydrogen ion receptor because of a very high threshold for the conversion to lactic acid, but that is not so sure and I wouldn't want to advertise it.

That system in a very curious way depends upon reflex afferents, and it does so in a way that I far from fully understand, so please accept that all I can give you is my own current terms as a very limited amount of knowledge which doesn't explain an awful lot that has come up here.

Pulmonary reflexes, of course, are of two kinds. There is the one major stretch receptor reflex which travels over the afferent fibers with the vagus nerve and enters the central structures and is called the Hering-Breuer inhibitory reflex; it is generated by full expansion of the lung. The early phase of the Hering-Breuer reflex is facilitatory and, in fact, stimulates tachypnea, so if there is any cutoff before full depth is reached, respiration is accelerated. A full, deep inspiration inhibits not only the breath that is being taken but also in some way changes the central generator so as to slow the overall rhythm of respiration, and this is readily observed by the fact that a deep breath inhibits not only that particular inspiration but also

the next period of expiration, which can't be explained as a simple inhibitory feedback cycle.

Within the tracheal wall are receptors which lead to the expiratory complex of the brain stem, and in all probability the push that Dr. Brackett observes is almost certainly secondary to stimulation of surface receptors in the tracheo-bronchial tree which so characteristically leads to the "hu-hu-hu" which can easily be induced by a variety of manipulations in experimental animals.

Chest wall receptors probably combine with pulmonary irritant receptors to account for the tachypnea that we so predictably see in either surgical or medical patients with severe disease, and Widdicomb localizes these within the subendothelial area. I am not sure whether their structural studies have gone further to give a precise anatomic description, although these are diffusely sensitive to ammonia, to surface irritation in the depths of the lungs, or to distension as occurs by infection or edema fluid. There are certainly also interstitial stretch receptors which are turned on as soon as that alveolar septal wall widens, which also is an accelerator of respiratory rate and which contributes to this well-identified tachypnea.

The final stimulus comes from a chest wall receptor which is in series with the intercostal muscle, and therefore, of course, contraction of the intercostal muscle against increased resistance contributes to acceleration of pulmonary ventilation.

I grant you that it is a small wonder that any of us ever manage to sort this out and have an oscillation of breathing. It should be remembered that what we once thought might be central neurogenic hyperventilation is an extremely rare matter.

Within the past 10 years, we have been able to find one well-documented example of primary central hyperventilation. This was in a child with a glioma of the pons. The respiratory rate during sleep at night in good health was 56. The PCO_2 never climbed above 12–14 mm Hg. The arterial PO_2 never fell on room air (during ambient activities) below 110 mm Hg. This condition went on for 5 weeks before the child finally began to deteriorate with the spread of the tumor. That has been the only patient I have ever been able to document in a satisfactory way of the disease that Gus Swanson and I erroneously diagnosed in 1954.

DR. KURZE: It might be of interest to give a brief report from the battlefields of Los Angeles, which I think has been going on consistently. On the map, it is more difficult to understand.

We have been interested in the potential therapeutic benefit of positive and expiratory pressures to elevate or what we think improve the blood gases in head-injured patients. We have recently studied 20 patients with a variety of intracranial pathology, traumatic, severe, coma scores of 8 or less in each instance. In each case, we measured (using Douglas Miller's Elastex evaluation) a 1 cc injection of lactated Ringer's into the ventricles, and we observed that if we had 2 torr rise following this, there was consistently a 50 percent to a 1500 percent rise in intracranial pressure when we used a 10 cm increase in end expiratory pressure. When we did not have a 2 torr rise, we found that we had no such effect. This has been consistent in each instance.

So, we therefore think that it probably is safe to use end expiratory pressures to increase or improve circulatory blood gases in the presence of pulmonary pathology associated with head injury. Whether it be primary or secondary is a chicken-and-egg sort of problem which we don't have any idea about solving. This point I think should be made.

The other point that was made by someone earlier we subscribe to, that this compliance must be measured on a continuum. You cannot assume that because it is this way at 1 hour, it is going to be that way 2 or 3 hours later.

DR. HARVEY SHAPIRO: I would like to suggest to Dr. Kurze and the rest of you that this PEEP panacea has a Pandora's box aspect. As he mentioned, what we are concerned about here is the fact that we are increasing the airway pressure which then will be variably transmitted, depending on the degree of lung pathology, to the central venous system.

In our neurosurgical patients, we are frequently employing diuretics and we are in a situation where we have a constricted, almost totally eradicated blood volume. In addition to that, we can have a drop in cardiac output which may be reflected in a change in the blood pressure. This is something we really hadn't thought too much about.

Like Dr. Kurze and his group, we have been very concerned that the transmission of the central venous pressure would increase the intracranial pressure. There is, however, a theoretical problem here, and that is that we are only talking about a 15 cm water application of pressure to this system. Therefore, if you sit the patient erect, 15 cm of water above heart level, you should to some extent attenuate these responses. We in fact did this in a series of animals. After witnessing variable results in the ICU, where we saw the same kind of rise Dr. Kurze talked about, in other instances we saw no increase in intracranial pressure but neurological degeneration when therapy was applied.

This is a series of cats with intracranial pressure balloons and no lung pathology other than that which might be introduced by our protocol of increasing intracranial pressure (Fig. 1). What you see here is the usual kind of clinical response. We have the normal or grouped responses running through here, the mean and standard error; we have plotted the intracranial pressure, and this is time after application of PEEP. Here is the positive end expiratory pressure pattern going from 5 to 10 to 15 to 10 and then to 0. Note what occurs here. The general trend is a great drop in the cerebral perfusion pressure. This occurs because of the blood pressure problem I alluded to earlier. This may be accompanied by a gain in intracellular pressure which is much greater than the gain added to the entire system in terms of simple hydraulics. In addition we noticed, even in animals that did not exhibit that marked increase in intracranial pressure, fairly frequent deterioration of the EEG trace.

There is another hazard, and it occurs at this point. This is where the PEEP is removed and we then get a retransfusion of blood to the central core, with an augmented cardiac output and an elevation in blood pressure. This is subsequently followed by a brain which may have been made to some extent hypoxic during this period, but a marked increase in pressure in some animals. This trend even shows across here in these other what we would call normal responding animals, and in fact a number of animals herniated during this particular procedure, which would be very commonly employed in ICUs where patients are taken from PEEP to ambient atmosphere in an effort to suction the endotracheal tree.

The problem is quite complex. What I think is very, very important to consider is the manner in which lung compliance interacts with the transmission of these pressures. Obviously, people improve with arterial oxygenation, and therefore it should not be withheld, but what has to be watched exceedingly carefully is the match be-

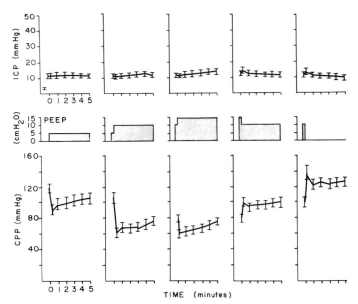

Fig. 1. Mean (± S.E.M.) changes in intracranial pressure (ICP) and cerebral perfusion pressure (CCP) during the progressive application and removal of PEEP in animals with normal lungs. The pattern of the PEEP appliation is indicated in the middle panel. The control ICP (± S.E.M.) obtained prior to inflation of an intracranial expansion balloon is indicated before zero time in the first panel.

tween the lung compliance; perhaps we should also look at the intracranial pressure compliance curve at this time so that where in the initial instance we have a situation where as the patient gets better and his lungs get better, we will be faced with this particular problem because of the transmission of pressure through to the peripheral cardiovascular system.

All of these systems now, I think, have to be very carefully considered when we apply very potent therapy, regardless of the etiology of the pulmonary picture we have seen so ably demonstrated today.

DR. BRACKETT: We follow Dr. Moss's work with great interest because of the important suggestion that these changes might be prevented by Dilantin, and we have attempted to reproduce his experiments and have encountered some difficulties.

First, in experimental animals on normal ventilation in the laboratory, we found over the years that it is very difficult to prevent these animals from shunting, and it requires a good deal of attention to their controlled ventilation to prevent shunting. So, it is of great interest to us that Dr. Moss's control animals did not develop any pulmonary difficulties.

The second difficulty we have had is that this is a patchy change in the lung and it is difficult to grade—at least we have had difficulty in grading the lung because some areas of the lung appear to be perfectly normal, biopsied from certain areas, and others may show the atelectatic changes. We have done about 27 dogs now, and as usual some had to be discarded initially for experimental errors. I simply want to report on 16 dogs, 2 controls and 14 hypoxemic dogs.

The initial dogs were done with a membrane oxygenator simply to try to control temperature a little bit better and to be able to control the PO_2 and CO_2 of the perfusate without having to vary those parameters in the ventilated gas. First, these animals were under very light anesthesia and were hyperdynamic a bit, so their cardiac output is a bit high to start with. The result of the hypoxemic perfusion and the control perfusion would drop the cardiac output modestly.

Second, there is an increase in pulmonary artery pressure in the hypoxemically perfused dogs.

There is a modest increase in wedge pressure. This is only modest, and it tends to sort of reconstitute itself toward the end of the 2-hour observation period. We have not made measure-

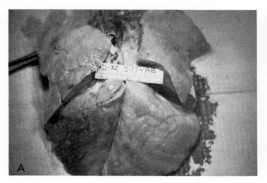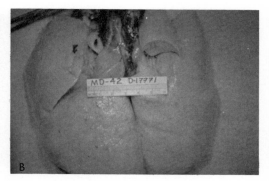

Fig. 2.   Supine (*a*) and prone (*b*) views of hypoxia perfusion animal.

ments of left atrial pressure because we didn't want to open the chest, but I did want to ask Dr. Moss whether or not he has measured left atrial pressures and, if not, what his data are to indicate that these animals in fact have pulmonary venular constriction.

There was no significant change in FRC either in the control or hypoxemic perfusates. If anything, it increased slightly.

Because the dogs hyperventilated, there was an increase in PaO_2. None of the animals developed a systemic hypoxemia.

It has been our experience in noncontrolled ventilation animals that they start with a somewhat increased shunt, venous admixture, but instead of increasing the shunt, if anything, decreased probably as a result of their hyperventilation of hyperpnea.

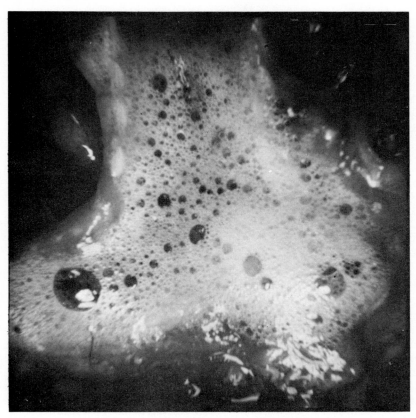

Fig. 3.   Pulmonary edema resulting from experimental head injury.

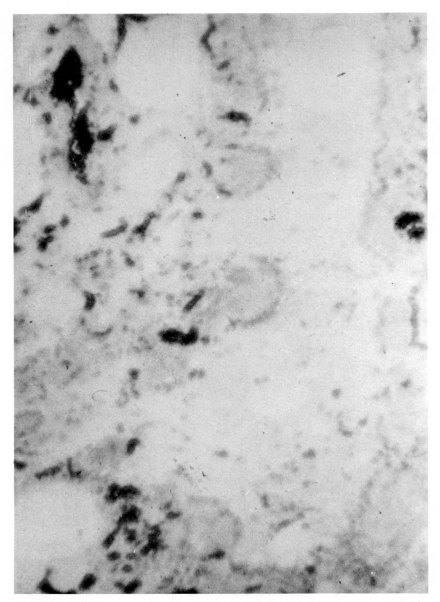

Fig. 4. Microscopic appearance of experimentally produced pulmonary edema resulting from head injury. The small bronchioles are filled with fluid without inflammatory response.

One animal out of the 16 showed significant changes in the lung.

But the usual picture—and this is the most severe of the animals—the lungs appeared like this (Figs. 2 and 3). This shows only moderate changes in this area (Fig. 4). We did find that if we biopsied from different areas the results might be quite different.

DR. DUCKER: Just very quickly, we have been trying to do what Dr. Moss mentioned, and we have been using rhesus monkeys because, as he rightly points out, they are a bit closer to us. We have been communicating fairly often with Dr. Brackett on the telephone, and the one thing that comes out (first of all, it must be the way we are doing it) is that it is different for different animals.

We have different blood pressures, different respiratory things in the monkeys, and we would like Dr. Moss to comment on that.

We have managed to produce a lung that looks like this with gross pulmonary edema. We have others that don't look as good as this. What we have done is the Moss preparation. We have taken atrial blood, used the coronary perfusion pump with filter, and perfused the common carotid in a rhesus monkey, as Dr. Moss has described. What we have been measuring is cerebral flow, intracranial pressure, systemic arterial pressure, perfusion pressure, A/V oxygen difference, tidal volume, rate, and rhythm. So, we were trying to see if there was a change in oxygen uptake and systemic parameters with this preparation. We have managed, as I said, to produce pulmonary edema in one animal, gross, like this.

On histology this is what it looks like. If we control the ventilation in these animals—these are spontaneously respiring—if we control the ventilation there is very little of this, and little or no congestion, but the thing that worried us was that measuring the oxygen uptake, and measuring the systemic oxygen, there was no difference between the control group and the spontaneously respiring group. Measuring the oxygen uptake continuously, we only find a falloff in the last 3 or 4 minutes, and I think to our mind this goes with Dr. Loudon's experiments, that what we are finding is that this is a terminal agonal thing and may have very, very little relevance to the clinical subacute thing that Dr. Becker was talking about.

DR. MOSS: First, as far as having work reproduced, probably the most frustrating thing is not to have it reproduced. The one group that has now reported line-to-line reproductions is actually an anesthesiology research group in Galveston. They sent a team up to Rensselaer Polytechnical Institute and spent a few days, and I spoke to Dr. Joseph Walker there. This will be the University of Texas in Galveston. They claim that they have a large number of dogs, every one of which has the lung lesions induced by cerebral hypoxemic perfusion. This was the only mechanism that gave them consistent results. They had tried all kinds of different things.

It is a frustrating procedure, trying to produce this in animals or in people. Dr. Plum was talking about going up mountains and hitting 55 mm Hg. With our dogs, if we were dealing with a common garden variety, not very healthy, worm-laden animals, 30 to 40 mm Hg was about what we found was adequate, but PO_2 alone is not enough to determine what oxygen delivery is. We found that with our healthier animals, with our beagles, which had hematocrits ranging from 42 to 55, we could not produce the lung lesions with hemorrhagic shock nor with perfusion using their venous blood. We found we had to drop their hemoglobin when we perfused them, and then we did the experiment which I think reconciles results from different laboratories in shocked lung work with dogs.

One school of thought said, follow this routine cookbook procedure: hemorrhage to 44 mm Hg, in lightly anesthetized heparinized dogs 2 hours, give him the lung back, and he has lesions always. The other group says, we never get it; there is no such entity.

Those who say there is no such thing are too rich, because in this day of tight money they have healthier dogs, purebred beagles, or well-conditioned mongrels. We took our beagles a week before and subjected them to hemorrhage and immediate volume rate expansion so that a week later their blood proteins, their blood volume, was normal. They couldn't restore their red cell mass. Hematocrits were ranging in the low 30s. These healthy young animals we then subjected to 40 mm Hg mean arterial, arterial hemorrhage under light barbiturate anesthesia with heparin for 2 hours, uniformly developed lung lesions.

We are in the same state. We are 125 miles apart, and I respect Watts' work, but we actually have no connection. I have been following his work closely, and he followed me on the program to comment on that presentation, saying he had reviewed his experience with hemorrhagic shock in dogs where they ranged in hematocrits from 5 to 50 with an exact parallel of this experiment, that those with the highest levels—they scrapped the experiment because they got nowhere and were frustrated. But as the animal was more anemic then, the lung lesions were produced with greater regularity and intensity, to the point where at the lowest level of hemoglobin the animals couldn't even continue the experiment because they expired with the lousy picture of lungs.

To answer the question about monitoring left ventricular dynamics, yes, we had half a dozen animals with preplaced left atrial catheters. There was no fluctuation for practical purposes in left atrial or pulmonary venous pressure. A maximum of 2 mm. This was in a random fashion.

Another half dozen animals I didn't mention had bilateral glomectomy. Carotid bodies were removed and this seemed to have no effect on the pattern.

Dr. Plum made the point that reimplanting a lung does more than simply denervate it, and that is true. However, we only worked with one lung. If you denervate both lungs, you are going to have a profound effect because of the loss of the efferents, the respiratory pattern changes; you get deeper, slower breathing; you are relying more on the chest receptors he referred to than the receptors within the lung.

This animal has an intact right lung, so his respiratory pattern as far as we can tell is indistinguishable from the normal control animal. His respiratory pattern is determined by his normally innervated right lung.

Also, in the use of Dilantin, these were animals not on respirators that were subjected to hemorrhagic shock rather than brain perfusion. We haven't continued our studies, priorities, and limitations, so we didn't try to find a protective effect of dephenylhydantoin with cerebral hypoxemia with perfusion. These were lightly anesthetized rats, lightly anesthetized dogs that were subjected to the standard regimen, the standard for the dog now being an anemic dog, and under those conditions we had the protection.

Again, to the question of what reimplantation of a lung does, if we wait between 1 and 2 months we know from other people's work there is regeneration of lymphatics. However, nobody has demonstrated any restoration of neural control in either direction. The Boston group has shown that you can get local responses in lung when you have your tracheal divider, your Carlins Y type tube when you denervate one lung, and when you respire that lung with nitrogen you get inhibition of blood flow through the lung as local response. This is lost, and you will not get it within 2 months.

I am not sure how the lung comes back into the control circuit. Eventually it seems to, whether it be a direct innervation or whether it becomes a heightened sensitivity to circulating catecholamines or something else, such as Cannon showed with the nicotinic membrane; I don't know.

Working now closer to 1 month than 2 months, minimizing mechanical and metabolic trauma to the lung (and this is just trickery), doing 100 or more animals a year every day, and the technicians doing it and doing it well, we are able to have essentially as close as we can get to a normal lung which is denervated, and it has had its lymphatics regenerated. I am not sure with the bronchial arterial supply, but that may also have been regenerated. We are working with animals with a lung that seems no longer to have the mechanical trauma in evidence a month later. The chest is closed, the animal is not respired.

I want to emphasize, too, that the respiratory distress syndrome, whatever the cause, has a wide spectrum, and I will agree that it is rare, thank heaven, that the bubbling pink frothy pulmonary edema is not common. However, again I want to emphasize that 85 percent of the GIs dying in Vietnam of their head injuries had a full-blown respiratory picture. So, it is not rare in its less severe form.

We are talking about drawing out the lungs, (this was alluded to) and fluid restriction, and its consequences were alluded to. Actually, there is a series of pressures, if we accept Starling and his concept. Oncotic pressure enters into the picture. Max Harry Wild runs the ICU at Los Angeles County Hospital, and he measures colloid osmotic pressure of plasma, and he also measures something that reflects pulmonary capillary pressure, the pulmonary artery wedge pressure, and he has reported on several occasions now that if the measured colloid pressure exceeds the measured wedge pressure (call it pulmonary capillary pressure) by 9 mm Hg or more, he never sees pulmonary edema. If it is 3 or 4 mm Hg or less, that is, the measured colloid pressure and subtracted from that something that reflects the capillary pressure, if that is 3 or 4 mm Hg or less, he universally sees pulmonary edema, and he uses this as a way of titrating his patients, not with water restriction but with restoration of the lost colloid, human albumin. He states 3 or 4 mm Hg differential or less, and it is universal pulmonary edema; 9 mm Hg or greater, and it never is. He also correlates survival and pulmonary function that way.

A universal finding in this situation is pulmonary congestion; the smallest cells are engorged with blood. A universal finding is increased pulmonary vascular resistance without knowing where. To me it is just logical. I haven't measured the sites of where the resistance occurs or rises, but it seems to me if you have precapillary resistance, you have a bloodless field. If you have postcapillary resistance, you have a tourniquet effect, an engorgement. So, it is logical to me that it would be postcapillary, as Watts Webb has reported and measured. I haven't made those measurements.

John D. Michenfelder, M.D.
Thoralf M. Sundt, Jr., M.D.

23

Anesthesia, Cerebral Metabolism, and Cerebral Ischemia

Since it was first recognized that anesthetics possess the potential to depress cerebral oxygen requirements, it has been postulated by many that anesthetics should provide a degree of cerebral protection in the event of oxygen deprivation. The variable effect of different anesthetics (and different anesthetic concentrations) on cerebral metabolic requirements for oxygen (CMR_{O_2}) is apparent in examining Table 1. These data were collected in a series of canine studies and, where comparison is possible, they are both qualitatively and quantitatively similar to that reported in humans. That a relatively large dose of thiopental reduces CMR_{O_2} to the same level as that occurring during moderate hypothermia (30°C) suggests that these two circumstances should result in similar degrees of cerebral protection. Such a protective effect for hypothermia is unquestioned, but data concerning barbiturate protection are less convincing.

If in terms of protection these circumstances are not similar, one possible explanation might be a different effect on the limited energy stores of the brain. However, several studies[1,2] have clearly demonstrated that energy stores are unaffected by anesthesia per se and are the same as that found in hypothermic brain (Table 2); thus, a similar degree of protection might be anticipated.

We examined this question by comparing the rates of cerebral energy depletion and lactate accumulation in dog brain immediately following onset of abrupt anoxia (decapitation) in hypo-

This investigation was supported in part by Research Grants NS-7507 and NS-6663 from the National Institutes of Health, Public Health Service.

thermic animals (30°C) and in normothermic animals anesthetized with different agents.[3] The unexpected result was that normothermic brain regardless of the anesthetic circumstance showed a similar rapid rate of ATP depletion and lactate accumulation, whereas hypothermic brain showed a significant slowing of these rates of a magnitude predicted by the Q_{10} of canine brain. These differences are most striking in comparing hypothermic dogs to dogs deeply anesthetized with thiopental (Figs. 1 and 2). Thus, despite similar CMR_{O_2}S and similar energy stores, the potential for cerebral protection is apparently not similar.

The following explanation is offered. With abrupt anoxia, measurable electrical activity from the brain is abolished within 10 to 20 seconds; this is true both at normothermia and hypothermia. Assuming anesthetic-induced alterations in CMR_{O_2} are entirely secondary to alterations in electrical function of the brain, then with abolition of that function, differences among anesthetics on cerebral energy requirements will disappear and the rate of energy utilization for maintenance of brain cell viability will be identical. By contrast, hypothermia presumably alters CMR_{O_2} by a direct effect of lowered temperature on rates of biochemical reactions. This effect should be operative both in the presence and absence of cerebral electrical activity and thus with anoxia and cessation of electrical activity, the rate of energy utilization will be slowed in accordance with the temperature. Thus, in the circumstance of oxygen deprivation sufficient to abolish electrical work done by the brain, hypothermia does protect but anesthetics do not.

Similarly, it should follow that in the circum-

Table 1

Effect of Anesthetics on
Canine CMR_{O_2}

Anesthetic Circumstance	Change in CMR_{O_2}, %
Halothane, 0.8%	−18
Methoxyflurane, 0.2%	−10
Cyclopropane, 20%	−15
Isoflurane, 1.4%	−20
Enflurane, 2.2%	−30
N_2O, 70%	+10
Fentanyl, 0.006 mg/kg	−18
Morphine, 2.0 mg/kg	−18
Ketamine, 2.0 mg/kg	+10
Thiopental, 15 mg/kg	−40
Hypothermia, 30°C	−45

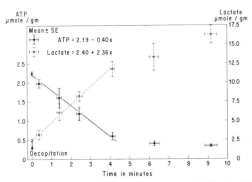

Fig. 2. The effect of a thiopental infusion (43 mg/kg/2 hr) on rates of ATP depletion and lactate accumulation following onset of cerebral anoxia. ATP is rapidly depleted to 25 percent of normal by 4 minutes while lactate accumulates to five times normal.

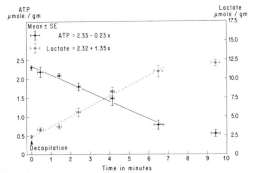

Fig. 1. The effect of hypothermia (30°C) on rates of ATP depletion and lactate accumulation following onset of cerebral anoxia (decapitation). A progressive and apparently linear decrease in ATP occurs in the initial 7 to 8 minutes until ATP is decreased to about 25 percent of normal. Lactate accumulates in a reciprocal fashion to about five times normal at 7 to 8 minutes.

stance of O_2 deprivation insufficient to abolish electrical work done by the brain, an anesthetic-induced reduction in that work should provide a degree of protection. This was demonstrated in a subsequent study wherein profound hypotension was induced (mean pressure = 25 mm Hg) but at a level insufficient to abolish the EEG.[4] In that situation, dogs pretreated with thiopental maintained their cerebral energy stores at a significantly higher level than did dogs not so pretreated (Fig. 3).

A logical extension of this hypothesis should be that anesthetics given in increasing concentrations would progressively inhibit CMR_{O_2} until such time as an isoelectric EEG is produced. Thereafter, further effects of anesthesia on CMR_{O_2} should not be demonstrable. This prediction was confirmed in a study wherein canine systemic circulation and oxygenation were supported by an extracorporeal circuit and progressively larger doses of thiopental were administered while CMR_{O_2} was measured and the EEG was monitored.[5] In these studies, CMR_{O_2}

Table 2

Effect of Anesthetics on Cerebral Energy State (Mean ± SE)

Anesthetic Circumstance	CMR_{O_2} ml/100 g/min	ATP μmol/g	Lactate μmol/g
Halothane, 0.8%; 37°C	4.65 ± 0.16	2.26 ± 0.03	2.20 ± 0.27
N_2O, 70%; 37°C	5.88 ± 0.17	2.23 ± 0.05	2.63 ± 0.19
Thiopental infusion			
46 mg/kg/2 hr; 37°C	2.89 ± 0.19	2.21 ± 0.02	1.78 ± 0.17
Hypothermia; 30°C	2.80 ± 0.16	2.29 ± 0.06	2.35 ± 0.20

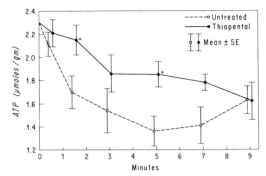

Fig. 3. The effect of thiopental (15 mg/kg) on the cerebral energy state during profound hypotension (25 mm Hg). ATP depletion in dogs pretreated with thiopental was significantly less than that seen in dogs not pretreated.

Table 3

Effect of 9.0% Halothane on Cerebral Energy State (Mean ± SE)

	Control	9.0% Halothane
ATP, μmol/g	2.33 ± 0.09	0.97 ± 0.11
PCr, μmol/g	4.96 ± 0.41	1.33 ± 0.58
Lactate, μmol/g	2.34 ± 0.16	13.31 ± 0.98
L/P	7 ± 1	55 ± 5

progressively decreased until an isoelectric EEG was produced; at that point, the CMR_{O_2} achieved a "basal" level and despite further doses of thiopental, no further CMR_{O_2} depression was observed (Fig. 4). In addition, at the termination of these studies, brain energy stores and lactate levels were normal.

We anticipated that this limitation on the CMR_{O_2} effects of thiopental would be common to all anesthetics. However, when halothane was studied using a similar protocol,[6] no "basal" CMR_{O_2} could be demonstrated and a progressive decrease was observed even after onset of an isoelectric EEG. Additionally, at the termination of these studies, cerebral energy stores were grossly depleted and lactate levels were markedly elevated (Table 3). This occurred despite the fact that cerebral blood flow (CBF) was well maintained, venous oxygen tension leaving the brain

was high, and distribution of CBF was homogeneous. We were forced to conclude that halothane at very high concentrations (2.5 to 9.0 percent) has a direct and potentially toxic effect on cerebral metabolic pathways.

The impact of these metabolic effects of anesthetics on ischemic brain is largely speculative as regards mechanisms. Nonetheless, anesthetic effects have been examined in a variety of animal models of cerebral ischemia in terms of effects on survival, neurologic function, and frequency and size of cerebral infarction. Smith et al.,[7] in a canine model of regional cerebral ischemia, reported that as compared to "awake" animals, barbiturate anesthesia was associated with significantly less frequent and smaller infarctions, whereas halothane anesthesia resulted in a high incidence of large infarctions. These observations are compatible with our metabolic studies which suggest a potential protective effect for barbiturates and a detrimental effect for halothane. However, Smith et al. believe that the differences they observed may be more related to the cerebrovascular effects than to the metabolic effects of these anesthetics. They suggest that in

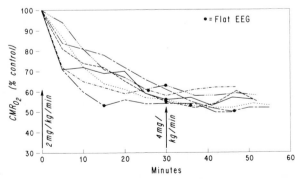

Fig. 4. The effect of massive doses of thiopental on CMR_{O_2}. CMR_{O_2} progressively decreases in each of 7 dogs until the EEG becomes isoelectric. At that point, a "basal" CMR_{O_2} is achieved and despite an increased infusion rate of thiopental, no further decrease in CMR_{O_2} occurs.

Table 4
Effect of Pentobarbital and
Halothane on Cerebral Energy State
2 Hours Following Middle Cerebral
Artery Occlusion (Mean ± SE)

	Pentobarbital, 40 mg/kg	Halothane, 1.0%
ATP, μmol/g	1.20 ± 0.11	0.92 ± 0.06
PCr, μmol/g	1.92 ± 0.37	1.53 ± 0.28
Lactate, μmol/g	9.99 ± 1.47	18.21 ± 1.21
L/P	27 ± 5	44 ± 2

regional ischemia, reduction in flow to normal brain will reduce cerebral blood volume and, hence, intracranial pressure and thereby encourage maintenance of collateral flow to the area of ischemia. An opposite effect is assumed for a cerebral vasodilator. Since barbiturates constrict normal cerebral vessels and halothane is a cerebral vasodilator, such a mechanism could account, at least in part, for their observations. Thus, there are at least two mechanisms whereby barbiturates might be protective and halothane detrimental in regional cerebral ischemia.

The work of Smith et al. might be criticized because the dog is probably not the best model for such studies due to the marked differences from humans in the potential for collateral cerebral blood flow. We therefore examined this question in squirrel monkeys, since the potential for collateral CBF in this animal is apparently similar to that of humans. In previous studies in the squirrel monkey, we have shown that occlusion of a middle cerebral artery (MCA) results ultimately in an area of infarction similar in relative size and distribution to that seen in humans.[8] However, if flow is reestablished after 2 hours of occlusion, approximately 50 percent of the animals do not infarct, whereas after 4 hours of occlusion, infarction is almost 100 percent.[9] This correlated with a series of metabolic studies demonstrating a progressive slow reduction in ATP and accumulation of lactate in the area of ischemia which was potentially reversible up to 4 hours following MCA occlusion.[9] Furthermore, regional CBF in the area of ischemia is reduced to about 40 percent of normal following MCA occlusion and is maintained at that level for at least 2 hours.[10] Finally, electrocorticograms taken from the region of ischemia show a progressive diminution in activity which correlates with the level of energy stores measured in the brain.[9] Thus, using this as a

model of regional cerebral ischemia, there appears to be a significant period of time (2 hours or more) during which therapeutic intervention might alter the usual course of progression to infarction. Furthermore, any favorable or detrimental effects of intervention should be apparent after 2 hours of MCA occlusion.

Accordingly, we compared the effects of 2 hours of MCA occlusion in animals anesthetized with either pentobarbital (40 mg/kg) or halothane (1.0 percent).[11] In acute metabolic studies, we found that depletion of cerebral energy stores and accumulation of lactate in the area of ischemia was significantly less in animals anesthetized with pentobarbital than in animals anesthetized with halothane (Table 4). In chronic studies, we found that mortality, neurological deficit, and frequency and size of infarction were again less in animals anesthetized with pentobarbital during a 2-hour period of MCA occlusion. These studies only demonstrated that there is a difference between pentobarbital and halothane anesthesia as regards their effect on regional cerebral ischemia. This difference might be accounted for by a protective effect of pentobarbital, a detrimental effect of halothane, or a combination of both.

To determine if there is a meaningful protective effect provided by barbiturate anesthesia, we designed a protocol intended to mimic the circumstances of acute stroke followed by a 48-hour period of intensive supportive care comparable to what might be available in a standard medical facility.[12] For these studies, we used the Java monkey since their larger body size (as compared to the squirrel monkey) greatly facilitated the intensive care measures that we instituted. Monitoring included direct arterial pressure, central venous pressure, EKG, EEG, repetitive blood gases, repetitive electrolytes, urinary output, fluid intake (intravenous), temperature (rectal), and minute ventilation. In all, 18 monkeys were studied; in these, the right middle cerebral artery was permanently occluded via a transorbital approach (under light halothane anesthesia). After occluding the MCA, halothane was discontinued and the animals were sedated with diazepam and paralyzed with pancuronium. Ventilation was controlled and adjusted to maintain normal blood gases. In 9 of the monkeys, 30 minutes after the MCA was occluded pentobarbital anesthesia was induced (14 mg/kg) and maintained (7 mg/kg/2 hr) for 48 hours. Except for pentobarbital anesthesia, the 2 groups of 9 monkeys each (control group and pentobarbital group) were maintained

Table 5

Survival, Deficit, and Infarction after 48 Hours of Intensive Care
Following Permanent MCA Occlusion

Control Monkeys				Pentobarbital Monkeys			
No.	Survival	Deficit	% Infarct	No.	Survival	Deficit	% Infarct
1	Yes	0	0	1	Yes	0, −1	3
2	No	−4	24	2	Yes	−2, −3	8
3	Yes	−2, −3	<1	3	Yes	0, −1	2
4	No	−4	100	4	Yes	0	0
5	Yes	0, −1	0	5	Yes	0	0
6	Yes	−2, −3	2	6	Yes	0	0
7	No	−4	4	7	Yes	−1, −2	5
8	Yes	−1, −2	18	8	Yes	0	0
9	Yes	−3	20	9	Yes	0	0

and monitored in an identical fashion for 48 hours. After 48 hours, all drugs were discontinued and following arousal, the animals were returned to their cages, observed for 5 days, and then killed. At necropsy, the brains were removed and stored in formalin for subsequent examination for infarction size and location.

In the control group, 3 animals could not be weaned from the ventilator and died in the immediate postintensive care period; all of these had large cerebral infarctions with massive edema. Of the remaining 6, 4 displayed a significant neurologic deficit with cerebral infarction, 1 had a transient deficit without infarction, and 1 had no deficit and no infarction (Table 5). In the pentobarbital group, all awoke and survived the 5 days of observation. Five had no deficit and no infarction, 2 had a transient deficit and small infarctions, and 2 had significant deficit with infarction. These differences in survival, neurological deficit, and size and frequency of infarction were significant at the 0.06 probability level.

From these series of studies, as well as the work of others, we conclude that barbiturate anesthesia does provide a limited, but real, degree of protection for ischemic brain. On a metabolic basis, we believe protection is limited to a circumstance of O_2 deprivation, which is insufficient to immediately abolish neuronal function (and not to a circumstance of total anoxia with abolition of function such as occurs following cardiac arrest). Apparently in acute stroke and presumably in head injury, there are areas of marginal perfusion wherein neuronal function, although altered, is not immediately abolished. In ischemia of this sort, barbiturates, by reducing the work of the neurons

and hence their energy and oxygen requirements, should be protective for as long as marginal perfusion is maintained and hopefully until adequate collateral circulation can be established. On a hemodynamic basis, barbiturates might be protective in the same circumstances by minimizing intracranial pressure increases and thus preventing progressive diminution in flow to areas of ischemia.

If applied clinically, the proper duration and depth of anesthesia is problematical. Reasonably, the depth of anesthesia should be the maximum consistent with stable systemic hemodynamics. This can probably best be ascertained by EEG monitoring; a logical EEG end point should be that of burst suppression which is indicative of a moderately deep level of anesthesia that is still compatible with adequate cardiac function. The proper duration of such an anesthetic is not established. We selected 48 hours because this is the period of developing edema following MCA occlusion in cats.[13] After 48 hours, edema spontaneously subsides in that species. If this is also true in humans, then 48 hours would seem to be the minimum desirable duration and perhaps 72 to 96 hours would be optimal.

The risk of a prolonged general anesthetic cannot be denied. These risks would be exaggerated in elderly stroke patients wherein multiple systems disease is likely. However, in young and otherwise healthy head trauma patients, these risks should be minimal. Except for the maintenance of a proper anesthetic depth, the care required for these patients should not differ significantly from that already in routine use in most intensive care facilities.

REFERENCES

1. Michenfelder JD, Van Dyke RA, Theye RA: The effects of anesthetic agents and techniques on canine cerebral ATP and lactate levels. Anesthesiology 33:315–321, 1970
2. Nilsson L, Siesjö BK: The effect of anesthetics on the tissue lactate, pyruvate, phosphocreatine, ATP and AMP concentrations, and on intracellular pH in the rat brain. Acta Physiol Scand 80:142–144, 1970
3. Michenfelder JD, Theye RA: The effects of anesthesia and hypothermia on canine cerebral ATP and lactate during anoxia produced by decapitation. Anesthesiology 33:430–439, 1970
4. Michenfelder JD, Theye RA: Cerebral protection by thiopental during hypoxia. Anesthesiology 39:510–517, 1973
5. Michenfelder JD: The interdependency of cerebral functional and metabolic effects following massive doses of thiopental in the dog. Anesthesiology 41:231–236, 1974
6. Michenfelder JD, Theye RA: In vivo toxic effects of halothane on cerebral metabolic pathways (in prep)
7. Smith AL, Hoff JT, Nielsen SL, Larson CP: Barbiturate protection in acute focal cerebral ischemia. Stroke 5:1, 1974
8. Sundt TM Jr, Waltz AG: Experimental cerebral infarction: retro-orbital extradural approach for occluding the middle cerebral artery. Mayo Clin Proc 41:159–168, 1966
9. Sundt TM Jr, Michenfelder JD: Focal transient cerebral ischemia in the squirrel monkey: Effect on brain adenosine triphosphate and lactate levels with electrocorticographic and pathologic correlation. Circ Res 30:703–712, 1972
10. Sundt TM Jr, Waltz AG: Cerebral ischemia and reactive hyperemia: Studies of cortical blood flow and microcirculation before, during, and after temporary occlusion of middle cerebral artery of squirrel monkeys. Circ Res 28:426–433, 1971
11. Michenfelder JD, Milde JH: The influence of anesthetics on the metabolic, functional and pathologic response to regional cerebral ischemia. Stroke (in press)
12. Michenfelder JD, Milde JH, Sundt TM Jr: Cerebral protection by barbiturate anesthesia and intensive care for 48 hours following permanent middle cerebral artery occlusion in Java monkeys (in prep)
13. O'Brien MD, Waltz AG, Jordan MM: Ischemic cerebral edema . . . distribution of water in brains of cats after occlusion of the middle cerebral artery. Arch Neurol 30:456, 1974

H. M. Shapiro, M.D., J. Lafferty, M.D.
M. M. Keykhah, M.D., M. G. Behar, Ph.D.
K. Van Horn, B. S.

24

Barbiturates and Intracranial Hypertension

In 1973 we reported that a short-acting barbiturate, thiopental, could effect rapid reductions in intracranial pressure (ICP) in neurosurgical patients during the induction of anesthesia and following ICP elevations elicited by anesthetic agents with cerebrovasodilating properties.[1] Intracranial tension reductions were greatest when the ICP was high and were frequently accompanied by increases in the cerebral perfusion pressure. The enhancement of perfusion pressure indicated that the intracranial hypotensive action of thiopental was to some extent independent of blood pressure reductions due to the barbiturate. A rationale for these observations was provided by the earlier studies of Pierce and his associates (1962) demonstrating that thiopental anesthesia markedly increased cerebrovascular resistance and decreased cerebral blood flow and metabolism.[2]

Following the intraoperative experience with thiopental, its effects were tested in a number of patients with persistent intracranial hypertension despite aggressive therapy with osmotic agents, steroids, and controlled hyperventilation.[3] Test doses of thiopental given to these patients could reduce the elevated ICP. However, the ICP reducing power was less and the changes in cerebral perfusion pressure accompanying these tests were quite variable. Subsequent doses of barbiturates were administered only to patients who reacted to the thiopental test with ICP reduction accompanied by improved or unchanged brain perfusion pressure gradient. In the extraoperative management of intracranial hypertension, a longer acting barbiturate, pentobarbital, was employed and hypothermia added to the protocol. The choice of the barbiturate-augmented hypothermia in head-injured humans was based on the speculation that the combination therapy might produce an additive or synergistic effect on cerebral circulatory and metabolic indices.

This hypothesis is currently being examined in a series of dogs. In one group (I), after control measurements are made in animals lightly anesthetized with pentobarbital (35 mg/kg given IP 4 hours previously), an additional dose of the barbiturate (35 mg/kg given IV) is administered (in divided doses to avoid reducing the mean blood pressure below 55 torr). This results in an isoelectric electroencephalogram (EEG) as recorded from epidural electrodes at a gain of 50 $\mu v/7.5$ mm. After cerebral circulatory and metabolic measurements are performed in this condition, hypothermia to 29.5°C is induced and the measurements repeated. In the second group (II) of animals, the order of the treatment is reversed.

Total cerebral blood flow was measured by discontinuous sampling of sagittal sinus and arterial blood flow during desaturation of radioactive krypton.[4] Arterial and venous gas tension, pH, and oxygen contents were determined to permit calculation of cerebral metabolic rate for oxygen ($CMRO_2$). Carbon dioxide was added to the inspired gases to maintain a temperature corrected $PaCO_2$ near 34 torr in the paralyzed animals maintained at a constant minute ventilation. Temperature was estimated from rectal and esophageal probes and temperature gradients between these points maintained at less than 0.6°C throughout the experiment.

The preliminary experimental data (3 dogs/experimental group) are summarized in Tables 1 and 2. The blood pressure was not pharma-

Supported in part by USPHS Grants # GMS 15430-07, and 215-16.

Table 1
Blood Gases (Mean ± SEM)

	pHa	PaCO$_2$ (torr)	PaCO$_2$ (torr)	PvO$_2$ (torr)	Ca-v O$_2$ (Vol %)
Control	7.37 ± .02	34.1 ± 2.1	153.8 ± 13.3	34.5 ± 1.5	6.77 ± .70
Group I					
Barbiturate	7.33 ± .01	32.1 ± 1.5	155.3 ± 7.8	39.5 ± 6.5	7.02 ± 1.3
Barbiturate/ hypothermia	7.33 ± .08	30.1 ± 3.1	190.3 ± 11.7	26.0 ± 2.0	9.79 ± 0.3
Group II					
Hypothermia	7.38 ± .01	37.4 ± 2.3	108.3 ± 24.7	24.5 ± 1.3	12.40 ± 1.6
Hypothermia/ barbiturate	7.38 ± .02	36.7 ± 1.6	124.0 ± 6.0	25.2 ± 1.4	9.21 ± 1.1

cologically supported, and mean arterial pressure ranged between 68 and 133 torr during measurement periods. The lower blood pressures were observed after administration of the EEG suppression dose of pentobarbital, and the lowest mean arterial tension was associated with the highest cerebral venous oxygen tension (PssO$_2$ = 39.5) in normothermic dogs. The largest mean arteriovenous oxygen content difference (12.4 vol%) was noted in hypothermic dogs immediately prior to EEG suppression with pentobarbital (Group II).

As shown in Table 2, pentobarbital depressed cerebral blood flow (CBF) by an average of 18 ml/100/g/min at normothermia in Group I. This was accompanied by a fall in blood pressure from a control of 135 torr to 75 torr. When hypothermia was induced in these animals, who had persistent isoelectric EEG recordings, a large increase in cerebrovascular resistance (CVR from 4 to 7.3 torr/ml/100 mg/min) occurred at an arterial pressure of 82 torr. A CVR increase of a similar magnitude was observed in Group II dogs cooled immediately after the control period. EEG activity remained relatively unchanged in these animals at 29.5°C.

When the EEG supression dose of pentobarbital was given to normothermic dogs, already

Table 2
Physiologic and Metabolic Variables (Mean ± SEM)

	BP (torr)	CBF ml/100 g/min	CVR (torr/ CBF)	CMRO$_2$ ml/100 g/min
Control	132.7 ± 6.7	39.6 ± 5.2	3.76 ± .62	2.97 ± .29
Group I				
Barbiturate	75.3 ± 10.3	22.8 ± 5.1	3.98 ± 1.6	2.70 ± .27
Barbiturate/ hypothermia	82.3 ± 11.6	11.91 ± 1.5	7.28 ± 1.8	1.26 ± .17
Group II				
Hypothermia	109.3 ± 6.2	15.6 ± 1.7	7.07 ± .40	1.28 ± .47
Hypothermia/ barbiturate	68.0 ± 6.1	10.9 ± 1.1	6.28 ± .60	.77 ± .16

under light barbiturate anesthesia, only a very small decrease in the cerebral metabolic rate for oxygen ($CMRO_2$) was found. This should be compared to the large $CMRO_2$ reduction due to the subsequent induction of hypothermia (Group I). Reversal of the treatment order (cold before pentobarbital) demonstrated that hypothermia again elicited a significantly greater degree of metabolic depression. Considering the overall lowering of $CMRO_2$ by both treatments, barbiturates reduced oxygen uptake by 16 percent and 23 percent, while hypothermia decreased $CMRO_2$ by 84 percent and 77 percent in Groups I and II, respectively.

Our preliminary findings indicate that large doses of pentobarbital do not greatly potentiate hypothermic-induced cerebral metabolic or circulatory changes in intact dogs already lightly anesthetized with barbiturates. If the control state had been established in awake dogs a larger effect of barbiturates on cerebral metabolism probably would have been demonstrated. However, cooling performed in the absence of premedication is accompanied by a variable amount of catecholamine release. The circulating catecholamines increase the basal metabolic rate via the mechanism of nonshivering thermogenesis. This increases tissue oxygen requirements and the animal's resistance to cooling. Although barbiturates do not seem to potentiate $CMRO_2$ depression or CVR elevation under established low body temperature conditions (as shown in the present work), they or other "lytic cocktails" are required for the rapid and smooth attainment of hypothermia. Barbiturates with their ability to quickly halve $CMRO_2$ in healthy brain and lower an elevated ICP may additionally reduce the potential for cerebral ischemia during the period required to attain significant temperature reduction.

Because we found that more than 75 percent of the total $CMRO_2$ reduction in our experiment was attributable to cold, our work is consistent with Michenfelder's findings indicating that hypothermia is superior to anesthetics in its ability to retard high energy metabolite depletion and lactate accumulation in ischemic brain tissue.[5] His work indicating that thiopental reduces $CMRO_2$ only insofar as it reduces brain electrical activity may explain our inability to show a larger pentobarbital related CBF and $CMRO_2$ reduction since our "control" EEG's already showed signs of light barbiturate anesthesia and had CBF and $CMRO_2$ values somewhat below awake values reported by

Table 3

Possible Mechanisms for Barbiturate/ Hypothermic Protection of Ischemic Brain

---

Reduced metabolic requirements
Improved CBF distribution
Intracranial pressure reduction
Modified inflammatory response
Other

---

others.[5] Should the results of the present study and Michenfelder's work be interpreted as indicating that barbiturates have no therapeutic role in the treatment of progressive intracranial hypertension or other cerebral ischemic states?

Barbiturates can reduce some types of intracranial hypertension and they can prevent cerebral infarction in certain experimental stroke models. Therefore, the therapeutic potential of barbiturates should not be lightly dismissed at this time. The pentobarbital dose used in our study exceeded that used by Smith et al. when they demonstrated protection against cerebral infarction after middle cerebral artery occlusion.[7] It appears that our problem is understanding how barbiturates work and under what clinical circumstances they could be utilized.

Table 3 suggests possible mechanisms by which barbiturates or hypothermia might prevent irreversible cellular changes in ischemic brain. Metabolic depression, whether achieved by anesthetics or hypothermia, has its limits if some basal nutrient supply to tissue is not maintained or if the period of anoxia is overlong.[8,9] Even in profound hypothermia to $15°C–20°C$ there is evidence for continued metabolism, EEG activity, and neuronal loss after 1 hour of circulatory arrest.[1,10] Since the clinical period of brain ischemia due to either an occlusive stroke or increased ICP far exceeds a time span measured in hours, factors other than a reduced metabolism may contribute to tissue survival.

In stroke and focal brain trauma drugs causing vasoconstriction of cerebral vessels, e.g., barbiturates, may improve the intracranial distribution of CBF. This would be analogous to the inverse cerebral steal attendant to a reduction in $PaCO_2$.[13] As previously shown, the vasoconstrictor properties of barbiturates can quickly effect a reduction in intracranial pressure presumably, by reducing intracranial blood volume.[1] There is experimental data suggesting that pentobarbital reduces the amount of cerebral edema following a cold lesion and barbiturates and hypothermia may also decrease cerebrospinal fluid secretion rates, further contributing to decompression of the intracranial compartment.[13,14,15] The combined sedative and blood pressure reducing actions of barbiturates may reduce that component of vasogenic cerebral edema which is dependent on the arterial pressure head.[14] Barbiturates and cold may possibly modify the inflammatory response to injury by lowering neurotransmitter formation

and release.[16,17] Without invoking hypometabolism, there still appear to be a number of possible ways in which barbiturates and/or hypothermia could offer protection to the damaged brain. Measurement of cerebral blood flow and metabolism in the controlled environment of the neurological intensive care facility should provide us with the information we need to evaluate the efficacy of barbiturates and hypothermia in head trauma.

REFERENCES

1. Shapiro HM, Galindo A, Wyte SR, et al: Rapid intraoperative reduction of intracranial pressure with thiopentone. Br J Anaesth 45:1057–1062, 1973

2. Pierce EC Jr, Lambertson CJ, Deutsch S, et al: Cerebral circulation and metabolism during thiopental anesthesia and hyperventilation in man. J Clin Invest 41:1664–1671, 1962

3. Shapiro HM, Wyte SR, Loeser J: Barbiturate-augmented hypothermia for reduction of persistent intracranial hypertension. J Neurosurg 40:90–100, 1974

4. Lassen NA, Munck O: The cerebral blood flow determination in man by the use of radioactive krypton. Acta Physiol Scand 33:30–49, 1955

5. Michenfelder JD, Theye RA: The effects of anesthesia and hypothermia on canine cerebral ATP and lactate during anoxia produced by decapitation. Anesthesiology 33:430–439, 1970

6. Michenfelder JD: The interdependency of cerebral function and metabolic effects following massive doses of thiopental in the dog. Anesthesiology 41:231–236, 1974

7. Smith AL, Hoff JT, Neilsen SL, et al: Barbiturate protection in acute focal ischemia. Stroke 5:1–7, 1974

8. Nilsson L: The influence of barbiturate anesthesia upon the energy state and upon acid-base parameters of the brain in arterial hypotension and asphyxia. Acta Neurol Scand 47:233–253, 1971

9. Michenfelder JD, Theye RA: Cerebral protection by thiopental during hypoxia. Anesthesiology 39:510–517, 1973

10. Reilly EL, Brunberg JA, Doty DB: The effect of hypothermia and total circulatory arrest on the electroencephalogram of children. Electroenceph Clin Neurophysiol 36:661–667, 1974

11. Fisk GC, Wright BB, Turner BB, et al: Cerebral effects of circulatory arrest at 20°C in the infant pig. Anesth Intensive Care 2:33–42, 1974

12. Soloway M, Nadel W, Albin M et al: The effect of hyperventilation on subsequent cerebral infarction. Anesthesiology 29:975–980, 1968

13. Clasen RA, Pandolfi S, Casey D, et al: Furosemide and pentobarbital in cryogenic cerebral injury and edema. Neurology (Minneap) 24:624–628, 1974

14. Clasen RA, Pandolfi S, Russel J, et al: Hypothermia and hypotension in experimental cerebral edema. Arch Neurol 19:472–486, 1968

15. Cevario SJ, Macri FJ: The inhibitory effect of pentobarbital Na on aqueous humor formation. Invest Ophthalmol 13:384–386, 1974

16. Osterholm J, Bell J, Meyer R, et al: Experimental effects of free serotonin on the brain and its relation to brain injury. J Neurosurg 31:408–421, 1969

17. Lidbrink P, Corrodi H, Fuxe K, et al: Barbiturates and meprobamate: Decreases in catecholamine turnover of central dopamine and noradrenaline neuronal systems and the influence of immobilization stress. Brain Res 45:507–524, 1972

Frank M. Yatsu, M.D.

25

Protective Effects of Barbiturates on Cerebral Ischemia

Brain damage associated with head trauma results from both its immediate shearing and disruptive physical forces and the secondary changes of edema and impaired microcirculation which initiate ischemic brain damage. The degree of neurological recovery following such head trauma depends on the extent of injury and also on the preservation of neural functions threatened by ischemic damage plus the operation of neural regeneration or "plasticity," an exciting area of current research. It is to the problem of secondary ischemic brain damage with head trauma and the means of averting its destructive effects that I address my comments.

Our research interest in ischemic brain damage is focused on our attempts to reduce its effect in experimental strokes. We believe similar ischemic pathogenetic mechanisms aggravate brain trauma and therefore propose that therapies, such as barbiturates, aimed at reducing ischemic brain damage with stroke are equally applicable to brain trauma.

Because preexisting experimental models of cerebral ischemia do not provide predictable and reproducible areas of ischemic brain damage, we developed a model of global cerebral ischemia. This was accomplished by combining hypotension induced with intravenous Arfonad plus hypoxia with 4 percent oxygen in awake, succinyl choline paralyzed rabbits. We found that with moderate cerebral ischemia, as defined by a 3-minute EEG, animals showed no detectable impairment follow-

ing extubation, while 2 minutes longer or 5 minutes of an isoelectric EEG resulted in irreversible brain damage to the rabbits which was demonstrated after the experiment by an inability to sustain their respiration or motor paralysis. Our published studies, which included an assessment of all major organs histologically including brain as well as platelet size and number and evidences for disseminated intramuscular coagulation, indicate that the brunt of ischemic injury is primarily upon the brain.[1]

On this model of global cerebral ischemia, we assessed oxidative phosphorylation and the energy charge of the adenylate pool and have concluded that the mechanism of energy synthesis, namely mitochondria, is not the vulnerable focus of brain to ischemia; rather, it is an energy-dependent process. Possible loci of vulnerability are processes such as Na-K ATPase and neurotransmitter metabolism.

Since our model offered an opportunity to evaluate stages of reversible and irreversible ischemic brain damage, which no preceding model had done from a functional view, we assessed the effectiveness of barbiturates in retarding ischemic damage. Previous studies using various volatile and nonvolatile anesthetics, as well as hypothermia, used survival time as the end point and did not assess the question of retarding irreversible ischemic damage directly.[2-4]

In our model,[5] following the onset of an isoelectric EEG, injection of 5 mg/kg of methohexital, a rapid-acting barbiturate, and the continuation of 5 minutes isoelectric EEG resulted in no detectable neurological damage. These dramatic findings were reported in 1972. After this, the use

This work was supported by the U.S. Health Service Grant NS10976 from the National Institute of Neurological Diseases and Stroke.

of barbiturates was applied to a model of focal cerebral ischemia by my colleagues in San Francisco, Dr. Julian Hoff and Dr. Alan Smith[6,7] and their colleagues. Their findings also support the concept that barbiturates reduce ischemic brain damage.

Bolstered by these findings and the conviction that retardation of brain metabolism would provide "lead time" until adequate circulation became available to ischemic tissues, we applied for and received permission from our Committee on Human Research to use barbiturates in stroke patients.

Since this innovative form of therapy for ischemic stroke requires careful monitoring, particularly of blood pressure and respiration, funds are needed to undertake a large-scale study in a randomized fashion. The first such barbiturate-treated stroke patient was reported by us to the Princeton Conference on Cerebral Disease[8] last year. This historic use of barbiturates in an acute stroke was in a 60-year-old patient who presented with progressive right-sided weakness including complete paralysis of his right hand and difficulty in speaking. Phenobarbital therapy was begun approximately 8 hours after onset. He was given 500 and 400 mg of phenobarbital, respectively, over the first 2 days treatment. By the fifth day, the patient showed near normal strength although he had difficulty in handwriting. Today the patient is neurologically normal. One patient, of course, does not make a series nor establish a form of therapy, since the patient may have recovered fully without barbiturates. The actual clinical benefits of barbiturates in ischemic strokes must await randomized studies.

From our experimental studies and those of others, plus our single stroke patient, we are convinced that barbiturates should be assessed clinically for their potential in retarding or preventing ischemic brian damage. There are two concerns in using barbiturates: The problems of (1) viability, and (2) monitoring.

1. *Viability:* Tissue that is ischemic but not dead is the only one that can be preserved if adequate sustaining circulation is provided. Thus, various parameters of viability must be marshaled to augment the clinical examination, for example, the use of evoked potential responses from light, sound, or pain.
2. *Monitoring:* These relate to potential complications of barbiturates such as hypoventilation. hypoxia, and hypotension and also to measures of cerebral blood flow (CBF), cerebral metabolism (CMRO$_2$), and intracranial pressure.

In order to gain insight into the molecular basis for the protective effect of barbiturates in reducing ischemic damage, we have been investigating the effects of barbiturates on preserving synaptosomal sodium-potassium ATPase. We[9] find that 5 minutes of ischemia is associated with impaired Na-K ATPase activity as monitored by Na-stimulated glucose oxidation. With this form of ischemia, our preliminary data show that phenobarbital restores ATPase activity to 95 percent of control from an impaired value of 81 percent. We also find with ischemia that an increase in synaptosomal Na-K ratio occurs. Whether this failure of Na-K ATPase activity and increased Na/K ratio accounts for brain edema, seen with both ischemia and head trauma, remains for future research.

In summary, we strongly believe that experimental studies support the concept that ischemic brain damage can be averted by a reduction of brain metabolism, particularly with barbiturates. With the difficult and complex problem of head injuries, multiple factors contribute to causing brain damage. One factor, ischemic injury, would appear to be remediable. Where adequate regional cerebral blood flow can be maintained or restored, and the patients are well monitored, reduction of cerebral metabolism with barbiturates offers promise of preserving brain function.

REFERENCES

1. Yatsu FM, Lindquist P, and Graziano C: An experimental model of brain ischemia combining hypotension and hypoxia. Stroke 5:32–39, 1974
2. Bain JA, Catton DV, Cox JM, et al: The effect of general anaesthesia on the tolerance of cerebral ischaemia in rabbits. Can Anaesth Soc J 14:69–78, 1967
3. Dhruva AJ et al: Fluothane as an anaesthetic adjuvant for prevention of hypoxic brain damage. (An experimental study.) J Exp Med Sci 5:1–7, 1961

4. Wright RL, Ames A: Measurement of maximal permissible cerebral ischemia and a study of its pharmacologic prolongation. J Neurosurg 21:567–575, 1964

5. Yatsu FM, Diamond I, Graziano C, et al: Experimental brain ischemia: Protection from irreversible damage with a rapid-acting barbiturate (Methohexital). Stroke 3:726–732, 1972

6. Smith AL et al: Barbiturate protection in acute focal cerebral ischemia. Stroke 5:1–7, 1974

7. Hoff JT et al: Barbiturate protection from cerebral infarction in primates. Stroke 6:28–33, 1975

8. Yatsu FM: Effect on lipid metabolism of reduction of the energy state. Ninth Princeton Conf Cerebral Vascular Diseases. Princeton, NJ, January 9–11, 1974

9. Yatsu FM, Liao C-L, Park OK: Impaired synaptosomal ATPase activity following ischemia. Am Acad Neurology Meeting, Miami, May 1, 1975

Edited by Javad Hekmatpanah, M.D.
and John Mullan, M.D.

Open Discussion

DR. PLUM: I think these are clearly important and of the greatest interest, but there is a very decided difference in both head injury and stroke between operating on a vessel and clamping it under anesthesia and then observing the natural history of that recovery from the treatment of occlusive vascular disease, which happens on the outside and then brings a patient to the hospital.

To evaluate some such techniques clinically would seem almost to be prohibitive in terms of expense and control of the variables that would be involved, and it is reminiscent of the wave of enthusiasm that followed Hubert Rosomoff's experiments on dogs, reported at the American Neurological Association in the 1950s, which saw a great many hypothermic blankets widely distributed in both surgical and medical neurological units, but which never somehow got into a second generation, particularly when Dr. William Field reported from Texas that of 11 patients with stroke treated with hypothermia, 10 died, which was a somewhat high mortality even for that rather serious disease.

I believe that to treat patients with such a procedure at the present time, before well-documented and exhaustive animal studies which simulate the clinical condition, is perhaps not in either the patient's nor our own best interests. I must say I do hope [Dr. Yatsu], that you will give us in a large number of subjects, with a suitable interval between the time of injury and the time of initiation of the treatment, something to go on as a lead because, as you imply, what you say is so terribly important.

DR. SHAPIRO: Obviously [Dr. Plum], we have been thinking the same things you have been thinking, and it is with trepidation and rather late that we would initiate this kind of therapy in a head injury patient. I think perhaps the whole question of hypometabolism and its attended vascular effects—and really the barbiturates and hypothermia are fairly similar to those effects, whether the mechanisms are the same or not remains to be determined—is really up for reevaluation at this time.

When Hubert Rosomoff did his work, we didn't have the current kinds of abilities to support patients in ICUs. We didn't have the thrust to do the things we can currently do. We didn't have the successes we now see in the coronary care unit and everyday kinds of medical performance. At least insofar as the head injury patients are concerned, those who we feel are slipping away as we watch them at the bedside—and I think we have enough information to know when we are losing (unfortunately we started late, not early, with the barbiturates)—it might not be unreasonable to consider those and hypothermia as well, realizing we are starting late rather than early, in view of what we can now do in terms of supporting patients.

DR. MITCHENFELDER: In our same series of Java monkeys we did 5 with hypothermia, 20°C, again identical to the control except for the hypothermia, and we started out to do 9 of them, but we abandoned it because 5 of them died at 36 hours during intensive care. We couldn't keep them going hemodynamically, and all 5 of them had massive edema, which surprised us. We wondered if it might be a reflection of viscosity at 20°C with the marginal collateral flow being shut down by the viscosity. The obvious way to get at that would be to hemodilute the animals and cool them. Certainly hypotension was not the same with barbiturates in that protocol.

DR. YATSU: I don't want to be in the position to have to defend the cause nor have to act as someone who is championing the cause. I don't think we are. It is almost a collusion that all three seem to be saying the same thing. I do think there is tremendous potential, and I would agree with [Dr. Plum] that we do need more and better ways of evaluating patients.

The whole question of viability still bothers me. We really don't know where we are in terms of the comatose, traumatic patient. Obviously, patients who are dead, a lot of the patients I think who have been treated, are so late that nothing could have been done anyway. So, viability still remains an important question.

DR. SHAPIRO: I don't think hypothermia is quite as fatal as you seem to imply [Dr. Mitchenfelder]. We have used it. Certainly we have used it alone for days without untoward complications. By that, I am talking about 20°C with ventilatory support. We have used it in combination with the barbiturates, and we have really had a very stable situation in the clinic. Whether or not it is efficacious in terms of what happens to the head, I think, is up for grabs. We agree, but it can be used and can be used in a stable, well-supported situation.

DR. LINDSAY SYMON: I have a number of comments. First, I suppose I must be getting just about as old as Dr. Plum because, like him, I had a sort of *deja vu* feeling as I heard the story of the barbiturates.

I think there are a number of problems in relation to the interpretation of these animal models, and the first of them is that middle cerebral ischemia either in the squirrel monkey or in the baboon does not produce the homogeneous area of ischemia in the middle cerebral fields. It produces a reduction of blood flow to less than 10 moles/100 g/min as of a 2-minute clearance with hydrogen flow only in the center of the middle cerebral fields, and by that I include the basal ganglia. Over quite a wide area it produces a reduction to about 25 percent of basal flow, which is about 12 to 15 mils/100 g/min, and over a much wider area it produces the sort of 40 percent reduction which Dr. Simp, who I believe at that time was using it in his study, would find.

One of the difficulties that one has in matching metabolic analyses in tissue to flow studies is that it becomes extremely important to decide which part of the tissue one has taken for analysis. I think this is something one has to be very careful about. I would like to ask Dr. Mitchenfelder how he did that.

The other thing is that it has been known since the time of Tompson and Smith that if you wish to increase the size of the middle cerebral deficit, the best way to do it from that of an infarct (and an infarct like that) is to lower the animal's systemic blood pressure. I was interested to hear Dr. Mitchenfelder briefly allude to a perfect match of blood pressure and PCO_2 and other variables in 2 animals anesthetized for 48 hours after middle cerebral occlusion by entirely disparate methods. This is very interesting, and I would like to know just how carefully the blood pressures were matched at the time of middle cerebral occlusion, and what the absolute levels of blood pressure were, thinking of this particularly

in relation to one of his series where, in fact, none of the animals recovered from middle cerebral occlusion. It is really quite unusual, because both Sutt and ourselves and many others have found this is really not a lethal procedure either at light halothane anesthesia.

DR. MITCHENFELDER: Regarding the tissue biopsy, of course we are aware that it is a rather sloppy approach to know whether you are getting the area of maximum ischemia. The only way we did it (and I grant it is sloppy) is by simply looking at the infarctions that develop in monkeys in whom the clip was not removed, identifying where the central core of ischemia most commonly occurs, but not consistently, as has been pointed out, and this is the area that is biopsied in the punch biopsy technique that takes about a 200 mg sample of brain and dumps it immediately in suction system. There is no question there has to be variability. If there were a better way to do it, I would like to hear how it might be done. If you look at the cortex of the brain, you obviously can't identify which is the most ischemic area for certain, at least in the depths.

The second point regarding blood pressure: Again we were very much aware of the importance of blood pressure control. At the time of clipping, the animals were all under 1 percent halothane, and the mean arterial pressure for both groups was in the high 90s. For the 48-hour period, there was obvious variability during the 48-hour period in blood pressure, but for the 18 animals, the 2 groups of 9 each, the grand mean arterial pressure for both groups was in the low 90s throughout the 48-hour period. We did arbitrarily decide to treat any drop in pressure below a mean arterial pressure of 60, and this was necessary in about 2 animals out of each group for transient vasopressor therapy. This was our arbitrarily selected minimum pressure of 60. The grand mean was in the 90s.

DR. JULIAN HOFF: You heard an allusion to Allen Smith and my dog studies in San Francisco. We did a series of baboons in which we occluded the middle cerebral artery and then had a survival time of 1 week after that. The two anesthetic groups were halothane and pentobarbital. Pentobarbital was given in different doses to try to get this dose response curve. It turns out that barbiturates do provide some protection in the size of the infarction.

These two groups, 90 mg and 120 mg/kg, are significantly different than this group, which is similar to the awake dog group in size of the infarction. This group is very difficult to manage as a viable preparation anesthetically. They have a lot of arrhythmias, and so I would certainly substantiate the fact that they need intensive care if you are going to get any sort of viability in this group anesthetized with a dose that seems to be protective.

The numbers are small, so I don't know if it is well enough substantiated to try it on humans. I have trepidations about that, so we haven't started on any head injury study. If we do, it will have to be in very large doses, and there will be a lot of work.

DR. DUCKER: This is just a comment, not a question. I was very excited when [Dr. Yatsu] had this stuff come out about a year ago, and we took it to our lab for those interested in trauma below the foramen magnum again, and in our standard model for spinal cord injury we tried to test this. We injured the cord in a threshold where we knew the animal would be paraplegic. We did this study based on two facts, one the protective fact with ischemia, and secondly we have shown that in severe spinal cord injury there is a progressive drop in blood flow; therefore, we thought ischemia was contributing to it.

We did not use those high doses Dr. Yatsu showed us, as far as 90 to 120 mg/kg. We used 50 mg/kg in the injured cord. These animals were not significantly different from the others, so in that limited trauma experiment on the spinal cord with that limited dose, which we thought was a healthy dose (at least I did), it was not helpful.

DR. OVERGAARD: May I return to clinical head injuries and barbiturates. We used phenobarbital as a routine treatment in all severe head injury cases, and especially in a group with decerebrate rigidity, also in other patients. I have plotted here the relation between the CBF unit and the S-E Fenemal, as we call it, and again CBF 10 and S-E Fenemal, and I will say the assumption that high doses of phenobarbital will reduce the cerebral blood flow doesn't hold.

We use high doses for we really intend to have a serum level between 30 and 70. Most of the patients are not about 30, but that was the intention. Often you have to give more than 1 g/24 hours to get the patient relaxed and to get serum levels like this.

We have plotted against the oxygen uptake of the brain during the CBF study. I think the best part is the one we have here, and this is only CBF 10 and $CMRO_2$, and all these studies were from day 0 to day 21. Some patients would decrease their oxygen uptake a few days after injury. After an initial level of about 1.5 they go down to about .09. If they go here with the first 3 weeks, they will survive with severe deficits. That means the higher mental functions are not working, but they can so behave in the population that 90 percent of the people will not discover that anything is wrong with them. If in the first week they have a $CMRO_2$ here, and above that, they will usually recover all their mental functions again.

Serum Fenemal and oxygen uptake do not correlate very well with each other, so if the high doses of barbiturate or serum phenobarbital really reduce blood flow in this group of patients, I wonder. We have tried to do studies with fast injections, and we couldn't detect any decrease in blood flow or oxygen uptake, but testing the new steroid drug, Tessen, it is the best drug for reducing intracranial pressure.

This is a young patient when arterial hypertension in the first hours or days was over 220. This patient was on respiratory treatment. We gave very high doses of serum barbital, and you see despite this she had a pronounced hyperemia of the brain, and in about 3 weeks she changed to an akinetic movement. At that time she had a high intracranial pressure. She couldn't absorb her ventricular fluid. Then suddenly she woke up and started talking.

DR. HEKMATPANAH: Would you recommend barbiturates for patients with severe head injuries?

DR. OVERGAARD: I would. This is 3 days after injury.

DR. MOSS: I hesitate to rise again, but it is with a different hat, to substantiate Dr. Mitchenfelder's idea of there being two different metabolic functions within brain cells for cellular integrity, maintenance, and function. We have been studying pathways of oxidative metabolism, the pentose phosphate pathway, and the Krebs cycle activity. We found under normal circumstances in two different species, rat and bovine, it looks like about one-quarter to one-third of the normal glucose oxidative metabolism goes by the glucose phosphate pathway.

About the difference between halothane and barbiturate, we find that barbiturate anesthesia, despite lowering total glucose oxidative metabolism, seems to about double the pentose phosphate activity. Halothane does not have that effect, and these two pathways differ in significance. The pentose phosphate pathway uses the hydrogen carrier NADP which now, when in reduced form, would be utilized in glutathione reduction or the pathway for ribose or nucleic acid pool maintenance.

DR. HASS: What tissue are you looking at?

DR. MOSS: We were looking at the rat brain, calf brain, in situ. We were looking at turnovers of 6-phosphogluconate.

DR. HASS: And you found a shunt, and you found it to be one-third?

DR. MOSS: It has been reported in Anesthesiology, Transactions of the New York Academy of Medicine and Diabetes, many years ago.

IV

Cerebral Microcirculation

William I. Rosenblum, M.D.

26

Effects of Trauma on Directly Visualized Microvessels

The paucity of studies concerning direct observation of cerebral microvessels in traumatized brain makes it possible for me to utilize this presentation as a means of suggesting the pathways that future efforts might fruitfully take. In spite of the small literature, I will not cite all available references but I will concentrate instead on those publications that seem to point the way toward fruitful paths, and to cry out for meaningful follow-up.

First, I must introduce my own bias, which is to say that I wish to know not only what the vessels are doing but also why. Thus far, studies of flow in tissue have provided a means of evaluating overall vascular resistance in the volume of tissue being observed, but a given resistance may be arrived at in many different ways, and different mechanisms may be called into play to bring about a given overall resistance. I want to know, for example, whether some larger arterioles, perhaps under neurogenic control, are dilated, while some smaller vessels perhaps under metabolic control are constricted, or visa versa. Or, instead, are all vessels maintaining a normal tonus, giving a net resistance equivalent to that achieved in either of the two preceding cases?

Since this information cannot be obtained, at present, from examinations of regional cerebral blood flow, I am forced to study the surface vasculature where hints concerning the mechanisms of vasuular control or malfunction can be obtained by direct observation of individual vessels. Arbitrarily, vessels with an internal diameter of less than 100 μ, are placed in the microcirculation. These are the vessels I shall discuss.

The difficulty with any literature concerning effects on an organs blood flow, of trauma to that organ, is that trauma to the tissue involves simultaneous trauma to both parenchyma and vessels. To me, it seems imperative to separate the effects of trauma to the vessels from the effects on the vessels of trauma to the surrounding tissue. I do not deny the value of knowing what happens to vessels and flow in the complex case where both vessels and parenchyma are injured. But I suggest that to understand why vessels behave as they do in such a case, one must study simpler cases where vessels are observed when injury is more or less restricted first to vessels and then to the surrounding tissue.

First, let us consider what happens when cerebral microvessels are injured. In 1925, Florey[1] observed "white bodies" or platelet-leukocyte aggregates adhering to the endothelium of injured microvessels on the cerebral surface. We will call these vessels which lie in the subarachnoid space, "pial" vessels, keeping in mind that such vessels include not only microvessels from 100 to approximately 10 μ I.D., but also larger vessels, including those at the circle of Willis. Florey's observations, and our interest, concerns the microvessels. For 35 years there was bare mention of the thrombotic phenomenon described by Florey. Then, again in Great Britain, Honour and co-workers[2,3] reported that heat, locally applied chloroform, or mechanical stimuli, produced local thrombi at the point of injury. These thrombi consisted largely of platelets. The local thrombi could fragment, and then reform, the fragments embolizing the distal circulation, and this phenomenon could repeat for hours.

This model provides a means of quantifying

microvascular thrombosis by measuring the number of embolic episodes per unit time or the number of emboli produced. The model can be used to test the effects of systematically or locally applied drugs in potentiating or preventing thrombosis or embolis.[2-5] To the best of my knowledge there are only four such studies of cerebral vessels.[2-5] A similar model, employing a laser beam to injure individual vessels, has been employed in the peripheral (i.e., extracerebral) microcirculation, by first sensitizing the vessel with an intravascular dye, supposedly acting as a heat absorbing target.[6-10] These studies add new ways of quantifying the model by measuring the time taken to form a thrombus after a standard insult, or by measuring the time required for complete occlusion of flow or total time of occlusion. In spite of the elegance of such models, and the ability to correlate drug effects in vivo, with in vitro drug effects on clotting parameters, there are, again, an extremely small number of such studies, perhaps reflecting, once more, the small number of workers who are really interested in direct observation of microvessels. Nevertheless, if local injury is capable of producing microthrombi and emboli, and if these phenomena can be altered by drugs like aspirin,[10] then the phenomenon is of obvious interest to those who wish to understand and treat impairment of cerebral blood flow and the progression of this impairment, following brain injury.

Please note that the thrombi to which we refer are formed without injury to brain parenchyma itself. However, Honour and co-workers[4] also described what they called "minor injury." Here no thrombi formed where the noxious stimulus was applied, *unless* a chemical agent was then locally applied to the same site. ATP, ADP, and other "tissue extracts" were effective. The implications for brain trauma are obvious, since adenosine is now known to be released from hypoxic brain.[11]

Serotonin or norepinephrine are released from injured or hypoxic brain.[12,13,14] These agents, or others, might be released from injured brain parenchyma and produce microthrombi and emboli in vessels that were rendered susceptible by what Honour termed "minor injury."

In addition to microthrombi, Honour observed a further phenomenon, namely vasospasm or arteriolar contriction on either side of the damaged site.[3] Moreover, agents that produced thrombi at sites sensitized by "minor injury," first produced constriction at those sites, with the

white thrombus appearing only after the constriction passed off. This plunges us directly into the problem of cerebral vasospasm in general.

Spasm is a frequent angiographic concomitant of subarachnoid hemorrhage, whatever its cause. Spasm is certainly observed in the angiograms of trauma patients, though whether it may be ascribed to hemorrhage in such patients, is unclear, at least to me. However, angiograms do not reveal the microvessels. There is a variety of opinion in the literature concerning the degree to which prognosis can be associated with angiographic spasm. There appears to be a consensus that prognosis is better related to blood flow. It is my belief that correlation with spasm would be improved if microvascular spasm could be monitored.

Spasm of microvascular vessels can definitely occur. This was demonstrated by Florey, again in 1925,[1] through local application of $BaCl_2$, a smooth muscle spasmogen. Again Florey's observation lay fallow, until I began in 1961 to use this technique as a routine means of testing contractile potential in the cerebral microcirculation.[15] Pial arterioles are now known to constrict greatly to a variety of stimuli, both physiological and nonphysiological.[16-19] In fact, smaller arterioles may be more sensitive to some stimuli than larger arterioles.[20] Of particular interest is the evidence that a variety of pathologic states may enhance vasoconstriction. For example, the threshold to serotonin seems reduced in experimental infarction.[21] Although this might result from a local elevation in perivascular serotonin released from injured tissue,[21] it might also result from a decrease in contractile threshold produced by a decrease in regional perfusion pressure, since reduced pressure has been shown to increase the sensitivity of pial arterioles to $BaCl_2$.[22]

In short, both intraluminal and extraluminal factors may enhance vasospasm. Intraluminal factors might be mechanical—for example, reduced pressure; or they might be chemical—for example, release of a material from aggregating or injured platelets. Extravascular factors would be chemical, released from brain tissue or from blood in contact with the tissue, and, as we will discuss shortly, they might be neurogenic. In experiments on extracerebral microvessels, an increased sensitivity to catechols has been demonstrated where endothelial damage has been so slight that no local thrombi formed.[7] Catechols have been reported to constrict pial arterioles, but in high concentrations.[16,17,18] It will be of great interest to see whether the response to extra-vascular norepinephrine is enhenced by damage to the vessel itself or by damage to surrounding brain. As for factors diminishing vasospasm, it is of interest that aspirin inhibits not only platelet aggregation at the site of injury in the extracerebral microcirculation but also inhibits vasoconstriction around the injured site.[10]

In any event, we must consider not only the enhancement or diminution of vasospasm by intravascular and extravascular factors but also the nature of "THE" primary spasmogen. At least we would assume so from the available literature, since for years, people have searched for the one substance in blood which produces spasm when that blood is introduced into the subarachnoid space. There is good evidence that one such material is platelet borne,[23] and serotonin has been considered a prime candidate.[23] Attempts at identifying the material have, however, definitely excluded serotonin.[24] More recent candidates might be one of the prostaglandins, for example, $F_{2\alpha}$, which have been shown by several groups to constrict cerebral arteries and arterioles.[19,25,26] Recently in work still unpublished, we have shown the prostaglandins of the B series also constrict pial arterioles. However, we have also suggested that, although there may be still unidentified or unproven spasmogens in blood, possibly synthesized by platelets, the search for a single agent may be ill conceived. Rather, we point out the possibility that several agents might act together to cause a summation of their effects.[19] Unfortunately there is virtually no work on the capacity of vasoactive agents to act either additively, or to potentiate, when applied in vivo to cerebral vessels. We hope these remarks will stimulate such work.

We have noted that direct observation of cerebral microvessels is only possible in the pial portion of the cerebral vascular tree. Will observations there, permit valid conclusions concerning parenchymal microcirculation? We wish to put the question differently. It is known that pial vessels respond, in general, in a manner that parallels the response of the cerebral vasculature as a whole, when the latter is monitored by blood flow measurements.[16,27] For example, the pial arterioles are easily dilated by increased CO_2 or lowered pH, and cerebral blood flow is increased by the same maneuvers. Either parenchymal arterioles behave, in many important ways, like pial arterioles, or else the control of cerebral circulation is often dominated by events in the pial vasculature. These hypotheses are not mutually exclusive. In any case, either of the hypotheses results in the conclusion that a study of factors controlling pial vascular diameters is vital to our understanding of factors controlling cerebral blood flow.[27]

Finally, we must discuss the possibility that neurogenic factors affect the cerebral microcirculation. Such a discussion is made relevant by publications which show that cerebral vasospasm may occur within 1 minute of head injury and that such spasm extends into the extracranial portions of the cerebral vascular tree.[28] The rapidity of response is compatible with a neurogenic response, though it does not preclude a metabolic response. However, the observation of extracranial vasospasm seems to rule out production of spasm solely by materials in the subarachnoid space. Either there is a wave of sympathetic activity along with the well-defined sympathetic innervation of the pial vasculature and the great vessels of the neck,[17] or else the constriction, initiated within the skull, is propagated along muscle cells within the media of contiguous vascular segments. These hypotheses are not mutually exclusive. Propagation within the media of large systemic arteries has been demonstrated by others.[29] In our own laboratory we have shown that sympathetic nerves to cerebral vessels do participate in generalized autonomic discharges. Thus, anesthesia and sham operations involving orbital exenteration and removal of bone to expose the brain result in depletion of norepinephrine from cerebrovascular nerves, even when there is no subarachnoid hemorrhage. Such a depletion of norepinephrine occurs in other perivascular nerves at the same time, for example, in the nerves to mesenteric arterioles. Parenthetically, this discharge of cerebrovascular nerves did not, by itself, result in pial vasospasm.[30] In pursuing the role of neurogenic stimuli in altering cerebrovascular dynamics following brain injury, it may be wise to repeat the angiographic studies that showed both rapid onset of spasm and involvement of neck vessels, since participation of the latter is such an important clue to the mechanisms that may be involved.

In conclusion, I would propose a five-point program pointing to the future.

1. The effects of trauma on cerebral vessels must be separated from the effects on the vessels of trauma to adjacent brain.
2. Attention must be directed to events occur-

ring within vessels (e.g., microthrombi and emboli). Attention must not be directed exclusively at alterations in vascular diameter.

3. We must study the possible interaction between microthrombi and/or platelet injury, on the one hand, and altered vasomotor tone, on the other. For example, materials like serotonin or prostaglandin, released by injured or aggregating platelets, could also produce vasoconstriction.

4. Materials released by injured brain may be vasoactive. One must study not only the response of normal vessels to such agents but also the response of injured vessels, since the responsiveness of such vessels may be abnormal. One must also investigate the possible interaction of multiple substances in the vicinity of such vessels.

5. One must consider neurogenic influences on cerebral vessels, even when these influences, by themselves, do not appear to cause major alterations in vascular tone.

REFERENCES

1. Florey H: Microscopical observations on the circulation of blood in the cerebral cortex. Brain 48:43–64, 1925
2. Honour AJ, Ross Russell RW: Experimental platelet embolism. Br J Exp Pathol 43:350–362, 1962
3. Honour AJ, Mitchell JRA: Platelet clumping in injured vessels. Br J Exp Pathol 45:75–87, 1964
4. Born GVR, Philip RB: Inhibition by adenosine and by 2 chloroadenosine of the formation and embolization of platelet thrombi. Nature 202:761–765, 1964
5. Born GVR, Philip RB: Effect of anaesthetic on the duration of embolization of platelet thrombi formed in injured blood vessels. Nature 205:398–399, 1965
6. Kochen JA, Baez S: Laser-induced microvascular thrombosis. Ann NY Acad Sci 122:728–738, 1965
7. Baez S, Kochen JA: Laser-induced microagglutivation in isolated vascular model systems. Ann NY Acad Sci 122:738–746, 1965
8. Grant L, Becker F: Mechanisms of inflammation II Laser-induced thrombosis. Arch Pathol 841:36–41, 1966
9. McKenzie FN, Svensjo E, Arfors KE: Effect of sodium pentobarbital anesthesia on platelet behavior in vitro and in vivo. Microvasc Res 6:194–201, 1973
10. Kovacs IB, Csalay L, Garay P: Laser induced thrombosis in microcirculation of the hamster cheek pouch and its inhibition by acetylsalicylic acid. Microvasc Res 6:194–201, 1973
11. Berne RM, Rubio R, Curnish RR: Release of adenosine from ischemic brain. Effect on cerebral vascular resistance and incorporation into cerebral adenosine nucleotides. Circ Res 35:262–271, 1974
12. Osterholm JL, Bell J, Meyer R, et al: Experimental effects of free serotonin on the brain and its relation to brain injury (pts 1, 2, 3,). J Neurosurg 31:408–421, 1969
13. Welch KMA, Meyer JS, Teraura T, et al: Is-chemic anoxic and cerebral serotonin levels. J Neurol Sci 16:85–92, 1972
14. Meyer JS, Stoica E, Pasew I, et al: Catecholamine concentrations in CSF and plasma of patients with cerebral infarction and hemorrhage. Brain 90:277–288, 1973
15. Rosenblum WI, Zweifach BW: Cerebral microcirculation in the mouse brain. Arch Neurol 9:414–423, 1963
16. Rosenblum WI: Cerebral microcirculation: A review emphasizing the interrelationship of local blood flow and neuronal function. Angiology 16:485–507, 1965
17. Rosenblum WI: Neurogenic control of cerebral circulation. Stroke 2:429–438, 1971
18. Rosenblum WI: Contractile response of pial arterioles to norepinephrine. Arch Neurol 31:197–199, 1974
19. Rosenblum WI: The constriction of pial arterioles by prostaglandin $F_{2\alpha}$. Stroke (in press)
20. Raper AJ, Kontos HA, Patterson JL: Response of pial precapillary vessels to changes in arterial carbon dioxide tension. Circ Res 28:518–523, 1971
21. Blair RDG and Waltz AC: Regional cerebral blood flow during acute ischemia. Correlation of autoradiographic measurements with observations of cortical microcirculation. Neurology 20:802–808, 1970
22. Rosenblum WI: Effect of hypotension on sensitivity of minute cerebral vessels. Arch Neurol 23:266–270, 1970
23. Zervas NT, Kuwayama A, Rosoff CB, et al: Cerebral arterial spasm: Modification by inhibition of platelet function. Arch Neurol 28:400–404, 1973
24. Kapp J, Mahaley MS, Odom GL: Cerebral arterial spasm. Pt 3. J Neurosurg 29:350–356, 1968
25. Yamamoto YL, Feindel RW, Wolfe LS, et al: Experimental vasoconstriction of cerebral arteries by prostaglandins. J Neurosurg 37:385–397, 1972
26. Pennink M, White RW, Cockarell J, et al: Role of

prostaglandin $F_{2\alpha}$, in the genesis of experimental vasospasm. J Neurosurg 37:398–406, 1972

27. Rosenblum WI, Kontos HA: Editorial: The importance and relevance of studies of the pial microcirculation. Stroke 5:425–428, 1974

28. Ekelund Z, Nilsson B, Ponten U: Carotid angiography after experimental head injury in the rat. Neuroradiology 7:209–214, 1974

29. Hilton SM: Local mechanisms regulating peripheral blood flow. In vascular smooth muscle Eichna LW (ed): Physiol Rev Suppl 5, 265–282, 1962

30. Rosenblum WI, Giulianti D: Participation of cerebrovascular nerves in generalized sympathetic discharge. Arch Neurol 29:91–94, 1973

Derek A. Bruce, M.D.

27

Cerebral Microcirculation Assessed by Regional Blood Flow Alterations in Damaged Brain

The one fifth of each breath
That keeps flesh firm on the bone, the old blood warm
Thought bright as young fish in the brain

Joan Swift

Major advances have been made in our understanding of the microvascular system leading to an expanded concept of the microcirculation as a functional organ. The techniques used have included direct observation of capillary flow and interstitial fluid movement and isogravemetric determination of alterations in fluid exchange. Brain capillaries are not visible on the surface of the brain in higher mammals making direct observation impossible. The ability to isolate the brain and retain its function while performing isogravemetric experiments to measure filtration constants is lacking. Further, the brain is a complex tissue with a capillary density that varies from gray to white matter and even within different layers of gray matter, making extrapolation of data from one small area to another exceedingly difficult.[13] The metabolic rates and cellular functions of the various components of the brain have not been fully clarified. Finally, the extracellular spaces of the brain are poorly defined in terms of size, composition and function.

Attempts to study the microcirculation in the brain have been based mainly on measurements of tissue blood flow and inference from these measurements about what is occurring in the tissue itself. X^e133, the most commonly used gas, gives a mean flow value for a core of tissue. The core is defined by the collimation of the gamma detector used to measure the radiation. In normal tissue the clearance of Xe from the brain can be broken down to give two exponents. A fast exponent which is taken to be gray flow and the second a slow exponent taken to be white flow. This is a grossly macroscopic way of learning about the microcirculation. Using small gamma probes and X^e133, or beta counting Kr^{85} blood flow from just the superficial layers of the brain has been measured. Further miniaturization of flow techniques with hydrogen microneedle probes and a microhydrogen generator and recorder system have shown that even within these small areas the flow can vary from 0–400 ml/100 g/min. With further application of these techniques our understanding of the cerebral microcirculation should progress.[2, 16, 17]

Studies of the cerebral microcirculation have been concerned with alteration in one major parameter, the blood flow. We shall see that this is of limited concern. The capillaries are primarily exchange organs and the level of flow through them necessary for adequate exchange is dependent on the capillary environment and cellular metabolism at least as much as capillary flow.[35]

A brief review of recent concepts of the microcirculation in organs other than the brain will help us in our discussion about the pathophysiological processes that may occur in the cerebral microcirculation. Our concepts of the microcirculation have to be expanded. Blood flow will deliver necessary nutrients to the tissue capillary interface. This is only a first step in the cellular receipt of this material. The nutrients must now pass through the capillary tissue interface, through the interstitial space, and across the interstitial space-cell membrane interface before they can be used by the cell. Thus, when we conceive of the microcirculation in modern terms, we consider not only the capillary beds and the blood flow but also the interstitial spaces and tissue flow. The present pore theory of capillary exchange conceives of a large population of small pores in the capillary endothelium of 40Å in size that permit rapid egress of small molecules, and a small population of large pores 1600Å in size permit limited egress of larger molecules. Transport of larger molecules also occurs by pinocytosis. Filtration through small pores is controlled mainly by the Starling hypothesis,[23] taking into account tissue fluid and tissue oncotic pressure. Alterations in filtration do not necessarily reflect a change in permeability. A permeability change may be due to either increased pinocytosis or enlargement or increase in numbers of the large pores. These pores may indeed be gap junctions between endothelial cells.[11,34]

Fung[18] showed that mesenteric capillaries are exceedingly resistant to mechanical compression and proposed that the mechanical properties of the capillary would vary with the interstitial matrix surrounding it. He conceived of the capillaries running in tunnels within the matrix of the interstitial space. Further research has shown that exchange and diffusion in a capillary bed are also dependent on the composition of the interstitial matrix.[12,21]

Weiderhelm has proposed a two-phase model of the ECS, with a colloid-rich and a colloid-free phase. The colloid-free phase is pericapillary and contains albumin and water. There is a tissue flow of water and filtered proteins from the arterial end of the capillary to the venous end with reabsorption at the venous end.[12,38] The colloid-rich phase is a mixture of acid mucopolysaccharides and small amounts of protein. The acid mucopolysaccharide matrix in the extracellular space largely excludes proteins because of the molecular interactions.[38]

Laurent[24] showed that because of this exclusive effect, the osmotic pressure produced by a mixture of protein (albumin) and the mucopolysaccharides would be greater than that predicted by simple addition of the individual osmotic effects. The expected tissue oncotic pressure predicted on the basis of mucropolysaccharide content of .1 percent in connective tissue would be

11 mm Hg.[38] This value would play a major role in tissue capillary exchange as predicted by the Starling hypothesis. In this view of the extracellular space lymphatic drainage would remove only the water and protein that actually penetrated through the colloid rich phase.

When edema forms secondary to hydrostatic events, increased capillary surface area, or increased capillary pressure, a new steady state is reached. The compensatory factors are an increase of protein poor lymph flow and a decrease in tissue oncotic pressure. Both are the result of increased fluid filtration. There is a small rise in tissue hydrostatic pressure but this is not felt to be important.[22] When edema is caused by permeability change, e.g., injury or histamine, increased lymph flow with increased protein content is seen.[11]

Let us now consider the cerebral capillary in light of the foregoing discussion. It has several unique features which force us to modify some of the concepts discussed above. There is essentially no leakage of molecules of the size of protein from brain capillaries. The barrier to these molecules has been shown to be the tight endothelial junction.[8] Since even quite small molecules such as mannitol also fail to cross the blood-brain barrier, pores, if present, must be considerably smaller than the 40Å noted in other tissue. As yet there is no proof of cerebral capillary pores, and molecules of 1300 MW have been shown to pass slowly through the tight endothelial junction under normal circumstances.[29] No large pores have ever been seen except in those areas of the brain, e.g., area postrema where fenestrated capillaries have been demonstrated and absence of the blood-brain barrier noted. Pinocytosis seems to play a small role under normal circumstances in capillary transport in the brain.[7] Morphologically, the cerebral capillary with its 80 percent investment by glial feet fulfills the criteria of a tunnel capillary. Physiologically, however, there is no pericapillary fluid space and no evidence of a pericapillary protein water tissue flow.[39]

The brain interstitum has also been shown to have a ground substance[26,31,41] of mucopolysaccharide, and there is evidence that interference with this ground substance improves movement of dyes through the neuropil[1] and also interferes with cerebral function.[40] Modern concepts are that there are two locations for the polysaccharide in the brain. One is intracellular mainly in neurons, the other is as a cell fuzz coat projecting from the cell membrane into the interstitum. Thus, unlike other tissues the interstitum in the brain, at least in the gray matter, is in large measure an extension of the cell membrane. Many functional roles have been proposed for this polyanionic sponge, from the maintenance of an aqueous phase at the synaptic membrane to ensure ease of ion flux, to a role in memory and learning.[36] (The amount of mucopolysaccharide is less in white matter,[26] and the extracellular space is greater.) This matrix of polysaccharide does not appear to interfere with the movement of noncharged molecules up to 44,000 (peroxidase) weight.[9] The role of acid mucopolysaccharides as osmotic molecules has been well demonstrated[28,38] and understanding the conformational changes induced in these macromolecules by other macromolecules or by partly charged ions is a continuing field of chemical research.[24]

We have in the brain two very different types of tissue. Neuropil with its extensive intercellular matrix, high capillary density, high blood flow and high metabolic rate. The tight capillary junctions and absence of the pericapillary space allow for the most intimate contact between the blood, the interstitial matrix and the cell serving to minimize diffusion distances. Despite the brain's high metabolic rate, its capillary density is less than that of heart or muscle.[14] It would seem that the microcirculation, capillary and interstitial, in the brain is organized to preserve even more rigidly than in other parts of the body a stable milieau in which the cells can function. It may well be that the organization of the intercellular matrix plays a significant role in cerebral function. This would be another reason for the very strict limitation of changes permitted to occur in the extracellular space of the brain. The role of the astroglia in this overview would be in part the biomechanical support of the capillary tunnel and in part as a back up cell to ensure constancy of the neuronal environment in the face of breakdown of the capillary and interstitial mechanisms. The second tissue, white matter, has a large extracellular space, less interstitial ground substance, a lower capillary density, blood flow and metabolic rate. It is easy to imagine that disturbances of the extracellular milieau under these circumstances would be less deleterious and better tolerated since intercellular exchange in the white matter is limited.

Let us now consider what might happen to the cerebral microcirculation in injury. The responses of the microcirculation are similar to a variety of insults. Rupture of capillaries with petechial hemorrhages have been noted frequently in the pathology of human head injury. The result of the petechiae will depend on their number, size, and location. Obliteration of the capillary network will lead to local ischemia and cell death. Thus, a few petechiae in the midbrain may cause an irrecoverable deficit, whereas many more petechiae scattered though the cortex may cause no neurological disturbance. Of greater potential therapeutic importance are the commonly seen accompanying events: venous dilatation and congestion and peripetechial edema. These are common accompaniments of microcirculatory trauma.

This edema, secondary to direct capillary injury, is associated with an increased permeability which has been shown to be due to leakage of protein between endothelial cells and/or increased pinocytosis. This would also be the mechanism of edema in a local contusion or cerebral laceration. High protein edema would be expected to spread poorly in the gray matter. The protein content of the fluid would be excluded by the mucopolysaccharide fuzz coat of the cells. Some water would tend to remain with the protein osmotic molecule as would smaller ions. The edema would be expected to travel as one since the movement would not be diffusional because of changes in the interstitial matrix induced by ionic effects, but bulk flow from the injured area toward a more normal tissue. On reaching white matter with its lesser content of mucropolysaccharides and larger tissue spaces, spread of edema would occur more diffusely.

The edema described above is similar to the edema produced by the classic cold lesion of the cortex. The pathology of this lesion has been shown to be leakage of the tight endothelial junctions.[4] Uncharged protein molecules of 44,000 (peroxidase) spread through the gray matter but there is no change in gray extracellular space.[3,4] The protein edema front spreads to the underlying white matter and throughout the white matter to the ependymal surface and the opposite hemisphere. The flow is bulk flow as protein and sucrose move at the same rates. As the edema spreads, the white matter is expanded. It is still unclear how the protein is reabsorbed. Does it enter the CSF and circulate to be absorbed through the arachnoid villi? If so, would ventricular drainage (the use of the CSF as a sink) help? Would obliteration of the CSF spaces by hemispheric swelling or displacement prolong the period of resolution? There has been little study of the microcirculation in this type of edema. CBF studies using krypton and Xe show decreased blood flow that correlates well with increased water content.

Edema with increased protein permeability is found after contusion, and around inflammation and tumors. The edema is commonly accompanied by a neurological deficit which resolves with clearing of the edema. Thus, permanent change has not occurred in the neuronal connections involved. Present concepts suggest that local tissue pressure rises causing occlusion of capillaries and ischemia. It is well-established that when the mitochondrial oxygen tension falls below a critical level maximum respiration will not occur and thus function might be interfered with. The tissue pressure theory is based on decreased blood flow measurements which correlate with increased water content in the tissue. All our flow measurements are in units of m/100 g/min. Increasing the volume of the tissue being looked at by the clearance probe without increasing the number of capillaries will lead to a measured flow in m/100 g/min which has decreased. This is a real anatomic event but does not necessarily imply a decreased oxygen delivery per metabolically active unit. Relatively small decreases in capillary distance, 3–5 μ, seem to be capable of restoring tissue oxygen profiles in hypoxia or exercise.[6,15] The expected responses to an increase in intercapillary distance caused by edema would be an increase in the number of open capillaries. This would have a much better effect on tissue oxygen profile than an increase in flow.[19] As edema continued, there would be a completely dilated microvascular bed. Further O_2 needs would require an increase in flow from the arterioles. Thus, local areas of edema might have compensation of tissue O_2 needs at the expense of a completely dilated vascular bed. The bed would then manifest a pressure dependent flow profile (lack of autoregulation).

A further factor in cerebral edema is the presence of protein in the extravascular space. Recent studies show that oxygen diffusivity can be halved by increasing the albumin content in the media from 0 to 5 g%. A similar change is seen with gamma globulin concentrations from 0 to 2 g%.[30] Thus, in edema with increased permeability and therefore increased protein content, the deleterious effects on neurological function may be a combination of increased distance for oxygen diffusion and a decreased oxygen diffusivity secon-

dary to the protein content of the edema fluid. The concept of the capillaries as tunnel capillaries makes their compressibility that of the surrounding brain, making it highly unlikely that this type of edema can cause mechanical occlusion of capillaries.

The second form of edema that can result from capillary disturbances is that resulting from an increase in the capillary hydrostatic pressure and therefore fluid filtration. This is not accompanied by increased permeability to protein but again seems to effect mainly the extracellular space of the white matter. This type of edema can occur as a result of loss of autoregulation.[34] This is also the kind of edema found in pseudotumor cerebri. From what was said above we would not expect this type of edema to interfere with brain function until it caused significant elevation of the intracranial pressure such that there was a diminution in cerebral perfusion pressure. We would also expect this type of edema to be relatively diffuse. The importance of this type of edema in the clinic is hard to establish because we lack the methodology to demonstrate it. In pseudotumor cerebri, however, neurological function is usually well preserved until very high ICPs are reached.

Other types of cerebral edema, those due to anoxia, cell poisons, and water intoxication, are primary at the cell and do not bear on this discussion. However, evidence that chronic edema associated with lowered blood flow can exist in the face of normal neurological function has been obtained in triethyl tin induced edema.[10] The tremendous increase in white matter volume can readily been seen (Fig. 1). This we believe is the reason for the decreased CBF/100 g of tissue. The blood-brain barrier in this form of edema is intact, and the normal function of the animal strongly suggests that oxygen delivery to each metabolically active unit, "nutrient flow," is adequate for tissue demands. This argues in favor of the above theory that protein and disturbance of the interstitial space due to more than just water accumulation are necessary for cerebral dysfunction in edema.

Other microcirculatory events, e.g., viscosity changes, capillary occlusion by cell aggregates, thrombosis, etc., have not been examined in the cerebral circulation, but pathological data does not speak to their importance. The response to local trauma in small vessels is white cell and platelet adherence, short-term thrombosis, and prolonged endothelial adhesiveness. These un-

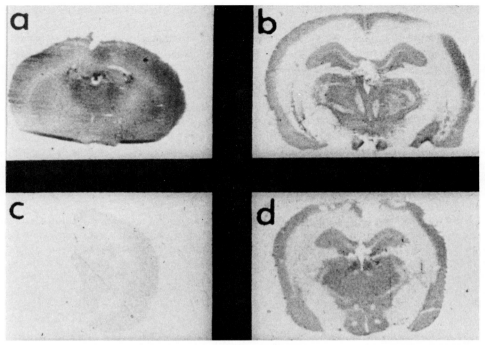

Fig. 1. Autoradiograph of rat brain following infusion of C^{14} antipyrine. (*a*) Normal control; (*b*) acute edema with low ICP; (*c*) acute edema with elevated ICP; (*d*) chronic edema. The edema induced with oral triethyl tin. In the acute cases 50 mg/l of water for 5 to 6 days; chronically 10 mg/l for 5 to 6 weeks. The rats with chronic edema (*d*) appeared to have normal behavior. Rats in (*b*) and (*c*) were very sick.

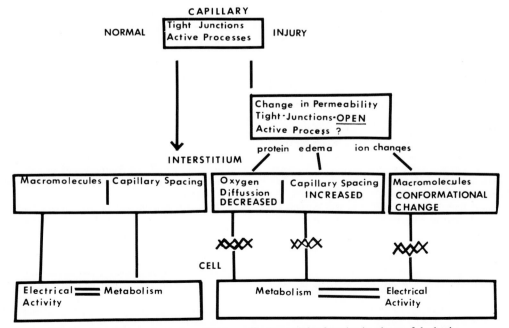

Fig. 2. Graphic representation of factors affecting cellular function in edema of the brain.

doubtedly occur and probably play a role in the changes that lead to edema in the brain. Indeed, the altered endothelial barrier may be caused by electrical charge changes leading to alterations in cell adherence and ion concentration.[25] Metabolic inhibitors have been shown capable of disrupting the barrier to protein and the role of metabolic processes in cell adherence has been pointed out.[32] These suggestions lend themselves to experimental verification. It is hoped that the use of extracellular markers, along with techniques of local flow and pressure measurements, oxygen profile, and neurophysiological recordings now available, will increase our understanding of the processes involved. The use of computerized axial tomography, both transmission and emission, to study the brain allow us to hope that markers can be developed that will be applicable in the clinic to study these processes in our patients. This will allow greater understanding of the pathophysiology and, we hope, lead to new and more specific treatments for the secondary events following head injury.

In summary, some recent concepts of the microcirculation and the importance of the interstitial space in exchange function have been briefly reviewed. An attempt has been made to see how these concepts might apply to the brain (Fig. 2). Emphasis has been placed on the interaction between the intercellular matrix and the capillary in edema. A tentative explanation for the lack of extracellular edema in the gray matter because of the interaction between the cell fuzz coats, water, and charged particles has been offered. In white matter, the larger spaces, and the organization of the tissue planes, the relative lack of polysaccharides allows expansion of the extracellular space. We suggest that cerebral dysfunction in proteinaceous edema is the result of increased capillary to cell distance for oxygen diffusion and decreased oxygen diffusivity because of the presence of protein in the fluid.

REFERENCES

1. Arteta JL: Effect of hyaluronidase on cat's brain. Proc Soc Exp Biol Med 91:440–442, 1956
2. Aukland K, Bower FB, Berliner RW: Measurements of local blood flow with hydrogen gas. Circ Res 14:164–187, 1964
3. Bakay L: The movement of electrolytes and albumin in different types of cerebral edema, in Biology of Neuroglia. Prog Brain Res 15:155–183
4. Baker RN, Cancilla PA, Pollock PS: The movement of exogenous protein in experimental cerebral edema. J Neuropathol Exp Neurol 30:668–678, 1971
5. Bondareff W: Electron microscopic evidence for the existence of an intercellular substance in rat cerebral cortex. Zellforsch Z 72:487–495, 1966
6. Bourdeau-Martini J, Honig CR: Direct measurement of intercapillary distance in beating rat heart in situ under various conditions of O_2 supply. Microvasc Res 1:244–265, 1969
7. Brightman MW, Klatzo I, Olsson Y, et al: The blood brain barrier to proteins under normal and pathological conditions. J Neurol Sci 10:215–239, 1970
8. Brightman MW, Reese TS: Junctions between intimately opposed cell membranes in the vertebrate brain. J Cell Biol 40:647–677, 1969
9. Brightman MW: The distribution within the brain of ferritin injected into cerebrospinal compartment. II. Parencymal distribution. Am J Anat 117:193–219, 1965

10. Bruce DA, Marshall LF, Graham DI, et al: The effect of triethyl tin sulfate on the behavior, blood flow, intracranial pressure and brain water content in the rat, in Lundberg N, Ponten U, Brock M (eds): Intracranial Pressure II, Berlin, Springer-Verlag, 1975, pp 280–284
11. Carter RD, Joyner WL, Renkin EM: Effects of histamine and some other substances on molecular selectivity of the capillary wall to plasma protein and dextran. Microvasc Res 7:31–48, 1974
12. Cosley-Smith, JN: The quantitative relationship between fenestrae in jejunal capillaries and connective tissue channels; proof of tunnel capillaries. Microvasc Res 9:78–100, 1975
13. Craijie FH: The architecture of the cerebral capillary bed. Biol Rev 20:133–146, 1945
14. Craigie FH: The comparative anatomy and embryology of the capillary bed of the central nervous system. Res Publ Assoc Res Nerv Ment Dis 18:3–28, 1937
15. Deimer K: Capillarization and oxygen supply of the brain, in Lubbers DW, Luft VC, Thews G, Witzel E (eds): Oxygen Transport in Blood and Tissue. Stuttgart, Thieme, 1968, pp 118–123
16. Feindel W, Yamamoto YL, Phillips K: Methodology of focal cerebral blood flow measurements by miniprobe scintillation and lithium-drifted silicon radioactive detector systems, in Russel R (ed): Brain and Blood Flow. London, Pitman, 1971, pp 29–33

17. Frei HJ, Wallenfang T, Poll W, et al: Regional cerebral blood flow and regional metabolism in cold induced edema. Acta Neurochir (Wien) 29:15–28, 1973

18. Fung YC, Zweifach BW, Intaglietta M: Elastic environment of the capillary bed. Circ Res, 19:441–461, 1966

19. Granger HJ, Shepherd AP: Intrinsic microvascular control of tissue oxygen delivery. Microvasc Res 5:49–72, 1973

20. Ingvar DH, Lassen NA: Regional flow of the cerebral cortex determined by Kr[85]. Acta Physiol Scand 54:325, 1962

21. Intaglietta M, DePlomb EP: Fluid exchange in tunnel and tube capillaries. Microvasc Res 6:153–168, 1973

22. Johnstone PC, Richardson DR: The influence of venous pressure on filtration forces in the intestine. Microvasc Res 7:296–306, 1974

23. Joyner WL, Carter RD, Raige, GS, et al: Influence of histamine and some other substances on blood lymph transport of plasma protein and dextran in the dog paw. Microvasc Res 7:19–30, 1974

24. Laurent TC: The exclusion of macromolecules from polysaccharide media, in Quintarecci G (ed): The Chemical Physiology of Mucopolysaccharides. Boston, Little Brown, 1965, pp 153–170

25. Lowenstein WR: Cell surface membranes in close contact. Role of calcium and magnesium ions. J Colloid Interface Sci 25:34–46, 1967

26. Margolis RV: Acid mucopolysaccharides and proteins of bovine whole brain, white matter and myelin. Biochem Biophys Acta 141:91–102, 1967

27. Meier-Ruge W, Gygax P, Iwangoff P, et al: The significance of pericapillary astroglia for cerebral blood flow and EEG activity, in Cervos-Navarro J (ed): Pathology of Cerebral Microcirculation. Berlin, de Gruyter, 1974, pp 235–243

28. Meyer FA, Silberberg A: In vitro study of the influence of some factors important for any physiolochemical characterization of loose connective tissue in the microcirculation. Microvasc Res 8:263–273, 1974

29. Mollgard K, Sorensen SC: The permeability of cerebral capillaries to a tracer molecule, alcian blue, with a molecular weight of 1390, in Cervos-Navarro J (ed): Pathology of Cerebral Microcirculation. Berlin, de Gruyter, 1974, pp 228–234

30. Navarri RM, Gainer JL, Hall KR: A predictive theory for diffusion in polymer and protein solution. AIChE 17:1028–1036, 1971

31. Pease DC: Polysaccharides associated with the exterior surface of epithelial cells, kidney, intestine, brain. J Ultrastruct Res, 15:555–588, 1966

32. Politoff A, Socolar SJ, Lowenstein WR: Permeability of cell membrane function; dependence on energy metabolism. J Gen Physiol 53:498–515, 1969

33. Renkin EM, Carter RD, Joyner WL: Mechanism of the sustained action of histamine and bradykinin on transport of large molecules across capillary walls in the dog paw. Microvasc Res, 7:49–60, 1974

34. Reivich M, Marshal WJS, Kassell N: Loss of autoregulation produced by cerebral trauma, in Brock M, Fieschi C, Ingvar DH, Lassen NH, Schuman K (eds): Cerebral Blood Flow, Clinical and Experimental Results. New York, Springer, 1969, pp 205–208

35. Rosenblum WI: Cerebral microcirculation: A review emphasizing the interrelationship of local blood flow and neuronal function. Angiology 16:485, 1965

36. Schmitt FO, Samson FE: Brain cell microenvironment. NRP Bull, 7(4): 1969

37. Stosseck K, Lubbers DW: Determination of microflow of the cerebral cortex by means of electrochemically generated hydrogen, in Russel R (ed): Brain and Blood Flow. London, Pitman, 1941, pp 80–84

38. Weiderhelm CA: The interstitial space, in Fung YC, Perrone N, Anliker M (eds): Biomechanics, Its Foundation and Objectives. Engelwood Cliffs, NJ, Prentice-Hall, 1972, pp 273–287

39. Wollam DHM, Miller JW: Perivascular spaces of the mammalian central nervous system. Biol Rev 29:251–283, 1954

40. Young IJ: Reversible seizures produced by neuronal hyaluronic acid depletion. Exp Neurol 8:195–202, 1963

41. Young IJ, Abood LG: Histological demonstration of hyaluronic acid in the central nervous system. J Neurochem 6:89–94, 1960

William K. Hass, M.D.

28

Cerebral Blood Flow and Metabolism after Experimental Brain Stem Trauma

Earlier in the conference I described to you in 45 patients with mild to severe head injury an inverse correlation between the level of cerebral oxidative metabolism (CMRO$_2$) and percentage of deaths attributable to the head injury itself. Also described was the resistance of this index of physiological function to hyperoxia, hypercarbia, and elevation of mean arterial pressure in selected patients in stupor or coma with or without brain stem signs.

Based on the observations of Ingvar et al. of a patient with destruction of the reticular core as a result of an infarct at the level of the superior colliculus who continued in a persistent vegetative state with a CMRO$_2$ of one-fourth normal for 3 years, we entertained the hypothesis that the brain stem dysfunction itself via depression of tonic stimulation by the reticular activating system accounted for a significant portion of the sharp and persistant decrease in CMRO$_2$.[1] It was postulated that the basic mechanism was a "switch" effect which possibly acted by sharply reducing total neural activity, thereby causing a sharp decrease in Na$^+$-K$^+$-ATPase activity and attendant O$_2$ utilization. In this regard, Whittam has demonstrated that at least 40 percent of a brain cell's production of ATP was utilized by the sodium-potassium stimulated membrane-bound ATPase system. Further, oxidative metabolism fell 40 percent when brain slices were exposed to ouabain. This work provided a rough estimation of the significant fraction of total energy of the brain

required to maintain the sodium-potassium pump.[2]

To test the concept that brain stem destruction by itself caused an *immediate* or *delayed* reduction in energy metabolism, multiple, large 2 × 2 mm steriotatic placed radio frequency lesions were placed in the mesencephalic reticular formation at the level of the Edinger-Westphal nucleus in awake rats. One hour before this, the animals had been placed on continuous ventilation and cu-rarized after briefly receiving a very small amount of ether for tracheotomy. A previously placed indwelling PE-50 arterial line permitted the measurement of mean blood pressure and arterial PO$_2$, P$_{CO_2}$, and pH. The EEG was monitored before, during, and after placement of the mes-encephalic lesions. Marked slowing of the EEG occurred. In lesioned animals, arterial blood gas and pH levels did not deviate significantly from normal values in lesioned, sham-lesioned, or control animals. One half-hour after placement of the radio frequency or sham lesions, brain samples were instantly obtained using a freeze blower technique. This technique described by Veech et al. permits recovery of 1 g of brain tissue *above* the site of the stem lesions as a thin homogenous pancake of tissue frozen within 1 second.[3]

Frozen samples were obtained from designated groups of 4 to 6 rats at zero time and at 15 and 30 seconds after decapitation. Control groups of 4 to 6 rats were similarly monitored and their brains were freeze blown at zero time or at 15 to 30 seconds after decapitation. Brain samples were analyzed for ATP, phosphocreatine and lactate by Lowry techniques.[4] Metabolite values in micro moles/gram at zero time were ATP 2.53

This project was supported by Grant No. NS07366 from the National Institute of Neurological Diseases and Stroke.

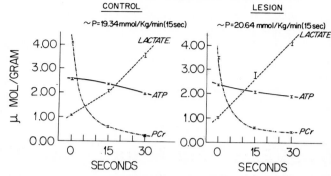

Fig. 1. Values for adenosine triphosphate (ATP), phosphocreatine (PCr) and lactate are shown to be essentially similar in control and mesencephalic RF acutely lesioned rats one half hour after placement of lesions both before and 15 to 30 seconds after decapitation.

± 0.03, phosphocreatine 4.07 ± 0.09, and lactate 1.07 ± 0.04. These values correspond very closely to those obtained by Veech et al.[3] The phosphocreatine values are higher than those found by Lowry in mice, probably because brain freezing takes place much more rapidly as a result of the freeze blowing technique than after immersion of a decapitated mouse head in liquid nitrogen. Zero time ATP, phosphocreatine, and lactate values in the RF lesioned animals were not significantly different from the controls. Metabolite values at 30 seconds after decapitation were approximately equal in all groups. High energy phosphate utilization calculated 15 seconds after decapitation in control and lesioned animals showed no significant differences. (Fig. 1)

These results suggested that the impairment of energy metabolism in patients with severe head

Table I

Regional Cerebral Blood Flow (rCBF) in Two Mesencephalic RF Lesioned Rats Compared to Two Controls One-Half Hour after Placement of Lesions Using a Modification of the ^{14}C-Antipyrine Technique for rCBF (No Significant Differences Are Observed in This Pilot Study)

Region	Normal (Reivich 1974)[5]	Normal (Study I)	Normal (Study II)	Lesion (Study III)	Lesion (Study IV)
Frontal cortex	—	0.74	0.67	0.68	0.56
Parietal cortex	0.63*	0.63	0.68	0.63	0.57
Occipital cortex	0.55	0.67	0.71	—	0.50
Thalamus	0.68	—	0.78	0.71	0.69
Caudate	0.60	0.64	0.67	0.60	0.61
Internal capsule	0.30	0.44	0.41	0.38	0.33
Cerebellar white	0.33	0.38	0.46	—	0.35
Cerebellar gray	0.65	0.70	0.63	—	0.64
Corpus callosum	0.32	0.41	0.46	0.38	0.31
Hippocampus	0.45	0.70	0.63	0.57	0.45
Mean arterial pressure	—	120	110	110	125
aP_{CO_2}	—	36	43	37	35

*Blood flow in milliliters/gram/minute.

injury was not an immediate or very early consequence of primary upper brain stem injury and disproves the "switch" hypothesis.

In addition, ^{14}C-antipyrine regional cerebral blood flow (rCBF) studies were performed in control and lesioned rats. Mean cerebral blood flows in control and lesioned rats showed no significant differences. Further, flow values for 10 regional areas in control rats showed a high degree of correlation with rCBF values reported by Reivich et al.[5] in rats, but contrasted with average cortical blood flows of 0.90 ml/g/min obtained by Eckloff et al.[6] in normocapneac rats using ^{14}C antipyrine and liquid scintillation counting rather than radioautography. (Table 1)

Thus, there was no immediate change in cerebral blood flow or metabolism due to brain stem lesions. The cerebral blood flow-metabolism couple is apparently maintained acutely. Similar results have recently been reported in dogs by Cucchiara and Mitchenfelder.[7]

Our very recent studies, however, suggest that two symmetrical RF lesions in the same mesencephalic reticular formation areas produce rats who can be maintained alive for 4 days or more on feeding via a stomach tube. They generally lie curled up, in a lethargic, stuporous state with extensor rigidity of the hind limbs in response to stimuli and appropriate running movements of the forelimbs in response to painful stimuli. When these animals' brains were freeze blown at 4 days, to our surprise *baseline* ATP and phosphocreatine values were reduced and lactate values were elevated.

The only present explanation we have for this phenomenon, which is now being carefully studied, is delayed multifocal or diffuse vasospasm, perhaps akin to that observed in human subarachnoid hemorrhage, creating significantly large areas of ischemia and correspondingly reduced baseline values for high energy phosphate compounds. We have, therefore, moved from the "switch" hypothesis to the concept that lesions in the brain stem set off a "cascade" of events which, via intrinsic vasogenic mechanisms possibly at the level of the microcirculation, causes persistent ischemia. These new observations in rats with brain stem injury after 4 days correlate with our observations in human head trauma and present us with what we believe will be an exciting model for the serial study of the changes in cerebral energy metabolism and blood flow which follow in the wake of an injury at a distance from the site of brain tissue studied.

REFERENCES

1. Ingvar DH, Sorander P: Destruction of the reticular core of the brain stem; a patho-anatomical follow-up of a case of coma of three years' duration. Arch Neurol 23:1–8, 1970
2. Whittam R: The molecular mechanism of active transport, in The Neurosciences. New York, Rockefeller Univ Press, 1967, pp. 313–325
3. Veech RL, Harris RL, Veloso D, et al: Freeze-blowing: a new technique for the study of brain in vivo. J Neurochem 20:183–188, 1973
4. Lowry OH, Passonneau SV, Hasselberger FX, et al: Effect of ischemia on known substrates and cofactors of the glycolyte pathway in brain. J Biol Chem 238:18–30, 1964

5. Reivich M: Blood flow metabolism couple in brain, in Brain Dysfunction in Metabolic Disorders. New York, Raven Press, 1974, pp 125–140
6. Eklof B, Lassen NA, Nilsson L, et al: Regional cerebral blood flow in the rat measured by the tissue sampling technique; a critical evaluation using four indicators C[14]-antipyrine, C[14]-ethanol, H[3]-water and xenon[133]. Acta Physiol Scand 91:1–10, 1974
7. Cucchiara RF, Michenfelder JD: The effect of interruption of reticular activating system on metabolism in canine cerebral hemispheres before and after thiopental. Anesthesiology 39:3–21, 1973

Carl Dila, M.D., Louis Bouchard, M.D.
Ernst Myer, M.S., Lucas Yamamoto, M.D.
William Feindel, M.D.

29

Microvascular Response to Minimal Brain Trauma

Many recent experimental studies of brain trauma have concentrated on changes found in rather extensive cerebral lesions involving cerebral edema or swelling, raised intracranial pressure, and alterations in cerebral circulation. Indeed, in clinical states these factors are often coexistent and interrelated. However, the very complexity and interrelationship of the many factors operative in cerebral injury have obscured the earliest changes, so that theories concerning the initial events in the pathogenesis of cerebral trauma have been inferred indirectly from observations made on extensive and far-advanced lesions.

The present study is concerned with the microvascular response of brain tissue to "minimal trauma," which, for present purposes, is defined as the least degree of trauma necessary to produce significant alterations in microregional cerebral blood flow. We have endeavored here to describe the cerebral equivalent of the cutaneous "triple response" described by Lewis,[1] a fundamental early and reversible response to mechanical brain trauma.

METHODS

In pentothal-anesthetized male mongrel dogs, a "minimal" lesion was made on the exposed cerebral cortex, using a spring-loaded mechanical impounder. In all experiments, the arterial pO_2

The work was supported in part by Medical Research Council of Canada Operating Grant MA 4949 (Carl Dila)

and systemic arterial blood pressure were maintained constant at normal values.

In 12 animals, the pattern of regional cerebral blood flow within the lesion was studied by means of serial fluorescein angiography[2] under conditions of normocapnia, hypocapnia, and hypercapnia. In an additional 5 animals, quantitative Xenon[133] microregional cerebral blood flow studies[3] were also carried out under normocapnic conditions. With each of these techniques, control studies were made prior to the creation of the minimal cerebral lesion, and the course of events was then observed for 1 hour following the lesion. At the conclusion of each experiment, the animal was sacrificed with an overdose of pentobarbital and the cerebral hemisphere was removed for histopathological study.

RESULTS

Grossly, the lesion produced by this method is sometimes indistinguishable from "normal" surrounding brain. There is no significant change in the caliber of the epicerebral vessels. In approximately 60 percent of cases, petechiae are seen grossly, and microscopic sections reveal petechiae within the cortical gray matter and the subjacent white matter. On fluorescein angiogram, "hang up" of the dye within the lesion in all experiments provides evidence of a break in the blood-brain barrier to protein.

The serial fluorescein angiograms were studied to determine the time of arterial and venous filling at the site of the lesion at intervals up to 1 hour posttrauma. Under normocapnic, hypo-

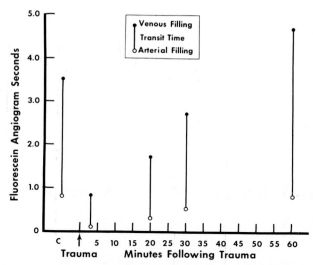

Fig. 1. Mean values of serial fluorescein angiograms in 12 experiments showing time of arterial and venous opacification up to 1 hour postminimal trauma.

capnic, and hypercapnic conditions, an identical pattern was observed: in the early period, up to 20 minutes posttrauma, there is a very rapid rate of arterial filling at the site of the lesion, and early draining veins are seen, resulting in a marked reduction in transit time through the lesion. In the period from 30 to 60 minutes posttrauma, this pattern reverts toward normal with respect to arterial filling at the lesion; there is, however, a delay in venous drainage of the lesion at 60

minutes, reflected in a prolonged transit time through the lesion 1 hour after trauma (Fig. 1).

In 5 animals, microregional cerebral blood flow studies using Xenon[133] revealed that the apparent "hyperemic phase" occurring early within a minimal cerebral lesion indeed represents a period of increased perfusion flow, followed by a restitution to the control values of rCBF during the period from 30 to 60 minutes following the lesion. In "other" areas of the hemisphere, at a

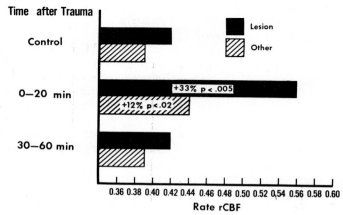

Fig. 2. Microregional CBF determinations using Xe^{33} clearance technique. In five experiments detectors were placed on the exposed brain at the site of the lesion and at a distance ("other").

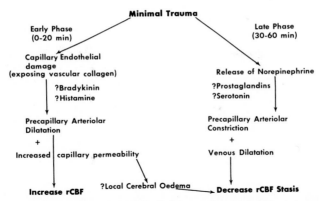

Fig. 3. Sequential pathophysiologic changes after minimal brain trauma.

distance from the lesion, there is also an apparent though less striking increase in rCBF following trauma (Fig. 2).

DISCUSSION AND SUMMARY

These data are consistent with earlier reports which under similar experimental conditions described "vasoparalysis"[4] or "loss of autoregulation"[5] and subsequently venous dilatation and stasis.[6] It seems clear that following a minimal mechanical trauma to the exposed cerebral cortex of the dog, a reversible or biphasic cerebrovascular response is observed. The increased rate of arterial filling and perfusion flow through the lesion within the first 20 minutes following trauma must be explained by dilatation of the precapillary (resistance) arteries and arterioles. During the period from 30 to 60 minutes following trauma, the restitution of the pattern and rate of regional cerebral blood flow to normal or even prolonged values implies the return of normal tone

and caliber of the precapillary resistance vessels or, perhaps, constriction of these vessels with simultaneous dilatation and stasis in the draining veins at the site of the lesion. This cerebrovascular response to minimal trauma is not modified by changes in arterial pCO_2 within the physiological range. The role of alterations of local tissue metabolites in the pathogenesis of this response must be determined, and consideration must also be given to the potential role of other vasoactive substances which might be locally released or carried to the area of the lesion, such as histamine or plasma bradykinins in the initial vasodilatory phase, and norepinephrine, prostaglandins, or 5-hydroxytryptamine (serotonin) in the later restitution or vasoconstrictive phase. The possibility of insipid local cerebral edema further contributing to the hemodynamic changes in the later phase must also be considered (Fig. 3). Appropriately designed experiments applying pharmacologic blocking agents in this experimental model may be used to test the various aspects of this hypothesis.

REFERENCES

1. Lewis T: The Blood Vessels of the Human Skin and Their Responses. London, Shaw, 1927
2. Feindel W, Yamamoto YL, Hodge CP: Intracarotid fluorescein angiography: a new method for examination of the epicerebral circulation in man. Can Med Assoc J 96:1, 1967
3. Yamamoto YL, Phillips KM, Hodge CP, et al: Microregional blood flow changes in experimental cerebral ischemia. Effects of arterial carbon dioxide studied by fluorescein angiography and Xenon[133] clearance. J Neurosurg 35:155, 1971
4. Marshall WJS, Jackson JLF, Langfitt TW: Brain

swelling caused by trauma and arterial hypertension. Arch Neurol 21:545–553, 1969

5. Reivich M, Marshall WJS, Kassell N: Loss of autoregulation produced by cerebral trauma, in Brock M, Fieschi C, Ingvar DH, Lassen NH, Schuman K (eds): Cerebral Blood Flow, Clinical and Experimental Results. New York, Springer, 1969, pp 205–208

6. Smith DR, Ducker TB, Kempe LG: Experimental in vivo microcirculatory dynamics in brain trauma. J Neurosurg 30:664–672, 1969

J. K. Vries, M.D.
R. Griffith, Ph.D.
D. P. Becker, M.D.

30

Continuous Observations of the Redox State of the Cortical Surface in Experimental Brain Injuries

The amount of ischemia which the brain can tolerate without irreversible damage is the subject of considerable controversy. The traditional threshold of 4 to 8 minutes is supported by extensive evidence in the literature.[2,3,6,9,13] Recently, however, Hossmann and his colleagues have demonstrated the return of metabolic and electrical activity in the brains of cats subjected to 60 minutes of complete ischemia.[7] The explanation for this difference in results is not immediately apparent. The experiments of Hossmann have been carefully controlled and extremely well documented. It is important to clarify this controversy because of its important prognostic and therapeutic implications.

In 1958, Chance and his co-workers developed a fluorometric technique for monitoring metabolic activity in vivo.[5] The technique was based on the fact that mitochondrial NAD shows a characteristic steady-state percentage of reduction, which is a function of the rate of oxidative phosphorylation and oxygen consumption.[4] Since NADH fluoresces at 468 mu when excited by ultraviolet light while NAD+ does not, measurement of tissue fluorescence at this wavelength provides continuous information about metabolic activity. This technique has been extended by Jobsis and his colleagues to demonstrate the relation between seizure activity in the cerebral cortex and metabolic activity, and by Rosenthal and Jöbsis to demonstrate the relation between cortical evoked potentials and metabolic activity.[8,10] We have used this technique in the present study to demonstrate the relationship between metabolic activity and spontaneous EEG activity in cerebral ischemia. A better understanding of this relationship may shed some light on the ischemic threshold controversy.

MATERIALS AND METHODS

Preparation of Animals

Adult cats weighing 2.5–3.0 kg were anesthetized with Nembutal 30 mg/kg given intraperitoneally. Cannulas were introduced into the femoral artery, the femoral vein, and the trachea. Each animal was placed on a volume respirator and spinalized via a cervical laminectomy. Blood pressure was maintained at a mean of 120 mm Hg after spinalization by a norepinephrine infusion. The following arteries or arterial trunks were ligated via a midline thoracotomy: the right and left internal mammaries, the right and left costocervicals, the right and left thyrocervicals, the left subclavian, the left vertebral, the left brachial, the mediastinal branch of the innominate, and the upper six intercostals on both sides. A special occlusive clamp was placed around the innominate in each animal, and a cannula was inserted into the right brachial artery. The right suprasylvian gyrus was then exposed via a 1 × 1 cm craniectomy. The dura was opened in a cruciate fashion and folded back over the bone edge to expose the cortex. A glass window was placed over the craniectomy site and sealed in place with dental cement.

Measurement of Fluorescence

The illumination from a 200 W mercury arc lamp was passed through a heat filter and the 366 mu line was isolated with an interference filter. The 366 mu line was projected on the cortex through the cranial window using an Ultropak optical system. A circular field 3.6 mm in diameter on the suprasylvian gyrus was observed with a Leitz microscope using a low power objective (3.8 X). Light incident on the cortex traveled up the barrel of the microscope to a beam-splitting prism. Ninety-five percent of the light went to an EMI 9524 photo multiplier tube equipped with an interference filter with peak transmittance at 468 mu. This registered the fluorescence. Five percent of the light went to an EMI 9524 photomultiplier tube equipped with an interference filter with peak transmittance at 366 mu. This registered the reflectance. The output from these photomultiplier tubes was amplified and written on chart paper. The output was also recorded on magnetic tape for computer analysis.

Recording the EEG

The EEG was recorded from screws in the skull which were in contact with the dura. The EEG signal was led into a Grass H1P511EF cathode follower and amplified by a Grass P511 preamplifier. It was displayed on an oscilloscope, written out on chart paper and recorded on magnetic tape for spectral analysis.

Monitoring Procedures

The blood pressure was monitored from both the femoral and brachial artery cannulas by means of Statham P-23 strain gauge transducers. Periodic blood gas determinations were made from the femoral artery cannula. The temperature was monitored via a rectal thermometer. During the course of the experiments the blood pressure was maintained at 120 ± 20 mm Hg, the pO_2 was maintained above 100 mm Hg, the pH was maintained between 7.35 and 7.40, and the temperature was maintained at $37.0 \pm .5°$ C.

Experimental Protocol

Animals were allowed to stabilize for 1 hour following completion of the surgical procedures. The fluorescence and reflectance were calibrated by adjusting their amplifiers to produce 1V of output on transition from no signal to baseline conditions. Saline was then injected into the brachial artery catheter and the ratio of the deflection in the fluorescence trace to the deflection in the reflectance trace was calculated. This ratio was used to correct the fluorescence trace for changes in blood volume in the field of observation.[8] A 25-minute baseline trace of the EEG, fluorescence, and reflectance was obtained at this point. Total cerebral ischemia was produced for periods of 1, 2, 3, 5, 10, 15, 30, or 60 minutes by closing the occluding clamp on the innominate artery. At the end of the ischemic period the clamp was opened and data for analysis was recorded for 120 minutes.

Data Analysis

Taped records of the EEG, fluorescence, and reflectance from successful experimental runs were analyzed by a Xerox Sigma computer utilizing a special program developed for this purpose. A continuous EEG power spectrum analysis was obtained through the use of a software filter system. The corrected fluorescence was calculated from the raw fluorescence and reflectance data using the correction factor mentioned earlier. Hard copies of the results of the computer analysis were written out on a Versatec line printer.

RESULTS

Twenty-four experiments were successfully completed and subjected to analysis. The response to clamping the innominate artery was similar in all animals. The fluorescence trace rapidly rose to a level about 150 percent of the baseline level, and the EEG activity ceased within 24 seconds. During the recovery phase after the innominate clamp was reopened, five patterns were identified which were a function of the duration of ischemia. The first pattern was seen in 1- and 2-minute animals. It consisted of a rapid drop in the fluorescence to a value 5 to 15 percent below the baseline, maintenance of this level for 1 to 2 minutes, and a gradual return to the baseline over 4 to 6 minutes. EEG activity returned in these animals in 30 to 60 seconds, and a normal spectral pattern was present within 1 to 2 minutes. The record of an animal subjected to a 1-minute period of cerebral

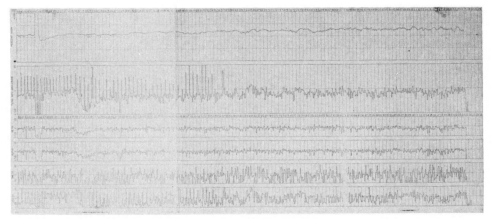

Fig. 1. The response of the corrected fluorescence and the spectrum of the EEG to a 1-minute ischemic insult.

ischemia is shown in Fig. 1. The second pattern was seen in 3-minute animals. The initial behavior of the fluorescence trace was similar to the 1- and 2-minute animals. However, after 4 to 6 minutes, the fluorescence trace overshot the baseline and remained elevated for about 10 minutes. Spontaneous EEG activity resumed at about 2 minutes in these animals, but a depression in the delta activity was present which persisted over 1 hour. The record of a 3-minute animal is shown in Fig. 2. The third pattern was seen in 5-minute animals. It consisted of a somewhat slower drop of the fluorescence to a level 5 to 10 percent below the baseline, persistance of this level for about 5 minutes, and a prolonged 5 to 10 percent overshoot of the baseline which lasted for over 30 minutes. EEG activity in these animals returned at

about 10 minutes. Marked depression in the delta range was present and mild alterations appeared in the higher frequencies. The record of a 5-minute animal is shown in Fig. 3. The fourth pattern was seen in 10- and 15-minute animals. It was characterized by a 5 to 10 percent undershoot which persisted for over 1 hour. In 4 of these animals, the EEG did not return within 120 minutes. In the 2 animals in which it did, the spectral analysis showed marked depression of the delta activity and a burst suppression pattern. It is interesting to note that EEG activity did not resume in these 2 animals until the fluorescence trace crossed the baseline. The record of a 15-minute animal is shown in Fig. 4. The final pattern was seen in 30- and 60-minute animals. The fluorescence trace was similar to that described

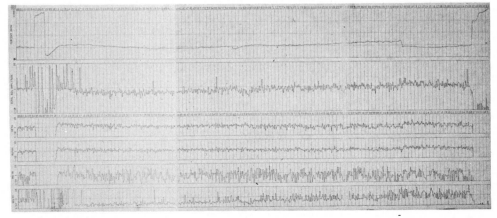

Fig. 2. The response of the corrected fluorescence and the spectrum of the EEG to a 3-minute ischemic insult.

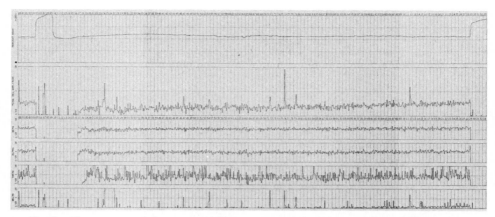

Fig. 3. The response of the corrected fluorescence and the spectrum of the EEG to a 5-minute ischemic insult.

for the 10- and 15-minute animals except that the initial drop below the baseline was markedly slowed. The EEG did not return within 120 minutes in any of the 30- or 60-minute animals.

DISCUSSION

The initial rise of fluorescence which occurs when the innominate is clamped reflects the fact that lack of oxygen at the mitochondrial level results in rapid reduction of NAD+ to NADH.[4,5,8] Loss of oxidative phosphorylation is associated with prompt cessation of the EEG. The factors responsible for inhibiting the EEG are not clear, however, since the intracellular phosphate energy charge is still relatively high at this point.[12] When circulation is restored, there is a rapid drop in fluorescence to a level of 5 to 15 percent below the baseline. This reflects the fact that ADP accu-

mulated during the ischemic period stimulates oxidative phosphorylation to rates higher than the baseline rate. This causes a higher percentage of the mitochondrial NAD fraction to become oxidized to NAD+. The fact that the fluorescence trace ultimately overshoots the baseline by 5 to 10 percent in animals subjected to ischemia of 3 minutes or greater indicates that the metabolic rates is lower than the baseline rate after the intracellular energy charge in these animals has been restored. This might occur as a result of substrate mobilization during the ischemic period, or it might indicate an inhibition of cellular metabolism. This latter hypothesis is supported by the fact that EEG activity in animals showing this phenomenon remains abnormal for a prolonged period of time. An even more interesting observation is the persistance of decreased fluorescence for periods of 1 hour or more in animals subjected to ischemic insults greater than 10 minutes. This

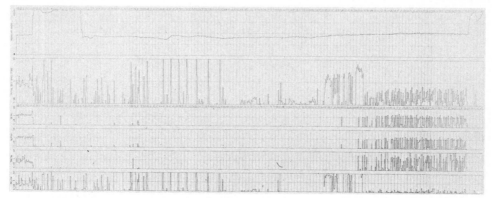

Fig. 4. The response of the corrected fluorescence and the spectrum of the EEG to a 15-minute ischemic insult.

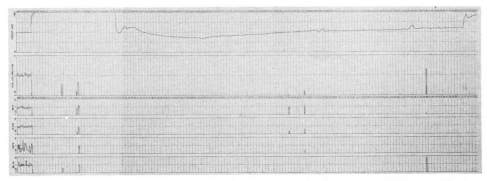

Fig. 5. The response of the corrected fluorescence and the spectrum of the EEG to a 30-minute ischemic insult.

suggests that the metabolic rate remains high far beyond the period of time necessary to restore intracellular energy charge in these animals. This could represent an uncoupling of oxidative phosphorylation, an increase in sodium potassium transport, or biosynthetic activity necessary to restore compounds catabolized during the ischemic period. It is interesting to note that the EEG activity shown in Fig. 4 did not return until this metabolic activity subsided. A final point worthy of note is the slow initial drop in the fluorescence in animals subjected to prolonged ischemia. In unpublished pilot studies, the authors demonstrated this could be overcome if the perfusion

pressure was increased from 120 mm Hg to 180 mm Hg. A perfusion pressure decrease to 90 mm Hg increased the phenomenon. This suggests that impairment of the microcirculation is present (no reflow) and that it is significant enough to have metabolic consequences.[1]

The results of this study suggest that a metabolic and electrical threshold is crossed when cerebral ischemia is prolonged beyond five minutes. Crossing threshold is characterized by prolonged unexplained metabolic activity in the cells, impairment of recirculation, and marked alterations in EEG amplitude and frequency content.

REFERENCES

1. Ames A III et al: Cerebral Ischemia: II. The no reflow phenomenon. Am J Pathol 52:437–453, 1968
2. Brierly JB, Meldrum BS, Brown AW: The threshold and neuropathology of cerebral anoxic ischemic cell change. Arch Neurol 29:367–372, 1973
3. Brown AW, Brierly JB: The earliest alterations in rat neurons after anoxia-ischemic. Acta Neuropathol 23:9–22, 1973
4. Chance B, Williams GR: Respiratory enzymes in oxidative phosphorylation. I–III. J Biol Chem 217:383–427, 1955
5. Chance B, Baltscheffsky H: Respiratory enzymes in oxidative phosphorylation. J Biol Chem 233:736–739, 1958
6. Grenell RG: Central nervous system resistance: I. The effects of temporary arrest of cerebral circulation for periods of two to ten minutes. J Neuropathol Exp Neurol 5:131–154, 1946
7. Hossmann KA, Sato K: Recovery of neuronal function after prolonged cerebral ischemia. Science 168:375–376, 1970
8. Jöbsis FF, O'Connor M, Vitale A, et al: Intracellular redox changes in functioning cerebral cortex. I. Metabolic effects of epileptiform activity. J Neurophysiol 34:735–749, 1971
9. Kabat H, Dennis C, Baker AB: Recovery of function following arrest of the brain circulation. Am J Physiol 132:737–747, 1941
10. Rosenthal M, Jöbsis FF: Intracellular redox changes in functioning cerebral cortex. II. Effects of direct cortical stimulation. J Neurophysiol 34:750–762, 1971
11. Schneider M: Critical blood pressure in the cerebral circulation, in Schade JP, McMenemey WH (eds): Selective Vulnerability of the Brain in Hypoxaemia. Oxford, England, Blackwell, 1963, pp 7–20.
12. Siesjö BK, Ljungren B: Cerebral energy reserves after prolonged hypoxia and ischemia. Arch Neurol 29:400–403, 1973
13. Weinberger LM, Gibbon MH, Gibbon JH Jr: Temporary arrest of the circulation to the central nervous system. I. Physiologic effects. Arch Neurol Psychiatry 43:615–643, 1940

Robert M. Berne, M.D.

31

Possible Role of Adenosine in the Regulation of Cerebral Blood Flow in Ischemia

Since the early 1960s evidence has accumulated to suggest that adenosine plays a role in the regulations of coronary blood flow and the observations of Deuticke and Gerlach[1] that ischemic brain also forms adenosine suggested that this nucleoside might also be involved in the regulation of cerebral blood flow. However, the studies of Byniski and Rapela[2] indicated that intraarterial infusions of adenosine produced negligible changes in cerebrovascular resistance. Recently the effect of adenosine on cerebral blood flow was reinvestigated since it seemed possible that adenosine did not cross the blood-brain barrier.[3] In dogs, ischemia was found to produce significant increases in cerebral adenosine levels as well as in the degradative products of adenosine, namely inosine and hypoxanthine and that these substances were released into the cerebrospinal fluid. Intraarterial infusion of adenosine confirmed the work of Byniski and Rapela,[2] but when the nucleoside was applied to the exposed superfused pial vessels of the cat, vasodilation was observed and the degree of vasodilation was roughly proportional to the concentration of adenosine in the artificial cerebrospinal fluid. In some experiments, the same pial arterioles were observed during intraarterial and topical administration of the adenosine. Only topical application elicited vasodilation.

Several experiments were conducted to determine to what extent adenosine crossed the blood-brain barrier. Intraarterial infusion of adenosine resulted in insignificant incorporation of the labeled adenosine into cerebral adenine nucleotides, whereas addition of the labeled nucleoside to the cerebrospinal fluid produced significant labeling of these compounds. Furthermore, an intravenous injection of adenosine in the rat resulted in a 20-fold greater incorporation of radioactivity in the cardiac than in the cerebral adenine nucleotides.

In another series of experiments, the effects of several interventions on adenosine production in brain tissues were carried out.[4] Electrical stimulation (5–10 V at up to 35 Hz) of the brain elicited a two- to threefold increase in the brain adenosine concentration. Reduction in brain perfusion pressure from 87 to 40 mm Hg produced a fivefold increase in cerebral adenosine levels. Moderate hypoxia (10 percent O_2 in the inspired air) gave a fivefold increase and severe hypoxia (5.5 percent O_2) gave a 10-fold increase in brain adenosine levels. Hyperventilation produced a twofold increase in cerebral adenosine levels whereas addition of CO_2 to the ventilating gas reduced the adenosine levels to below control values. Finally, lactate, pyruvate and cyclic AMP paralleled the changes in adenosine but the changes in cyclic AMP were small relative to those observed in tissue slices.[5]

From these observations, it can be concluded that adenosine is formed in brain tissue under a variety of conditions in which the oxygen supply fails to keep pace with the oxygen demand. In contrast to heart and other tissues, the adenosine does not readily escape into the venous blood, and hence there is probably little depletion of high energy phosphate stores in the brain. Our findings are compatible with a role for adenosine in the regulation of cerebral blood flow but the interrelationship between CO_2 and adenosine and the magnitude of the role of these two factors, as well as other possible metabolites remains to be elucidated.

REFERENCES

1. Deuticke B, Gerlach E: Abbau freier Nucleotide in Herz, Skeletmuskel, Gehirn und Leber der Ratte bei Sauerstoffmangel. Arch Ges Physiol 292: 239–254, 1966
2. Buyniski JP, Rapela CE: Cerebral and renal vascular smooth muscle responses to adenosine. Am J Physiol 217:1660–1664, 1969
3. Berne RM, Rubio R, Curnish RR: Release of adenosine from ischemic brain. Effect on cerebral vascular resistance and incorporation into cerebral adenine nucleotides. Circ Res 35:262–271, 1974
4. Rubio R, Berne RM, Bockman EL, et al: Relationship between adenosine concentration and oxygen supply in rat brain. Am J Physiol (in press)
5. Sattin A, Rall TW: Effect of adenosine and adenine nucleotides on the cyclic adenosine 3′,5′-phosphate content of guinea pig cerebral cortex slices. Mol Pharmacol 6:13–23, 1970

William E. Adams, M.D., M. Gary Hadfield, M.D.
Donald P. Becker, M.D., William F. C. Rigby, B.A.

32

Functional Alterations of Traumatized Synaptosomes

Acute mechanical brain injury may result in loss of consciousness, pronounced neurological deficits, or prolonged coma with minimal, if any, accompanying morphological changes. In these states the integrity of brain energy metabolism may be only minimally impaired.[9] Ischemic injuries have also been shown to have normal energy metabolism while brain electrical activity and neurological function remain severely depressed.[12] This information caused us to inquire into the integrity of neurotransmitter function following mechanical brain injury.

Ward,[23] in 1950, first published results suggesting the neurotransmitter acetylcholine played a role in central nervous system (CNS) trauma. The catecholamine pathways in the CNS were then documented in animals[1,5,6,11,22] and humans.[8] The literature regarding CNS trauma and neurotransmitters is quite confusing. The studies dealing with spinal cord trauma are concerned with two measurements of various neurotransmitter materials in the traumatized tissue and some of the studies suggest that the release of this material leads to further tissue damage.[10,14,16,17,18] Delatorre,[7] however, showed no alteration of catecholamine concentrations in traumatized spinal cords. The studies dealing with brain trauma have also measured various concentrations (levels) of neurotransmitters in the traumatized tissue and is just as confusing. Various authors have found elevated levels of various transmitters in the traumatized tissue,[2,3,15,24,25] while other authors find decreased levels.[7,13,20]

This caused us to question the integrity of neurotransmitter function following mechanical brain injury. This is a kinetic study of synaptosomal uptake of the neurotransmitter norepinephrine (NE) following an acute mechanical brain injury.

METHODS

Adult male Sprague-Dawley rats (250–350 g) were used. Trauma was inflicted by using the accelerating-decelerating device (Fig. 1) adopted from the original model of Sano.[19] All traumatized animals were subjected to the same force and all normal control animals were inserted into the device and allowed to fall, but not allowed to strike their heads. The animals were decapitated and the crude synaptosomal preparation of Axelrod, Snyder, Coyle, and others,[21] with minimal modifications, was obtained.

The whole brain, including the cerebellum and brain stem, was removed and weighed. The brain was then homogenized in 10 volumes of ice cold 0.32 M sucrose in a motor driven Polytef (teflon) pestle-glass tube system (0.25 mm clearance). The brain homogenate was centrifuged at 800 g for 10 minutes to remove nuclei, vessels, and debris. The supernatant was stirred to a uniform solution. Two hundred lambda of the supernatant suspension was then added to nylon test tubes which contained 3.8 cc Krebs-Henseleit solution with 1 percent glucose in which the calcium concentration was lowered by 50 percent, ascorbic acid (0.2 mg/ml), ethylenediaminetetra acetic acid (0.05 mg/ml) and varying concentrations (.5, .66, 1, and 2×10^{-7} M) of H^3-NE. All procedures prior to incubation were carried out at 0–4°C.

This mixture was then incubated in a Dubnoff

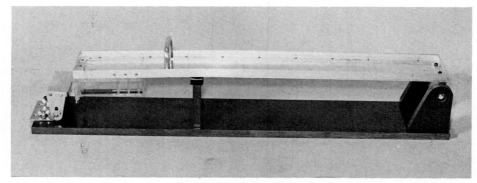

Fig. 1. Accelerating-decelerating head injury device. The animal is placed in the plexiglass container under the upper arm. The weight and height of the fall is the same for every traumatized animal.

metabolic shaker at 37°C. At the end of the incubation period the mixture was centrifuged at 39,-000 g for 30 minutes, washed with ice cold normal saline and centrifuged again at 39,000 g for 30 minutes.

The pellet was then dissolved in 10 cc of Triton X-100 in Toluene. The radioactivity was determined by using a liquid scintillation spectrometer.

Triplicate samples were used in all experiments. Medium samples were taken in order to calculate tissue: medium ratios, and triplicate samples were obtained at 0°C in order to determine the degree of passive diffusion.

RESULTS

Preliminary experiments were carried out to determine that the incubation period and tissue concentration were on the linear portion of the uptake curve. The accumulation of H^3-NE by normal and traumatized synaptosomes was subjected to Michaelis-Menten kinetics. Figure 2 is a graphic analysis of a double-reciprocal plot for the accumulation of H^3-NE. The normal animals yielded a Km value of 8.9×10^{-7}M and a V max of 0.958 m u mols/g tissue/4 minutes. Though values are not available in the literature for whole brain preparations, our values for Km and V max compare favorably with reports in a variety of normal discrete brain regions.

The traumatized animals cannot be analyzed by this method because their accumulation of H^3-NE was not a linear function. A graphic demonstration of accumulation as plotted against H^3NE concentration (Fig. 3) demonstrates this nonlinear relationship. This also demonstrates that accumulation is greater, at every concentration, in the traumatized group as compared with the normal controls. There was no significant

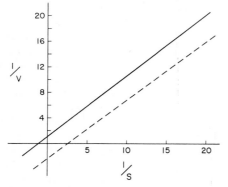

Fig. 2. Graphic analysis of reciprocals of H^3-NE concentrations and its uptake by whole brain homogenates. V = mu mols/g tissue/4 min. S = [NE] $\times 10^{-6}$ M.

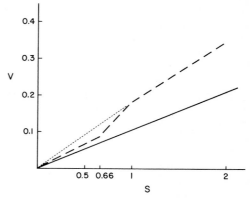

Fig. 3. Graphic analysis of H_3-NE concentrations and its uptake by whole brain homogenates. V = mu mols/g tissue /4 min. S = [NE] $\times 10^{-7}$ M.

difference in passive diffusion between normal and traumatized animals.

DISCUSSION

This is the first report of alteration of a neurotransmitter function following trauma. We have shown increases in NE uptake following trauma at every concentration studied. The exact way in which trauma alters the kinetics of synaptosomal uptake will have to await studies in myelin free preparations where a much broader range of NE concentrations can be studied. On the other hand, it is possible that trauma alters uptake in a manner that does not adapt itself to analysis according to Michaelis-Menton kinetics.

On the basis of the present data, however, it appears that both the uptake velocity and the membrane affinity for norepinephrine are increased following acute trauma. This very rapid reentry of neurotransmitter could alter neuronal function since reuptake is thought to be a principal mechanism for inactivating neurotransmitters. The question then is, How does trauma produce this increased uptake? We feel there are several possibilities.

1. Trauma may produce a primary release of neurotransmitter material. If this occurred, we could see a greater uptake as a result of this acute depletion. An electron-microscopy study published by Brown[4] in 1972 indeed describes a decrease in the number of synaptic vessicles present in axon terminals and presynaptic bulbs in animals sacrificed following mechanical trauma. This lends support to this hypothesis.
2. Trauma may alter the uptake sites to make more sites available or to increase the efficiency of sites present.
3. Or, trauma may damage the synaptosomal membrane so that it becomes "leaky." We did not find significant alterations in passive diffusion between the normal and traumatized animals, however, and we therefore tend to doubt this as a serious possibility.

At the present time, we tend to favor the first hypothesis but can easily see how severe trauma could damage the membrane and lead to further alterations in neurological function.

Further investigations of this type are necessary if we are to unravel the true pathophysiology or pathobiochemistry of head trauma.

REFERENCES

1. Anden NE, Dahlstrom A, Fuxe K, et al: Ascending nomamine neurons to the telencephalon and diencephalon. Acta Physiol Scand 67:313–326, 1966
2. Berman ML, Murray WJ: Effect of intrathecal epinephrine on rabbit spinal cord. Anesth Analg (Cleve) 51:383–386, 1972
3. Bowen FD: Alterations in catecholamines in local cerebral cortex lesions. Experientia 28:1082–1083, 1972
4. Brown WJ, Yoshida N, Canty T, et al: Experimental concussion. Am J Pathol 67:41–57, 1972
5. Cohen DL, Aladek JR: Evidence for the limited spread of intracerebrally applied serotonin. Brain Res 45:630–634, 1972
6. Dahlstrom A, Fuxe K: Evidence for the existence of monamine-containing neurons in the central nervous system. L. Demonstration of monamine cell bodies in the brain-stem neurons. Acta Physiol Scand 62:1–55, 1964
7. de la Torre JC, Johnson CM, Harris LH, et al: Monamine changes in experimental head and spinal cord trauma: Failure to confirm previous observations. Surg Neurol 2:5–11, 1974
8. de la Torre JC: Catecholamines in the human diencephalon: A histochemical fluorescence study. Acta Neuropathol 21:165–168, 1972
9. Elkelund L, Nilsson B, Ponten U: Carotid angiography after experimental head injury in the rat. Neuroradiology 7:209–214, 1974
10. Hedeman LS, Shellenberger MK, Gordon JH: Studies in experimental spinal cord trauma, Part I: Alterations in catecholomine levels. J Neurosurg 40:37–43, 1974
11. Karkari S, De Crescito V, Tomasula JJ, et al: Histochemical changes in feline spinal cord following intraspinal norepinephrine injection. J Histochem Cytochem 21:408–409, 1973
12. Marshall LF, Durity F, Graham DI, et al: The pathophysiologic, morphologic, metabolic, and flow consequences of severe experimental intracranial hypertension. Second Int Symp Intracranial Pressure, Lund, 1974
13. Matlina ESh, Rakhmanova TB: Adrenalin, noradrenalin, dopamine, and dopa in the blood and other tissues of albino rats following head injury. Biull EkSP Biol Med 63:55–57, 1967
14. Osterholm JL: The pathophysiological response to

spinal cord injury. The current states of related research. J Neurosurg 40:5–33, 1974

15. Osterholm JL, Bell J, Meyer R, et al: The neurological consequences of intracerebral serotonin injections. II. Trauma induced alterations in spinal fluid and brain. III. Serotonin-induced cerebral edema. J Neurosurg 31:408–421, 1969

16. Osterholm JL, Mathews GJ: A proposed biochemical mechanism for traumatic spinal cord hemorrhagic necrosis. Successful therapy for severe injuries by metabolic blockade. Trans Am Neurol Assoc 96:187–191, 1971

17. Osterholm JL, Mathews GJ: Altered norepinephrine metabolism following experimental spinal cord injury. I. Relationship to hemorrhagic necrosis post-wounding neurological deficits. J Neurosurg 36:386–394, 1972

18. Osterholm JL, Mathews GJ: Altered norepinephrine metabolism following experimental spinal cord injury. II. Protection against traumatic spinal cord hemorrhagic necrosis by norepinephrine synthesis blockade with alpha-methyltryosine. J Neurosurg 36:395–401, 1972

19. Sano K, Hiroshi H, Kamano S: Steroids and the blood-brain barrier with reference to astrocytic cells, in Reulen HJ, Schurmann K (eds): Steroids and Brain Edema. Berlin-New York, Springer, 1972, pp 177–193

20. Shirinyan EA: Catecholamine metabolism in the tissues of guinea pigs after head injury. Biull EkSP Biol Med 71:46–49, 1971

21. Snyder SH, Coyle JT: Regional differences in H³-norepinephrine and H³-dopamine uptake into rat brain homogenates. J Pharmacol Exp Ther 165, 1969

22. Ungerstadt U: Sterotoxic mapping of the monamine pathways in the rat brain. Acta Physiol Scand 367:1–47, 1971

23. Ward A: Atropine in the treatment of closed head injury. J Neurosurg VII: 398–402, 1950

24. Weitzman ED, Rapport M, McGregor P, et al: Sleep patterns of the monkey and brain serotonin levels. Science 160:1361–1363, 1968

25. Welch KMA, Meyer JS, Teraura T, et al: Ischemic anoxia and cerebral serotonin levels. J Neurol Surg 16:85–92, 1972

Edited by Michael O'Connor, M.D.
and Thomas Langfitt, M.D.

Open Discussion

In acute experiments, the disassociation between the frequency of the EEG and the apparent metabolic rate, as described by Hass in animals with brain stem lesion, is in contradistinction to what is generally thought to be true, namely that the metabolic rate is lower when low frequency activity dominates the EEG. Initially it was thought that cortical blood flow was the same in delta wave sleep as it was in the awake animal. However, differences were subsequently demonstrated by the antipyrine technique. Therefore, one might have expected to find regional differences in flow in Hass' study. There are no apparent differences in regional flow between lesioned and control animals (Table 1, p. 210). Regional changes in metabolism were not evaluated in this study.

This interesting work then points strongly toward a preservation of metabolic rate inspite of EEG slowing following a high brainstem lesion. There is relatively little data available concerning the metabolic effects, especially the regional metabolic effects of such a lesion. Hopefully, this study will mark the advent of increased investigation in this area.

Minimal or threshold brain injury as described by Dila as an experimental tool has the disadvantage that rarely is a threshold stimulus encountered in the clinical situation. However, it has the distinct advantage of permitting evaluation of initiating events and thus possibly of distinguishing between the primary and secondary effects of the trauma.

The study by Vries and collaborators demonstrates clear differences in both electrical and metabolic recovery following variable periods of cerebral ischemia. The origin and the effects of these differences are important to the understanding of the irreversible damage resulting from prolonged ischemia.

With regard to the electrical phenomena, it is interesting to note the selective suppression of delta activity in Figs. 2 and 3, pp. 219, 220. Higher frequency activity usually has a more focal distribution and may be dependent on a fairly restricted superficial portion of the brain. Therefore, these changes may reflect increased vulnerability of longer, more complex neuronal pathways. Such interpretations, however, are hazardous due to our poor understanding of the origins of the EEG.

An interesting technical point is the occasional, rather marked discrepancy between the visual interpretation and the computer analysis of the EEG. Personal experience by one of us (O'Connor) suggests a trend toward a computer overestimation or a visual underestimation of the higher frequency activity. Such variations are probably dependent on the computer program used. There are two problems that make interpretation of the fluorometric data somewhat difficult. The first deals with the artifact induced in the fluoresence transient by changes in vascularity of the field. Appropriate corrections have been made in the fluorescence traces in this report for small changes in hemoglobin content in the field. It is possible, however, that there may be slight changes in the waveform of the fluorescence transient with more extreme changes in vascularity.

The second difficulty arises from the fact that the NADH concentration is a result of a dynamic equilibrium. Therefore, on a long-time scale, it is difficult to say whether a rise in NADH is due to decreased oxidation or increased production (substrate activation) of NADH.

In the discussion of the paper by Berne, the question arose as to how much of the vasodilatation with hypoxemia or oligemia is due to increased hydrogen ion concentration and how much might be due to the increased concentration of adenosine. Another issue was whether there was a link between hydrogen ion concentration and adenosine.

Plum pointed out that Siesjo has shown that there is a progressive rise in blood flow with anoxia before there is a detectable rise in tissue lactate. Berne noted that studies in the heart have shown that the reactive hyperemia produced by a brief period of ischemia is paralleled by changes in adenosine concentration in heart tissue. Similar studies have not been done in the brain.

Pickard cited evidence that low-dose infusions of nonadrenaline increase cerebral blood flow and oxygen and glucose consumption after disruption of the blood-brain barrier by a modification of Rappaport's technique using hypertonic urea. Pickard's own work has shown that hypertonic urea alone does not change cerebral blood flow or brain oxygen and glucose consumption. Since adenosine does not penetrate the blood-brain barrier, a technique such as this one might be useful in evaluating the effects of adenosine administered intravenously. Pickard also suggested that when evaluating various "spasmogens," one might consider more fundamental factors related to contraction, specifically ionized calcium. He pointed out that the control of intracellular ionized calcium concentration is highly complex involving membrane pumps in sarcoplasmic reticulum and mitochondria, sodium-calcium exchange in the membrane, and a calcium permeability mechanism. The role of prostaglandins as well as many other agents should be studied in terms of intracellular calcium metabolism.

Flamm noted that agents that produce aggregation of platelets, such as norepinephrine, ADP, and some of the prostaglandins also are associated with vasoconstriction. In contrast, agents that inhibit platelet aggregation, such as adenosine, isuprel, aspirin, and tricyclic antidepressants are associated with vasodilatation. He added that many of these agents appear to exert their effect by a similar mechanism, namely an increase in cyclic AMP in the vascular smooth muscle, produced either by stimulation of adenylate cyclase or by inhibition of phosphodiesterase.

Commenting further on the mechanism of vasodilatation, Flamm cited evidence that cyclic AMP increases the sarcoplasmic binding of intracellular calcium and also decreases smooth muscle cell permeability to calcium thereby preventing the coupling of actinomycin. He expressed the opinion that in experimental cerebral vasospasm cyclic AMP in vascular smooth muscle could be manipulated in order to prevent or reduce the vasospasm.

Berne cited experimental work by others demonstrating that adenosine is almost as effective as catecholamines in increasing cyclic AMP levels in brain slices. He repeated these studies in intact animals and was able to increase cyclic AMP but not to the degree that occurred in brain slices. The effect on slices was about 30-fold greater.

Berne added that there has been a dispute on the role of prostaglandins in the coronary circulation and that some investigators have postulated that prostaglandins contribute to autoregulation in the brain and the kidney. However, Berne was unable to verify this hypothesis in his studies of the heart. There is also evidence from Berne's lab that prostaglandins release adenosine in the heart.

Regarding the mechanism of action of adenosine, he expressed the opinion that adenosine may act through changes in calcium permeability. Aminophyllin, for example, accelerates the influx of calcium and produces contraction. This can be opposed in frog sartorius by the administration of adenosine. In guinea pig atrium, if the fast sodium exchange is blocked or partial depolarization is induced with potassium, then the calcium current can be eliminated with physiological concentrations of adenosine. Addition of adenosine deaminase results in the immediate return of calcium current. Therefore, there is some evidence that the effect of adenosine may be mediated through calcium rather than through cyclic AMP.

Adams hypothesized that there is increased release of norepinephrine following trauma or that trauma may alter the uptake sites at the synaptosomal level. Tissue levels of catecholamines in traumatized central nervous tissue and their role in progressive ischemia have been controversial. Kobrine commented that he had data contradicting Osterholm's theory of catecholamine mediated spreading ischemia of the white matter. In animals rendered permanently paraplegic with a 600 g cm impact to the spinal cord, he found an increase, not a decrease in flow in the lateral white matter at the level of the lesion. Because of observations from Ransohoff's laboratory that histamine is increased in traumatized spinal cord, Kobrine investigated the effect of antihistamines, which block both the H_1 and H_2 receptor sites, on the vascular response to cord trauma. He found that in animals treated with chlorpheniramine and meperidine, the white matter hyperemia was abolished.

Rosenblum pointed out that in experiments in which peroxidase is used to evaluate the status of the blood-brain barrier, antihistamines are commonly given to prevent an anaphylactic reaction to the peroxidase. In light of Kobrine's data, this may have significant effects. That is, if part of the response to trauma is hyperemia, and this is blocked by antihistamines, then the data obtained from animals treated with antihistamines to prevent anaphylactic reaction will not be truly representative of the tissue reaction of trauma. Brightman pointed out that in mice and in one strain of rat, anaphylactic reactions to peroxidase do not occur.

V

Pressure-Volume Relationships

Discussion Editors:
Romas Sakalas, M.D.
Donald Becker, M.D.

33

A. Marmarou, Ph.D.
K. Shulman, M.D.

Pressure-Volume Relationships—Basic Aspects

THE INTRACRANIAL COMPLIANCE

The intracranial compartments which include blood, brain, and CSF are normally in a state of pressure and volume equilibrium. An increase in volume of one intracranial compartment must be accompanied by a decrease in one or more of the other compartments so that the total volume remains fixed. When this volume alteration involves the CSF space, the fluid pressure of the CSF is changed, and the magnitude of pressure change will depend on the amount of volume and the rate at which the interchange takes place. The change in CSF volume per unit change in pressure defines the "extensibility" of the CSF space, and within the rigid skull, this extensibility is provided by the resilient properties of the vasculature. In physical terms, the extensibility is quantified by a compliance ($\triangle V/\triangle P$) which is equivalent to the slope of the CSF volume versus pressure curve obtained by adding known amounts of fluid into the CSF space and recording the rise in pressure.

Many inanimate containers have "ideal" elastic properties. Such properties include a coefficient of compliance which does not vary with time and is constant for all degrees of expansion of the container. In such an "ideal" container, pressure varies linearly with volume and the slope of the volume pressure curve, or compliance is a constant. Pressure and volume in the cerebrospinal fluid compartment are not linearly related. For equal volume increments the $\triangle V/\triangle P$ ratio, or compliance decreases as pressure increases. This was first demonstrated by Ryder and Evans[1] in 1953, who described the general form of the curve as "hyperbolic." They also concluded that when the volume equilibrium was disturbed, the induced pressure and net seepage of fluid into or out of the cerebrospinal fluid space was in the direction to return the pressure to its original value.

Our studies have confirmed this nonlinear relationship between pressure and volume. Our analysis of the hydrodynamics involved in this process support Ryder's concept of dynamic equilibrium in that when intracranial compliance is measured by addition or withdrawal of fluid from the CSF space, the reaction is completely reversible and both pressure and volume return to their original resting level. Thus, the pressure-volume curve, in addition to providing an index of compliance, can be interpreted as a graphical representation of all possible equilibrium points and transient changes of CSF pressure. For this reason, the P-V curve is of fundamental importance in the understanding of mechanisms leading to sustained elevations of the ICP. A stable intracranial pressure is analogous to a point (Q_1) of the exponential CSF pressure-volume curve which remains stable (Fig. 1). Small perturbations in volume such as those produced by vascular pulsation will cause the point to shift back and forth on the trajectory described by the P-V curve. The corresponding changes in pressure can be evaluated by projecting onto the pressure axis. A permanent increase of intracranial pressure level represents a shift of the operating point to a new location of the curve (Q_2). The same perturbations in volume at raised ICP will result in an increase of the magnitude of pulsations due to the increased slope. Compliance then is not uniform throughout the range of pressure. As volume is measured the slope tends toward the pressure axis which accounts for the increased pulse pressure observed at high levels of ICP. The numerical value for compliance ($\triangle V/\triangle P$) will then depend upon the point of the curve or the pressure at which it is evaluated.

THE PRESSURE-VOLUME INDEX (PVI)

We have taken advantage of the fact that in an exponential process, there is a unique relationship between the slope ($\triangle V/\triangle P$) and pressure P. By plotting pressure data on a logarithmic axis against volume, the resulting $\triangle V$-logP curve can be approximated by a straight line (Fig. 2). The slope of the straight line was defined by us as the pressure-volume index (PVI).[2] Compliance at any pressure (P) can be computed by dividing (P) into the PVI (c = .4343 PVI/P).

In more practical terms, the PVI can be defined as the amount of volume (milliliters) necessary to raise the CSF pressure by a factor of 10 and thus does not require specifying equilibrium pressure level when describing the degree of intracranial extensibility.

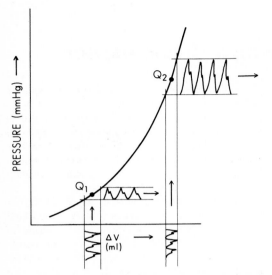

Fig. 1. A stable intracranial pressure is analogous to a point (Q_1) of the exponential CSF pressure volume curve which remains stable. A sustained increase of ICP represents a shift of the operating point to a new location of the curve (Q_2). Magnitude of pulsatile components increase as compliance is reduced.

PRESSURE-VOLUME CURVE

The pressure-volume curve is obtained by inserting known volumes into the CSF space and measuring the corresponding rise in pressure. In this process, the rate of volume addition must be considerably higher than the rate of CSF absorption to avoid errors due to normal compensation. However, the rate of injection must be below that level which causes vasodilatation and alteration of the original resting pressure. In our work with animals, the maximum rate of injection does not exceed 0.1 ml/sec. The peak pressures are then plotted on a semilogarithmic scale against volume

and the PVI is extrapolated from the slope of the curve. With this technique, the pressure rises abruptly and gradually returns to equilibrium which satisfies the physiological restriction of a completely reversible reaction.

The technique of CSF volume alterations described here involves a reversible, reciprocal exchange between vascular and CSF compartments; an increase of CSF volume is accompanied by a decreased intracranial blood volume, while brain tissue volume remains fixed. This model of a reversible reaction can be contrasted with a nonreversible model, such as the tissue response to balloon expansion studied by Langfitt.[3] Both produce exponential curves; the difference in curve configuration can be explained by the fact that the expanding balloon simulates a permanent increase in brain mass which must be compensated by a reduction of both blood and CSF compartments. As balloon volume reaches a critical point of expansion, loss of CSF compensation occurs. The end point is a sustained elevation of pressure which, in the steady state, is nonreversible.

DISTRIBUTION OF COMPLIANCE

The value of compliance obtained by the addition or removal of CSF volume represents the combined storage ability of both cerebral and spinal compartments. We have found in the cat that two-thirds of the available compensatory reserve is contained within the cranial compartment. Lofgren and Zwetnow[4] studied compliance distribution in dogs and reported a 50 percent contribution by the spinal axis above 20 mm Hg ICP. Lim and Potts,[5] in studies of dogs with aqueduct stenosis, reported that 52 percent of total

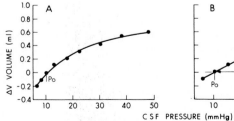
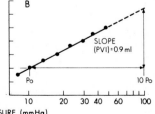

Fig. 2. By plotting pressure on a logarithmic axis, the resulting V-logP curve can be approximated by a straight line. The slope of this straight line segment is defined as the Pressure Volume Index (PVI) and is numerically equivalent to the amount of volume (milliliters) necessary to raise pressure by a factor of 10.

compliance was attributed to the combination of infratentorial and spinal compartments. Combining the results of these studies with out data, we estimate a compliance distribution of 48 percent supratentorial, 20 percent infratentorial, and 32 percent spinal.

Distribution in man can be derived from pressure studies by Gilland[6] of patients with spinal block and results of infusion tests by Katzman.[7] Our calculations, based on the analysis of this data, show that the total PVI in humans is approximately 30 ± 5 ml with a two-thirds to one-third distribution between cerebral and spinal compartments.

We reviewed the earlier work by Ryder et al.[1] with great interest since it represents the only study found in the literature where pressure-volume characteristics were obtained in humans over a pressure range of 2.5 to 118 mm Hg. The PV studies were performed using the bolus injection technique in a series of 30 patients with diverse intracranial disorders. The initial resting pressure averaged 11.9 mm Hg (S.D. = 8.08). The volume added ranged from 7 to 45 ml (mean = 20.6, S.D. = 10.9 ml) resulting in induced peak pressure of 10.3 to 118 mm Hg (mean = 51.8, S.D. = 23.6). The pressure-volume index (PVI) calculated from the response to bolus injection averaged 31.6 ml (S.D. = 14.4 ml). In a more recent study by Cohadon et al.[8] involving 8 normal patients, the limits of the pressure-volume curves were closely approximated by the exponential relationships $P m H = e^{.048v}$ and $P = e^{.060v}$. By our calculations, the exponential equations are equivalent to a PVI range of 38.4 to 48.3 ml.

Miller et al.[9] have studied the volume-pressure ratio (VPR) in head injured patients and have examined the relationship of the VPR to the resting level of the ICP. The VPR, introduced by Miller, is obtained by inserting a fixed increment of volume (1 ml) into the CSF space and computing the ratio of pressure to volume ($\triangle P/\triangle V$). This ratio ($\triangle P/\triangle V$) defines the magnitude of "elastance" (reciprocal of compliance) associated with the resting pressure at which it is measured. In an exponential process, the relationship of VPR measured at pressure P to the pressure-volume index (PVI) is given by the equation VPR = P/.4343PVI. If the shape of the pressure-volume curve remains fixed, the PVI is a constant and the VPR will vary linearly with pressure as a natural consequence of the exponential curve. With this concept, changes in the overall pattern of in-

tracranial elasticity are indicated only when VPR deviates from normal values at equal levels of pressure.

CALCULATIONS OF OUTFLOW RESISTANCE

The response of pressure to bolus injection serves a dual purpose. The initial rise in pressure is used to calculate the pressure-volume index (PVI) as compliance, while the rate of return provides data for calculating the resistance to fluid absorption.[10] The outflow resistance parameter (Ro) is a quantitative index and is a direct measure of the impedance offered to the egress of CSF. An increase in the resistance of fluid absorption increases the recovery time to equilibrium. The value of outflow resistance obtained from the response to bolus injection is similar to values measured by other methods and the single injection technique has been applied in determining the distribution of absorption between cerebral and spinal compartments.

It is our concept that the outflow resistance (Ro) in combination with a measure of intracranial compliance are the major parameters which determine both steady-state and transient characteristics of the ICP. Under normal circumstances, resistance remains fixed for elevations of pressure. In this case, the ICP will remain stable at a resting level determined by the absolute value of R. If the PVI or intracranial compliance is reduced so that resistance is no longer independent of pressure, a loss of dynamic equilibrium occurs resulting in a progressive increase of ICP.

CLINICAL APPLICATION

Our protocol for clinical evaluation is designed to provide data for the evaluation of both intracranial compliance and resistance to absorption. The protocol is subdivided into six segments. In the first segment, the resting VFP is monitored for a period of 10 minutes. The resting record is examined and average VFP is determined. During a period of stable VFP an amount of fluid is removed to reduce the VFP by 5 mm Hg, and sufficient time is allotted for pressure to return to the original resting level. From the removal data, the intracranial compliance (PVI) is calculated. This allows us to estimate the peak pressure that would result in response to bolus additions of fluid and clinical judgment is used to determine the amount of volume to be added by bolus injection. The rate of injection does not exceed 1 ml/2 sec. Sufficient time is allotted for pressure to return to equilibrium after each injection. Data extracted from the response to bolus injection is then used for calculation of intracranial compliance and outflow resistance throughout the range of pressure. In the final segment, fluid is removed at a fixed rate of 0.3 ml/min to circumvent the absorption mechanism and provide an estimate of venous exit pressure. The information derived from these studies form the basis of a separate report.

SUMMARY

The exponential variation of pressure to volume relationship complicates the quantification of intracranial compliance. As pressure increases, the intracranial contents become more rigid and compliance varies throughout the range of pressure. It is therefore necessary in the application of this concept to distinguish between changes of compliance which occur as a natural consequence of increased pressure and changes in the shape of the entire curve. By plotting pressure-volume data on a logarithmic pressure versus linear plot, the exponential curve can be approximated by a straight line. The slope of this line on a semilog is equal to the PVI and can be defined as the amount of fluid volume (milliliters) necessary to raise pressure by a factor of 10. The PVI in a random population of neurosurgical patients ranged from 10 to 50 ml. As the brain becomes more rigid, storage ability decreases and the pressure-volume index is reduced. The quantitative measurement of intracranial compliance and impedance to egress of fluid adds new information to aid in the understanding of the biomechanical processes leading to sustained elevations of the ICP.

REFERENCES

1. Ryder HW, Espey FF, Kimbell FD, et al: Mechanism of the change in CSF pressure following an induced change in the volume of the fluid space. J Lab Clin Med 41:428–435, 1953
2. Shulman K, Marmarou A: Pressure volume considerations in infantile hydrocephalus. Dev Med Child Neurol 13:90–95, 1971
3. Langfitt TW, Weinstein JD, Kussel WF: Cerebral vasomotor paralysis produced by intracranial hypertension. Neurology 15:662–641, 1965
4. Lofgren J: Pressure-volume relationships of the cerebrospinal fluid system. Univ of Goteborg, 1973
5. Lim ST, Potts DG: Ventricular compliance in dogs with and without aqueductal absorption. J Neurosurgery 39:463–473, 1973
6. Gilland O.: CSF dynamic diagnosis of spinal block. II: The spinal CSF pressure-volume curve. Acta Neurol Scand 41:487–496, 1965

7. Katzman R, Hussey F: A simple constant-infusion manometric test for measurement of CSF absorption. I. Rationale and method. Neurology 20:534–544, 1970
8. Cohadon F, Noillant A, Richard I, Vanderdressche M: Volume pressure relationship in clinical and experimental conditions of raised ICP. Proc 2nd Int Symp Intracranial Pressure, Lund, June 1974
9. Miller JD and Garibi J: Intracranial volume pressure relationships during continuous monitoring of ventricular fluid pressure, Brock M, Dietz H (eds): in Intracranial Pressure. Berlin, Springer, 1972, pp 270–274
10. Marmarou A, Shulman K, LaMorgese J: A compartmental analysis of outflow resistance. J Neurosurg 43:523–534, 1975

Open Discussion

DR. MARMAROU: We find that when the intracranial pressure is raised by artificial means; namely, infusion or additional volume to the cerebrospinal fluid space, the imedance to outflow remains constant and does not change with pressure. It is only when we induce changes in pressure by balloon compression or some similar method that we see the changes in outflow impedance.

DR. HUNT: Our data, obtained by fluctuating an animal's arterial blood pressure by pumping blood in and out of the aorta in a period shorter than 4 to 6 seconds so that autoregulation does not have a chance to occur, show that in the physiological range there is a dynamic pressure-flow relationship. What changes is the intercept of the baseline, which represents the critical closing pressure. We think a great deal of the autoregulatory mechanism is the adjustment of the critical closing pressure without dilation and without constriction in the cerebral vessel.

MR. SYMON: Although I am familiar with the work mentioned, the interaction between such things as the CO_2 response and the autoregulatory curve or between other vasodilators and the autoregulatory curve can only be explained if the autoregulatory curve is a function of progressive relaxation of vascular resistance, and not in terms of critical closing pressure.

MR. SYMON: Dr. Marmarou, did you derive your pulse data from animals or from your prediction?

DR. MARMAROU: All of the data you see in terms of the compliance measurements in outflow resistance were obtained from animals and checked with the dynamics as predicted by the computer study.

34

J. Douglas Miller, M.D., Ph.D., F.R.C.S (Glasgow),
F.R.C.S (Edinburgh)

Clinical Aspects of Intracranial Pressure-Volume Relationships

Relationships between raised intracranial pressure, cerebral blood flow, and neurological dysfunction are hard to define precisely because the factors of time and concomitant brain shift also operate. Thus, all patients with high intracranial pressure do not demonstrate neurological dysfunction, and some unconscious patients with severe brain damage have normal intracranial pressure.[2] Nevertheless, sustained intracranial hypertension is a declaration of failure in the system for volumetric compensation and demands treatment. The relationship between changes of volume and changes of pressure in the craniospinal axis plays a central role in determining the frequency and the extent to which intracranial pressure increases in patients with a wide array of brain disorders, tumors, hemorrhage, ischemia, inflammation, and injury. This pressure-volume relationship is therefore of fundamental importance to the management of such patients. This review focuses on measurements of intracranial pressure in patients with head injury, considering aspects of diagnosis, prognosis, and treatment largely from a practical standpoint including physical and ethical constraints on systems for assessing pressure-volume relationships.

MONITORING OF INTRACRANIAL PRESSURE

The part played by intracranial hypertension in determining the clinical course and outcome of patients with severe head injuries can be understood only if there is a continuous record of intracranial pressure (ICP) which is accurate and detailed and which commences as soon after the injury as possible. It is now clear that pressure must be monitored from the supratentorial compartment, from the epidural or subarachnoid spaces, or from the lateral ventricles.[5,6] The record must be displayed in a form which is easy to interpret by nursing staff, normally a strip

This work was supported by a Grant from the Secretary of State for Scotland's Fund for Medical Research.

chart recording. The chart should be observed frequently and staff told to look for a trend of rising pressure, sustained levels of high intracranial pressure defined as pressure in excess of 15 mm Hg, or pressure waves. The waveform of most clinical significance is the A-wave or plateau wave, since these are indicative of a decompensated situation.[15] In fact, these are rather infrequent in patients with head injuries, being most commonly observed in patients with tumors or benign intracranial hypertension.[2,15] The important factors concerning waves are the frequency, maximum height, and the duration of intracranial hypertension during each wave.

Intracranial pressure should never be considered in isolation; observers must be taught to look for any apparent relationship between high intracranial pressure and neurological changes, such as extensor posturing, and for changes in other variables such as arterial pressure and respiration during sudden changes in intracranial pressure. Simple impedance-monitoring devices are available which greatly facilitate observations of respiration in parallel with intracranial pressure.[20] Other factors which can be related to intracranial pressure are the state of body hydration, body temperature, and artefacts caused by body movement which should be marked on the chart recording by observers or filtered out by the data processing system.

Detection of high intracranial pressure is clearly of value. Observation of persistently low intracranial pressure with absence of pressure waves is also of considerable value in determining the management and, to some extent, the outcome of head injuries. Agents, such as steroids and hypertonic solutions which have a small but definite risk of side effects, can be safely withdrawn, and in patients who are deeply unconscious with extensor rigidity the probability that a severe degree of primary intrinsic brain damage is present, rather than secondary changes due to tentorial herniation, is increased.[1]

It must be emphasized, however, that a low or normal intracranial pressure is never a guarantee that no space-occupying process is occurring in the craniospinal axis. Continuous monitoring of intracranial pressure can never supplant diagnostic measures which identify degrees of brain shift and herniation, such as echo encephalography, plain x-rays (if the pineal gland is visible), computerized axial tomography, angiography, or ventriculography.

CAUSES OF RAISED INTRACRANIAL PRESSURE IN HEAD INJURY

As important as the height of ICP is, the source of the change in pressure, partly because this determines whether or not there is accompanying brain shift and/or ischemia and partly because different mechanisms have differing influences on the intracranial volume-pressure relationships, as seen below. Increases in intracranial pressure originate basically from additions to the volume of the intracranial constituents of brain tissue volume, brain water volume, and CSF and intracranial blood volumes. Extraneous volume in head injury is represented by accumulation of epidural, subdural, or intracerebral hematomas or formation of pus in abscesses. An increase of CSF volume, hydrocephalus, is usually a late complication of head injury when of the communicating type; obstructive hydrocephalus is a rather uncommon complication of acute brain compression by hematoma. An increase in brain water content, cerebral edema, is widely described in head injury, but there is very little factual evidence of its true frequency because to measure brain water content tissue sampling is needed. Computerized axial tomography may now yield this information.

The most labile contributions to intracranial hypertension are from increases in cerebral blood volume. These may be due to arterial dilatation (active) or distension (passive) or to venous obstruction, which permits blood to accumulate in the low pressure venous capacitance system. Causes of arterial dilatation relevant to head injury are hypercapnia, hypoxia, anesthetic or sedative drugs, pyrexia, and (REM) sleep. These potential causes of raised ICP depend on retention of cerebrovascular responsiveness. When brain damage is extensive and severe, this responsiveness may be lost, and in this circumstance blood volume may increase with rising arterial pressure because of arterial distension.[4] Normally, autoregulatory cerebral vasoconstriction prevents the head of arterial pressure from being transmitted through the vascular bed. As vascular tone is lost, the cerebrovascular net becomes more vulnerable to surges of arterial hypertension. Large passive rises in intracranial blood volume and pressure now occur, which may be accompanied by an increase in edema fluid.[3] Cerebral blood flow may fail to increase because venous obstruction also develops, causing an increase in total cerebrovascular resistance despite the loss of arteriolar tone.

All of the above mechanisms have in common an augmentation of the volume of the contents of the craniospinal axis. The factor which determines in an individual patient the magnitude of the resulting increase in ICP is the configuration of the pressure-volume curve and the points on the curve spanned by the change in volume.

INTRACRANIAL PRESSURE-VOLUME RELATIONSHIP

There is a logarithmic or exponential relationship between additions to intracranial volume and the resultant intracranial pressure (Fig. 1). This general rule has been verified in experimental animals with expanding intracranial balloons, in children with hydrocephalus, and in adults suffering from many different types of brain disorders including head injury.[4, 16, 17, 22] The expression $\Delta P/\Delta V$ would in a static system represent inverse compliance and has been called elastance by Löfgren and Zwetnow, using a term formerly found in respiratory physiology.[11] The precise shape of the curve described by this expression is subject to great variation and may indeed change from time to time in an individual patient. Shulman suggests that with the use of a logarithmic pressure scale, the curve will be reduced to a straight line function, whereas Löfgren and Zwetnow make a clear differentiation between low pressure and high pressure elastance with a breakpoint occurring when intracranial pressure is about 15 mm Hg. The latter proposal is based on experimental data, the former on hydrocephalus in infants, but the practical implications are clear no matter what the precise mathematical function that describes the pressure-volume relationship. When the pressure-volume curve is at the low elastance or slowly increasing stage, then fairly large increases in intracranial volume can be tolerated without causing much rise in intracranial pressure. When the high elastance phase or the steeply rising portion of the pressure-volume curve has been reached, comparatively small increases in intracranial volume may cause massive rises in intracranial pressure. The clinician managing a patient with a head injury wishes to know at which point on the pressure-volume curve his patient lies. Straightforward monitoring of intracranial pressure will not yield this information directly.

A solution to this can be provided by the clinician by deliberately attempting to alter intracranial volume in a controlled way and plotting the resultant pressures over a wide range so that the configuration of the entire pressure-volume curve is defined. It would then be clear when the patient's resting intracranial pressure was superimposed on that curve whether he would be liable to large or small increases in ICP if there was a given addition to intracranial volume. If one considers patients with head injury, however, this procedure may be neither feasible nor ethically advisable to carry out. Such a procedure implies changes of CSF volume, and the only way in which CSF volume can be changed over a wide range is by injection of fluid into or withdrawal from the subarachnoid space using a cisternal or lumbar puncture.[14] In a patient who may be suffering from a supratentorial expanding lesion such as a temporal lobe contusion, this type of procedure would be quite wrong because of the danger of subsequent coning. If the fluid exchange is to be conducted using an intraventricular catheter, it may be possible to inject an adequate volume of fluid to explore the upper range of the volume-pressure curve, but it is unlikely that an equivalent volume of CSF could be aspirated from the small ventricles. To increase intracranial pressure in such a situation would again be ethically inadmissible.

It is questionable, however, whether it is necessary to delineate the entire pressure-volume curve. The essential information is whether intracranial pressure is liable or not to increase greatly with addition of a given volume as might occur during respiratory obstruction or increasing brain edema. This concept led the author to propose a simpler test to study intracranial pressure-volume relationships some 3 years ago, which has been in regular use in the University Department of Neurosurgery in Glasgow for 3 years. The test consists of the injection of 1 ml fluid into the intraventricular catheter system in a time of 1 second and measurement of the immediate change in ventricular fluid pressure.[10] An

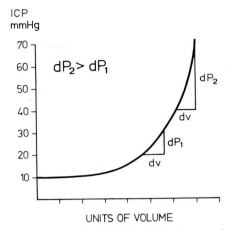

Fig. 1. Theoretical intracranial pressure-volume curve. As the subject moves up the steep portion of the curve, uniform increments of volume (dV) cause greater increases in pressure ($dP_2 > dP_1$). It follows that in theory there ought to be a positive correlation between resting intracranial pressure (ICP) and the response of pressure to a uniform change in volume.

increase of 0-2 mm Hg/ml is considered a normal finding; a rise of 3 or more mm Hg/ml represents abnormally increased intracranial elastance. As a safety precaution, prior to injection of fluid, the operator must determine that it is possible to aspirate at least 1 ml of CSF from the lateral ventricle; with this precaution any intracranial pressure wave which is triggered off by the 1 ml injection can be quickly aborted.[17] We have in recent publications entitled this measurement "the intracranial volume-pressure response" (VPR). Based on repeatability and variability tests in patients with intraventricular catheters for recording the intracranial pressure, a change in the VPR of 2 mm Hg or more in any individual patient can be considered significant.[18] Several studies have been carried out to examine the changes in the VPR related to diagnosis and treatment in patients with head injuries and other sources of raised intracranial pressure.

INTRACRANIAL VOLUME-PRESSURE RESPONSE IN PATIENTS WITH HEAD INJURY

In an initial survey of the volume-pressure response in patients with a variety of neurosurgical conditions, a loose relationship was found between resting intracranial pressure and the

Table 1
Findings in 16 Patients with Severe Head Injury

Principal Diagnosis	Resting ICP mmHg	$\Delta P/\Delta V$ mmHg/ml	Brain Swift on Angiography	Immediate Outcome
1. CSF rhinorrhea meningitis	7	1.0	None	Dead (meningitis)
2. Primary brain (stem) injury	7	2.4	No midline: slight temporal swelling	Sev. disabled
3. Primary brain (stem) injury	10	0.7	None	Vegetative
4. Primary brain (stem) injury	10	1.0	None	Sev. disabled
5. Primary brain (stem) injury	10	1.0	None	Vegetative
6. Cerebral contusion	10	1.6	2 mm midline: sl. temporal swelling	Mod. disabled
7. Cerebral contusion	10	1.9	2 mm midline	Good recovery
8. Primary brain (stem) injury	16	1.2	None: slight temporal swelling	Mod. disabled
9. Burst temporal lobe	17	7.2	5 mm midline: sev. temporal swelling	Good recovery
10. Intracerebral hematoma	24	5.0	6 mm midline: lge subfrontal swelling	Dead (compression)
11. Extradural hematoma	25	13.7	16 mm midline	Good recovery
12. Burst temporal lobe	35	2.9	3 mm midline: mod. temporal swelling	Sev. disabled
13. Extradural hematoma	35	6.0	6 mm midline	Dead (compression)
14. Burst temporal lobe	39	3.9	5 mm midline: mod. temporal swelling	Sev. disabled
15. Acute subdural hematoma	60	5.7	9 mm midline: sev. temporal swelling	Dead (compression)
16. Acute subdural hematoma	68	5.0	7 mm midline: sev. temporal swelling	Dead (compression)

height of the volume-pressure response.[17] There was, however, a considerable scatter of data. Subsequent studies have shown that when the lateral ventricles are large, the relationship between VPR and the baseline level of intracranial pressure breaks down, so that in these patients high levels of intracranial pressure are not necessarily associated with large values of VPR.[18]

We have studied in greater detail 16 patients with head injuries in whom continuous monitoring of intraventricular pressure was carried out and in whom it was also possible to obtain valid measurements of the volume-pressure response and to

make an assessment of brain shift by carotid angiography.[19] Details of these patients are shown in Table 1 but the findings can be summarized as follows. There is some relationship between the height of the intracranial pressure and the level of the volume-pressure response which is significant (Spearman rank correlation coefficient 0.735; $P < 0.01$). If the level of the volume-pressure response was compared with the degree of brain shift using a ranking system to place these in order of severity the correlation was even better (Spearman rank correlation coefficient 0.925; $P < 0.001$). This difference in correlations is because some of the patients who had only moderately increased ICP had extreme levels of brain shift and very high values for the VPR. These patients had intracranial hematomas—the most striking example being a boy who had a very large epidural hematoma with little associated brain swelling.

The limited studies which we have performed before and after surgical decompression indicate that the VPR reduces not just in parallel with the fall in intracranial pressure, but in several instances falls to an even greater extent.[17] This dissociation between the change in the VPR and the change in intracranial pressure will be referred to later.

PHYSIOLOGICAL FACTORS INFLUENCING BRAIN ELASTANCE

Studies in experimental animals with artificially raised intracranial pressure and in patients suffering from intracranial hypertension from causes other than head injury have shed light on the way in which physiological variables may affect intracranial pressure-volume relationships.[7-11,17,18,21] These findings will almost certainly find an application in the diagnosis and management of patients with head injury and are therefore worth describing briefly. Variations in arterial carbon dioxide tension will alter intracranial pressure through changes in cerebral blood volume, and as stated, the extent of increase of intracranial pressure produced by a given increment of volume will depend on the elastance value operating in that patient's brain at that time. Data from both experimental studies and some clinical data now indicate that changes in arterial PCO_2 do not in themselves alter brain elastance.[10] The volume-pressure response changes pari passu with the change in intracranial pressure.[9,21] Thus, if a rise in arterial PCO_2 increases cerebral blood volume by 10 ml and this, in turn, increases the intracranial pressure by 20 mm Hg, then a corresponding reduction in volume of 10 ml of CSF should bring the intracranial pressure back to its starting point. It is likely, but not yet proven, that all other agents which alter intracranial pressure by changing cerebrovascular resistance and cerebral blood volume, such as hypoxia, volatile anesthetics agents and all drugs which cause respiratory depression will also fail to alter the relationship between ICP and the volume-pressure response or intracranial elastance.

In contrast, alterations in arterial blood pressure have a more complex effect on intracranial elastance.[10] When intracranial pressure is normal, alterations in the blood pressure, up or down, have no effect. When intracranial pressure is increased, however, even to a moderate degree (>20 mm Hg), then there is a steep increase in the volume-pressure response with rising arterial pressure.[8] The implication of this is that once intracranial pressure is raised then arterial hypertension renders the brain tighter and more liable to severe superadded increases in ICP with even modest additions to intracranial volume. The converse also appears to hold true—that reduction of arterial pressure in the presence of raised ICP reduces elastance values.

There is some experimental evidence suggesting that intracranial elastance will rise sharply when it is cut off from the capacitance of the spinal compartment.[12] This could happen clinically during tentorial herniation or tonsillar herniation.[5,13] These experimental findings remain to be confirmed in clinical practice.

INFLUENCE OF TREATMENT OF INTRACRANIAL HYPERTENSION ON THE VOLUME-PRESSURE RESPONSE

Hyperventilation with hypocapnia is a well-established way of controlling intracranial hypertension. The change in arterial PCO_2 does not, however, alter the volume-pressure relationship, such that the reduction in ICP afforded by the reduction of a given cerebral blood volume produced by vasoconstriction will be instantly negated if an equivalent volume is added to the intracranial contents due, for instance, to an increase in cerebral edema, or to expansion of an intracranial hematoma.[9,21]

Intravenous mannitol and presumably other hypertonic agents have a rather different effect, in that there is a much greater reduction in the volume-pressure response than of the intracranial pressure itself.[9,18] This implies that even though there is a certain reduction in ICP due to removal of a given volume of brain water by the hypertonic agent, the subsequent addition of that same volume due for example to an increase in an intracranial hematoma will not result in intracranial pressure rising to its former value (Fig. 2). Diminution of this effect of mannitol with time may explain some instances of rebound of intracranial pressure to higher than previous levels.

Steroid therapy with powerful gluco-

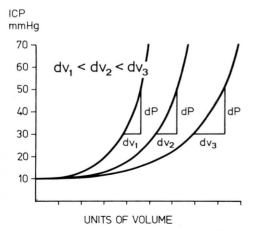

Fig. 2. Theoretical pressure-volume curves to show that as the curve flattens and moves to the right, it takes a greater addition to intracranial volume to produce a uniform rise in pressure.

corticoids provides an even more extreme example of the difference between the effect of the agents on ICP and on the volume-pressure response or elastance. After 24 hours of treatment with steroids in suitable patients, there is little discernible effect on resting intracranial pressure, although intracranial pressure waves are usually diminished in frequency, and there is a clearly apparent clinical response. At this stage we have demonstrated an unequivocal reduction in the volume-pressure response.[18] These data have, however, been gathered from patients with brain tumors and benign intracranial hypertension, and how applicable this is to patients with head injury in whom steroids have, to say the least, a questionable beneficial effect, is not known.

PRACTICAL IMPLICATIONS OF MEASURING INTRACRANIAL PRESSURE-VOLUME RELATIONSHIPS

If a regime is adopted in which intracranial pressure is monitored continuously and the volume-pressure response elicited at intervals,

then four main situations can arise. Intracranial pressure may be low (<15 mm Hg) and the elastance values may also be low VPR < 2 mm Hg/ml). This indicates a safe position with adequate intracranial compensatory reserve, and if it is present in a patient who is deeply unconscious with pronounced neurological impairment, it indicates severe primary brain damage.

The patient may have a low intracranial pressure and high elastance values (VPR > 3 mm Hg/ml). Despite the normal intracranial pressure, this patient must urgently be screened carefully for evidence of a mass lesion and brain shift by whatever means are available including, if necessary, carotid angiography. It is in this type of patient that the ideal behind the rationale of ICP monitoring is attained, namely the desire to detect incipient intracranial hypertension and prevent it before it occurs.

A paient may have high intracranial pressure (>25 mm Hg) with high elastance values. This patient requires treatment of intracranial hypertension urgently, and this should again include a measure aimed at detecting brain shift as the highest values of VPR we have encountered have been in patients with mass lesions.

Finally, on some occasions high intracranial pressure may be seen along with low values of intracranial elastance, and in such circumstances we would now suspect a severe degree of hydrocephalus.

The addition of this simple stress test to examine intracranial pressure-volume relationships to the continuous monitoring of intracranial pressure appears to add substantially to the information which ICP monitoring can yield. Although studies in head-injured patients performed thus far have been limited in extent the evidence strongly suggests that the information which these measurements provide will prove useful not only in understanding of the pathophysiology of events which occur after a head injury but also in the direct sense of helping the clinician make management decisions about his patients.

REFERENCES

1. Jennett WB, Johnston IH: The use of intracranial pressure monitoring in clinical management, in Brock M, Dietz H (eds): Intracranial Pressure. Berlin, Springer, 1972, pp 353–356
2. Johnston IH, Jennett WB: The place of continuous intracranial pressure monitoring in neurosurgical practice. Acta Neurochir 29:53–63, 1973
3. Klatzo I: Pathophysiological aspects of brain edema, in Reulen HJ, Schurmann K (eds): Steroids and Brain Edema. Berlin, Springer, 1972, pp 1–8

4. Langfitt TW, Weinstein JD, Kassell NF: Cerebral vasomotor paralysis produced by intracranial hypertension. Neurology 15:622–641, 1965

5. Langfitt TW, Weinstein JD, Kassell NF, Simeone FA: Transmission of increased intracranial pressure. I. Within the craniospinal axis. J Neurosurg 21:989–997, 1964

6. Langfitt TW, Weinstein JD, Kassell NF, Gagliardi LJ: Transmission of increased intracranial pressure. II. Within the supratentorial space. J Neurosurg 21:998–1005, 1964

7. Leech PJ, Miller JD: Intracranial volume-pressure relationships during experimental brain compression in primates. I. Pressure response to changes in ventricular volume. J Neurol Neurosurg Psychiatry 37:1092–1098, 1974

8. Leech PJ, Miller JD: Intracranial volume-pressure relationships during experimental brain compression in primates. II. Effects of induced changes in arterial pressure. J Neurol Neurosurg Psychiatry 37:1099–1104, 1974

9. Leech PJ, Miller JD: Intracranial volume-pressure relationships during experimental brain compression in primates. III. The effect of mannitol and hypocapnia. J Neurol Neurosurg Psychiatry 37:1105–1111, 1974

10. Löfgren J: Effects of variations in arterial pressure and arterial carbon dioxide tension on the cerebrospinal fluid pressure-volume relationship. Acta Neurol Scand 49:586-598, 1973

11. Löfgren J, Von Essen C, Zwetnow NN: The pressure-volume curve of the cerebrospinal fluid space in dogs. Acta Neurol Scand 49:557–574, 1973

12. Löfgren J, Zwetnow NN: Cranial and spinal components of the cerebrospinal fluid pressure-volume curve. Acta Neurol Scand 49:575–585, 1973

13. Löfgren J, Swetnow NN: Influence of a supratentorial expanding mass on intracranial pressure-volume relationships. Acta Neurol Scand 49:599–612, 1973

14. Lorenz R, Grote E: Relations between cerebrospinal fluid pressure, elasticity of the dura and volume of the CSF, in Brock M, Dietz H (eds): Intracranial Pressure. Berlin, Springer, 1972, pp 265–569

15. Lundberg N: Continuous recording and control of ventricular fluid pressure in neurosurgical practice. Acta Psychiatr Neurol Scand 36:(Suppl 149)1–193, 1960

16. Miller JD, Garibi J: Intracranial volume-pressure relationships during continuous monitoring of ventricular fluid pressure, in Brock M, Dietz H (eds): Intracranial Pressure. Berlin, Springer, 1972, pp 270–274

17. Miller JD, Garibi J, Pickard JD: Induced changes of cerebrospinal fluid volume. Effects during continuous monitoring of ventricular fluid pressure. Arch Neurol 28:265–269, 1973

18. Miller JD, Leech PJ: Effects of mannitol and steroid therapy on intracranial volume-pressure relationships. J Neurosurg 42:274–281, 1975

19. Miller JD, Pickard JD: Intracranial volume-pressure studies in patients with head injury. Injury 5:265–269, 1974

20. North JB, Jennett S: Impedance pneumography for detection of abnormal breathing patterns associated with brain damage. Lancet 2:212–213, 1972

21. Rowed DW, Leech PJ, Reilly PL, Miller JD: Hypocapnia and intracranial volume-pressure relationship. Arch Neurol 32:369–373, 1975

22. Shulman K, Marmarou A: Pressure-volume considerations in infantile hydrocephalus. Dev Med Child Neurol (Suppl 25) 13:90–95, 1971

Open Discussion

DR. BRUCE: It is interesting how well what Dr. Marmarou is doing with his models correlates with what Dr. Miller finds in patients. By affecting the vessels in the volume-pressure response there is a very good correlation between ICP and VPR because there is interference with what it is that is responsible for the change in compliance, whereas when Dr. Miller effects the reason for the raised pressure, which, for example, may be edema, he finds ICP and VPR dissociated.

The other thing that is important in Dr. Marmarou's paper is that when there is a shift where interference with venous drainage is more likely, this is where Dr. Miller had the best correlation with the volume-pressure response.

DR. TINDALL: The other day I pointed out a group of people who did not have mass lesions. They had been excluded by angiography. I ask you to consider the issue of whether or not intracranial pressure measurements in this group of patients are really helpful to the clinical situation.

DR. KURZE: In our experience with 42 patients who were well monitored for 7 to 8 days, none developed a mass lesion. Based on the incidence of intracranial hematomas (after head injury in patients screened by angiography) we would have to monitor approximately 106 patients before we would find one hematoma. Therefore, it would not be unusual to make pressure observations and not diagnose a hematoma. I think we have to be very careful about putting all our weight on one variable. We need to look at all variables.

DR. JENNETT: I would like to follow that remark because I think it is just the very opposite that the value of pressure measurements come in. In patients who look fairly good but have focal lesions or perhaps a shift demonstrated on an angiogram; or with the EMI scanner, the discovery of a lot of lesions a lot sooner, we will not know whether the lesions are surgically important because we won't have any norms to go by. I think we will find pressure the most useful single method of knowing whether or not we have a situation that needs dealing with.

I am sure pressure measurement is the single most important laboratory investigation. It should be added to whatever accuracy we already have from clinical data; Dr. Becker's paper showed

very clearly exactly the kind of application I had in mind. That it is not useful as a single measure is shown by a number of the most severe head injuries; namely, the shearing lesions which cause gross brain stem dysfunction, which are usually not associated with any increase in pressure at all. People who advocate applying measures to reduce pressure in all cases of severe head injury will find themselves trying to reduce the pressures of these patients who don't have a raised pressure. We should know whether or not the patient has increased pressure for a rational approach to management.

CHAIRMAN BECKER: Measuring the volume-pressure response in patients with elevated intracranial pressure with head injury and who do not have a shift can be very helpful in deciding treatment. We often say, Should we treat pressures at 25 or 30 mm Hg? If you know that with .25 ml fluid injected into a patient with a pressure of 25 mm Hg there is a rise to 50 mm Hg, that patient then is in an extremely critical situation. That patient demands some therapy to lower his intracranial pressure at that point. However, if you can inject a full 1 cc without a significant VPR, you feel a little more secure and less pushed to institute therapies which are difficult to use and may be risky.

DR. COLLINS: However, many physicians find that the increased danger of ventricular measurements is not necessary, since they find their hands and eyes tell them when they are in trouble as accurately as you do. Would you comment on the accuracy of your information as compared to your clinical judgment without it?

DR. MILLER: The clinical signs of edema or raised intracranial pressure are, by and large, the clinical signs of coning. The actual signs of raised intracranial pressure just don't exist. We know that patients with benign intracranial hypertension can run pressures of 90 mm Hg. The patients are sitting up in bed and are perfectly well although their optic nerve head is at risk. So, I don't think there is any way you can make a clinical judgment. What you can judge clinically is to what degree of coning the patient is suffering from, but this is a late stage.

CHAIRMAN BECKER: I would like to add to Dr.

Miller's response to Dr. Collins' question, How does measurement of ICP compare to clinical judgment without it? Are we justified in measuring pressure? The answer to this question has become confused because clinicians often compare ICP levels in patients with more chronic conditions such as pseudotumor cerebri or brain tumor with patients who have acute brain insults. These two situations must be discussed separately.

In patients with chronic slowly progressive states such as pseudotumor or brain tumor, ICP may be very high, even up to 70 to 90 mm Hg while the patient remains relatively alert, even with a mean blood pressure only 10 to 30 mm Hg higher than ICP. In this situation the blood flow autoregulatory state must have readjusted gradually to a new level to provide adequate cerebral perfusion. Thus, in states of very slowly elevating ICP, the brain can tolerate very high levels of ICP, and clinical correlations may not be good.

The situation is quite different in patients with acute brain insults. In our experience, patients with acute mechanical brain injury or recent aneurysm rupture are quite sensitive to rising ICP. It is the general rule that these patients begin to show neurological deterioration as their ICPs begin to rise over 30 mm Hg, and they will usually improve when their ICP is reduced below this level. The critical level of ICP is variable, and some patients will demonstrate progressive neurological dysfunction even with ICP levels in the 20–25 mm Hg range, only to improve when ICP is reduced to 10–15 mm Hg.

One important clinical advantage of ICP measurement in this acute situation is the aid it provides in understanding the intracranial problem associated with any neurological progression or lack of improvement. For example, if we know a patient has no major mass lesion from contrast studies, and he is comatose and not improving, or worsening, we must ask why? Is it due to intrinsic brain damage, vasospasm with decreasing blood flow, or could it be secondary to brain swelling and rising ICP. With continuous ICP monitoring, greater insight is immediately provided, and more informed decisions are possible.

35

Distribution of Pressure within the Cranial Cavity and Its Significance

Phenomena associated with raised intracranial pressure are widely known in neurosurgery, and long-standing clinical observation has taught us that in the last phases of an expanding intracranial mass, be it a rapidly expanding lesion such as an intracranial hematoma or a more gradually expanding lesion such as a brain tumor, there are displacements of the brain from its normal relationship to the skull and the intercompartmental septa within it. These displacements have been most widely recognized in relation to the two main foramina through which the neuraxis passes—the tentorial hiatus and the foramen magnum—although shifts of brain in relation to an expanding mass are as varied as the brain tumor or hematoma itself. The classical displacements are easily reproduced experimentally by, for example, an expanding extradural balloon. The typical triad of subfalcine herniation, uncal herniation, and displacement of tonsils through the foramen magnum has been repeatedly demonstrated.[1] The pathological importance of herniation, either with deformation of the upper brain stem from uncal displacement or with medullary compression from impaction of the tonsils in the foramen magnum, is also widely accepted, but despite the universal consensus attending these phenomena, the understanding of the relationship between intracranial pressure and intracranial shifts is still open to debate.

We must first consider the available compartmentalization of pressure within the intracranial space (Fig. 1). The three main portions of pressure within the intracranial space are pressures within the CSF spaces, pressures directly within the vascular system, and a third pressure which has only recently been measured—actual brain tissue pressure.

PRESSURES WITHIN THE CSF SPACE

Measurement of pressure within the CSF spaces was the first to attain clinical usefulness and acceptance. Cushing[2] attributed the introduction of lumbar puncture to Corning in 1885, and the work of Masserman[3] and Merrit and Fre-

mont-Smith[4] established the average cerebrospinal fluid pressure in the lateral recumbent position, that most generally used in clinical practice, as about 11 mm Hg. The range between 11 and 13 mm Hg may be regarded as normal, but above 14.7 mm Hg, CSF pressure must definitely be regarded as raised. When the CSF spaces are in free communication, simultaneous pressure measurement taken from the cerebral ventricle, cisterna magna, or lumbar sac show levels which in the lateral position are substantially equal, allowing for the differences in the level of the various needles. When the patient is erect, however, the intraventricular pressure has been established to be subatmospheric,[5,6,7] while the CSF pressure in the lumbar sac rises to between 26 and 44 mm Hg.[8] The normal zero level of pressure in the erect position has been stated to be at the level of the cisterna magna or the upper cervical theca.[5,6,8] Converse effects arise if the patient is tilted head down.

VASCULAR PRESSURES

Cerebral arterial pressure has been successfully measured in a number of animals, and in major branches of the middle cerebral artery in the baboon it has been found to be some 80 percent of mean arterial blood pressure,[9] and to be between 80 and 90 percent of femoral arterial pressure in similar vessels in the macaque.[10] There are relatively few recordings of cerebral arterial pressure in humans, but Bakay and Sweet's work[11] indicates that the levels of cerebral arterial pressure in larger primates hold also for humans. Sequential pressure measurements by Stromberg and Fox[12] in branches of the same pial arterial network yielded differences in pressure between the smallest (10–25 μ) and the (largest 260 μ) of only some 5 to 15 mm Hg, indicating that there was not a great pressure drop along the vessels of the pia, and suggesting that the above-quoted levels may be representative of pial arterial pressure although not necessarily of close arteriolar pressure, since brain arterioles lie entirely within the substance of the cortex. Direct

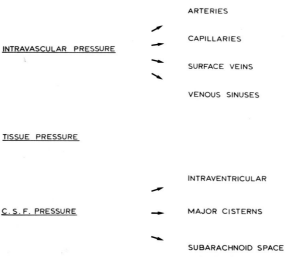

Fig. 1. Compartmentalization of pressures within the cranium.

measurements of the arteriolar, capillary, and venular pressures in the substance of the brain have not, to the author's knowledge, been made. On the venous side, cortical venous pressures measured in the baboon in circumstances of normocapnia have been recorded as 14 mm Hg (S.D. 0.24). The considerable changes in cortical venous pressure induced by either vasodilatation or vasoconstriction have been noted.[13] In general, however, the relationship between cortical venous pressure and ventricular fluid or central subarachnoid space pressure is a linear and constant one, as demonstrated by Rowan et al.,[14] who found a positive intercept of 2.5 mm Hg on the cortical venous pressure axis when plotted against ventricular fluid pressure. This small but significantly positive pressure intercept has been confirmed in the author's laboratory (Fig. 2), where the positive intercept appeared slightly greater, possibly because of the circumstances of the preparation where a period of extensive opening of the skull interrupted the relationship in the lower levels before the preparation reverted to a true closed skull state. In humans, the mean cerebrospinal fluid and dural-sinus pressures were reported by Shulman et al.,[15] and in their measurements at a cerebrospinal fluid pressure of 10 mm Hg, pressure in the sagittal sinus averaged 6.6 mm Hg and, at the torcular Herophili, 3.4 mm Hg. The gradient between cortical venous pressure and sagittal sinus pressure is thus fairly abrupt, and there is fairly strong evidence that cortical venous pressure is significantly higher than the central

space pressure, the presumed explanation being that if this were not the case, cortical veins would collapse and the circulation would cease.

BRAIN TISSUE PRESSURE

Direct tissue pressure measurements are a much more recent innovation. They depend on the introduction of wick catheters.[16] Using this technique, brain tissue pressure has been measured by several groups,[17-20] and, in general, the measurements have shown the interstitial fluid pressure or brain tissue pressure (the term used depends on the authors) to be positive and, on the average, 1–4 mm *below* the central CSF space pressure. The usual value under resting conditions for interstitial fluid pressure has been between 3 and 6 mm Hg. One group[21] claims to have measured consistently negative pressures in the centrum semiovale of dogs, but this finding has not been confirmed. These findings, however, are somewhat at variance with the general clinical neurosurgical experience, which is that brain tissue pressure is higher than pressure in CSF pathways under normal circumstances. Brain immediately bulges through when the pia is incised, for example, indicating that even under normal circumstances the brain is held under tension by the elastic network of fibers associated with blood vessels and with the pia matter itself. The experiments of Schettini et al.[22] indicate that cerebral tissue pressure appears significantly higher than

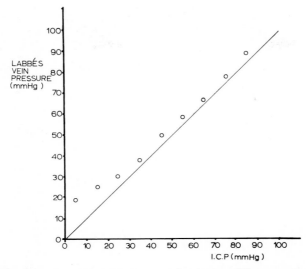

Fig. 2. Plot of Labbé's vein pressure against intracranial pressure in 6 animals during rising intracranial pressure induced by CSF infusion. There is a significant difference between the Labbé's vein pressure and the line of identity, the positive intercept being 10.6 mm Hg. It is probable that the deviation of the venous pressure from the line of identity at lower levels relates to the extensive opening of the skull necessary in the making of the preparation. The skull is artificially reclosed before infusion, but intracranial pressure takes some little time to rise.

CSF pressure. The fairly widely accepted figures for the relationship between ventricular fluid pressure and cortical venous pressure would also suggest that the intracapillary pressure within the mantle of the brain itself, which has never been directly measured, must lie at a level higher than that of cortical venous pressure and, therefore, correspondingly above central CSF space pressure. If this were not so, then the circulation would cease. However, the relationship between brain tissue pressure and CSF pressure must be regarded as still uncertain.

EVIDENCE OF DIFFERENCES IN PRESSURE SIMULTANEOUSLY RECORDED IN THE INTRACRANIAL SPACE

Evidence of focally abnormal pressure in the intracranial space is almost as old as clinical neurosurgery. There can be few neurosurgeons who have not met the pathologically thin bone overlying a temporal tumor or observed the grossly deformed skull with thinned bone overlying an infantile subdural hematoma (Fig. 3) or an arachnoidal cyst. This type of bony abnormality of the skull occurring in the absence of generally raised intracranial pressure can only be explained by an uneven dissipation of pressure within the head, presumably indicating that pressure is raised focally relative to the remainder of the intracranial space. Measurements of pressure differentials between portions of the supratentorial space under such conditions have yet to be made clinically. Differential pressure measurements between supratentorial and infratentorial spaces, however, or between the supratentorial space and the lumbar theca, have been made on numerous occasions, although there is no clear agreement as yet as to their time relationship to the development of foraminal or tentorial cones. Thus, Smythe and Henderson[23] demonstrated that pressure differences of about 8 mm Hg indicated a probable fatal outcome from tentorial herniation. A study using modern equipment and isovolumetric pressure recording in the lateral ventricle and the upper cervical subarachnoid space by Kaufmann and Clark[24] indicated that when intraventricular CSF pressure exceeded the cervical subarachnoid pressure by more than 10 mm Hg, significant transtentorial and/or tonsillar herniation had occurred. A more recent study by Soni[25] in Cardiff using a differential pressure

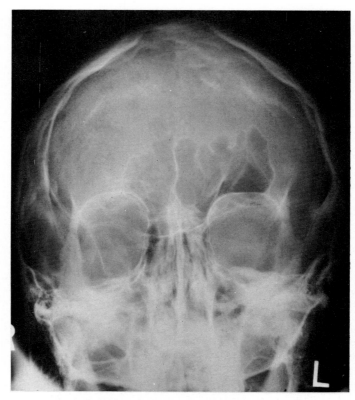

Fig. 3.   Antero-posterior radiograph of the skull in a patient with an infantile
subdural hematoma on the left side. The elevation of the sphenoidal wing and bulging
of the temporal fossa are evident.

transducer connected to both ventricle and
cisterna magna, indicated that a difference of up
to 12 mm Hg was compatible with life and did not
necessarily indicate the presence of tentorial
herniation. Soni further showed that there were
slow cyclical changes in pressure in the two compartments, which were not necessarily isometric.
Although further work will be necessary before
the acceptance of such a large pressure differential between supratentorial and infratentorial
space in the presence of patent CSF channels can
be accepted, it seems clear that at this time the
presence of difference in pressure between supratentorial and infratentorial space need not immediately imply the presence of a pressure cone.
Conversely, it is also clear from the clinic that it is
not necessary to have grossly raised intracranial
pressure for a pressure cone to be present. This is
particularly true in temporal lobe tumors, where
the uncus is frequently herniated despite the fact

that the intracranial pressure has never been
recorded as raised. It is also evident in patients
with space-occupying lesions in one-half of the
posterior fossa, where one tonsil may descend
while the other remains in normal situation. Large
pineal shifts may be demonstrated without
foraminal impaction. We must, however, remember that the measurement of normal intracranial or CSF pressure on one or two occasions in the course of the management of a
neurosurgical patient does not mean that the intracranial pressure is invariably normal,[26] and,
indeed, part of the value of Soni's contribution was
to indicate that during cyclical variations in intracranial pressure, differential pressures could
vary in extent quite widely.

The sequence of pressure change, displacement, and distortion of the brain was established
by Langgfitt et al.[27] when he showed the ease with
which the tentorial incisura could be obstructed in

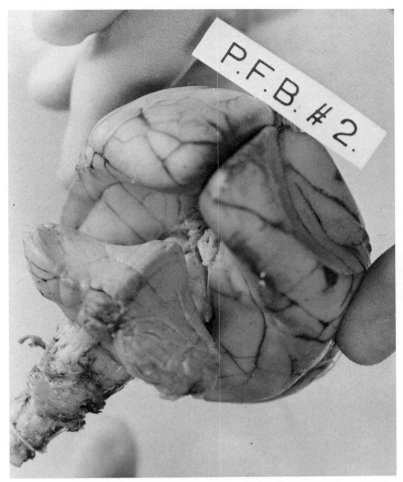

Fig. 4. The uncal and foraminal cones induced by the expansion of a supratentorial balloon over the posterior part of the right hemisphere. The impression of the balloon is evident. The rupture of the pia over the right uncus can be seen, and the extensive descent of the lower part of the tonsils into the upper cervical theca is apparent.

the monkey by an acute extradural space-occupying lesion, and these findings were emphasized by Weinstein, also in Langfitt's group,[28] when a rapid herniation of the occipital lobe and marked caudal displacement of the tectum was documented during the inflation of an epidural space-occupying lesion. Similar findings have been reported more recently by our own group,[1] in this case in the baboon with a fibrous tentorium, and, in contrast to Langfitt's original views, it is clear that a rapidly expanding supratentorial lesion may produce herniation both through the tentorium and the foramen magnum (Fig. 4).

EVIDENCE OF PRESSURE DIFFERENTIALS WITHIN A SINGLE COMPARTMENT

A good deal of recent experimental work has attempted to answer the question; Do gradients of pressure exist between portions of one intracranial compartment at any given time? As in most other fields of experimental physiology, the debate has centered on differences in methodology. Thus, Johnston and Rowan,[29] measuring subarachnoid space pressure, have consistently failed to find evidence of pressure differentials

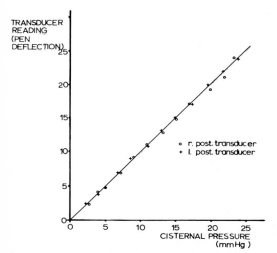

TRANSDUCER
READING
(PEN
DEFLECTION)

o r. post. transducer
+ l. post. transducer

CISTERNAL PRESSURE
(mmHg)

Fig. 5. Comparison of recording from a right and left intracranial pressure transducer plotted against cisternal pressure during the elevation of intracranial pressure induced by the inhalation of CO_2. The identity of pressures measured by the two transducers is apparent.

between one side of the supratentorial compartment and the other in the presence of a rapidly expanding space-occupying lesion on one side. The fact, however, that they were measuring in the subarachnoid space presumably indicates that immediate equilibration of pressures throughout that space was likely and that, by the very nature of the technique, pressure differentials between one side of the head and the other could not be measured. It has become clear that, to measure pressure differentials, some measurement of brain tissue pressure is required. Even here, however, there is no consistent agreement in the reports so far at hand. The experiences of our own group in a series of 6 baboons may be briefly summarized here. Epidural pressure transducers[30] were placed through trephine holes bilaterally in frontal and parietal zones, an epidural balloon was placed in the post parieto-occipital zone on the right side through a separate trephine hole, and the balloon inflated at a constant rate of 0.2 ml/min by a Palmer slow-infusion pump which ran continuously from the start of the inflation of the balloon, except during episodes of blood flow determination by hydrogen clearance, when the rate of inflation of the balloon was adjusted to maintain the level of intracranial pressure constant. Extradural pressures were calibrated against

cisternal pressure initially and also by the substitution of current deflection in a previously made in vitro calibration graph. Extradural pressure calibrated in this way correlated well with cisternal pressure measured at the same time, providing that accurate coplanar placement of the extradural transducer was ensured and dural indentation avoided.[1] Before balloon inflation, intracranial pressure was raised between 30 and 50 mm Hg by the inhalation of CO_2, and the extradural pressure recordings correlated with both the cisternal pressure and against each other. Figure 5 shows that such elevations of pressure were recorded accurately and equally on the two sides of the head and that differential pressures did not develop under these circumstances. At the beginning of the experiment, with cisternal pressures of about 10 mm Hg, there was no significant difference between the recordings of the four transducer sites. By the time the left posterior transducer, which as the one furthest from the balloon was taken as reference, had reached a recording of 30 mm Hg, significant differences between the right- and left-sided mean transducer pressures had developed, the right-sided mean being 39.4 mm Hg (S.D. 8.2) and the left-sided mean, 31 mm Hg (S.D. 4.0, $p < 0.01$). As the intracranial pressure continued to rise reaching a left posterior transducer level of 70 mm Hg, the mean left-sided extradural pressure of 69.5 mm Hg (S.D. 5.1) became significantly different from the right-sided pressure of 83.5 mm Hg (S.D. 10.7, $p < 0.001$). With pressures approaching peak values, pressures remained significantly different on the two sides, the highest pressure recordings in the 6 animals having a mean of 120.2 mm Hg (S.D. 39.9), comparing with the mean right-sided pressure of 147.2 mm Hg (S.D. 42, $p < 0.01$). The plot of the data from 5 animals which showed a definite differential pressure between right and left side is shown on Fig. 6, the regression line having a high level of significance ($r = 0.994$) and being significantly different from the line of identity ($p < 0.001$) compared with the left posterior transducer. Interestingly enough, the single example where differential pressures were not seen turned out to have an unusual balloon placement. Thus, Fig. 7 shows the average displacement of brain induced by the epidural balloon, and Fig. 8 the displacement in an animal where the balloon transgressed the midline, and where the plot of right-sided transducers against the left posterior transducer is indistinguishable from the line of identity. The earliest recording of pressure differentials between one side of the supratentorial compartment and the other must, however, be credited to Weinstein,[28] who demonstrated that the inflation of an intracerebral balloon in one hemisphere led to a rise in intrahemispheric pressure on that side compared with the other, the cerebral tissue pressure being measured by loose balloons placed in the tissue. Little has been made of this observation, presumably because of the admitted potential damage to the tissue which such devices involve. However, the exponents of the wick methodology have also numerous publications to suggest that pressures within the two hemispheres need not necessarily be the same. Thus, Brock et al.[31] demonstrated inequalities of tissue pressure following embolization of one hemisphere although the higher pressure, up to 120 mm Hg differential, was not necessarily consistently on the side of embolization. In 8 animals, the epidural pressure rose more on the affected side, while in 12, it was the nonembolized hemisphere which developed the higher pressure. In a recent report from Shulman,[18] cotton wick tissue probes measured interstitial fluid pressure in the brains of cats during the infusion of mock CSF into one cerebral hemisphere or during the expansion of an epidural balloon. He noted that under these circumstances, interstitial fluid pressure rose on the side of infusion or compression and that with balloon expansion interstitial fluid pressure also exceeded CSF pressure. Similar findings were reported by Reulen[20] who, using multiple wick measurements in relation to a cold injury in one frontal lobe, demonstrated raised pressures that were highest adjacent to the lesion and falling gradually toward the distant opposite areas. Pressure differences between corresponding recording sites in the injured and uninjured hemispheres could amount to 8 to 13 mm Hg, and tissue pressure in the area of edema was significantly higher than CSF pressure. With experimentally induced vascular lesions, both O'Brien and Waltz[32] and Dorsch and Symon[33] showed that, following the establishment of a large ischemic lesion in either the cat or monkey, significant differences in epidural pressure could be recorded over the surface of the two hemispheres, the side of the infarction being invariably the higher. Brock and his colleagues[34] further demonstrated differences in tissue

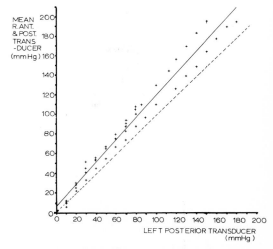

Fig. 6. Composite of plot of meaned right-sided intracranial pressure (obtained from two transducers) plotted against a left posterior transducer pressure in experiments in which the intracranial pressure was raised by the inflation of a right occipital balloon (five experiments). The significance of the slope is down. The deviation from the line of identity is significant (p < 0.001).

pressure between injured and noninjured cerebral hemisphere with a unilateral cryogenic lesion or with traumatic intracerebral hemorrhage. The levels of difference could be between 1 and 12 mm Hg, the injured side being invariably the higher.

In contrast to these reports, however, significant differences in brain tissue pressure were not thought to occur in acute experimental infarction in cats and monkeys by Tulleken et al.[35] who, again using wick methodology, embolized the middle cerebral or carotid artery or infarcted the hemisphere by clipping the main middle cerebral artery. They concluded that marked degrees of pressure gradient could be produced by a rapidly growing intracerebral volume such as an epidural balloon, but that no significant tissue pressure gradient could be recorded between the two hemispheres even up to 20 hours following middle cerebral occlusion, although the tissue pressure showed definite increase some 6 to 8 hours after clipping of the middle cerebral artery. Similar conclusions were reached by Halsey et al.[19] although the baseline drift of their catheter tip transducer (Miller instruments) appeared too great for much reliance to be placed on their measurements.

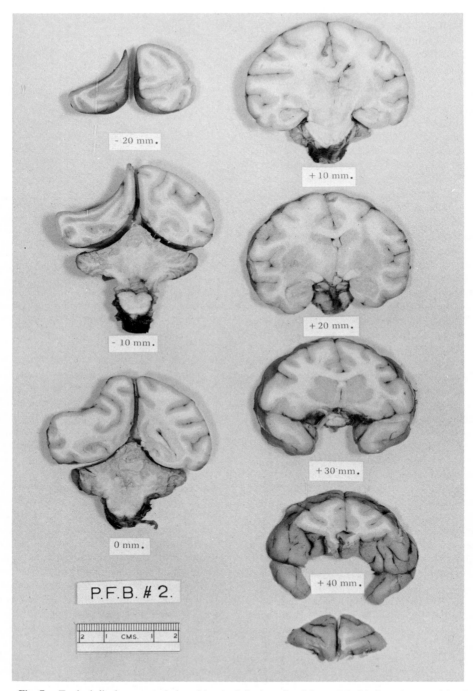

Fig. 7. Typical displacements induced by the inflation of a right occipital balloon in one of the five experiments whose data made up Fig. 6.

256

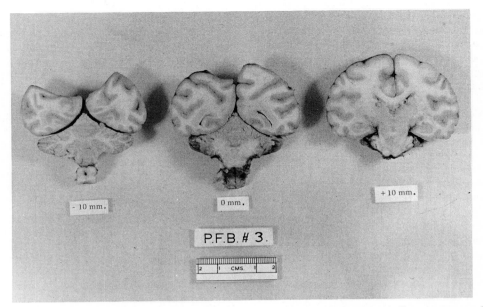

Fig. 8a. Selected brain displacements from one animal in whom the occipital balloon transgressed the midline and lay in the occipital region almost equally on the right and left sides of the midline. The absence of subfalcine herniation is evident in this figure.

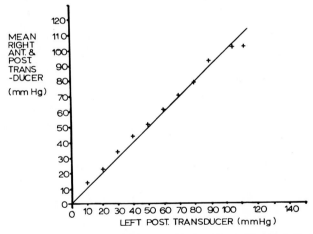

Fig. 8b. Plot of right-sided mean transducer measurements against the left posterior transducer pressure in the animal shown in Fig. 8a. No differential pressures were obtained in this instance.

THE SIGNIFICANCE OF INTRACRANIAL PRESSURE DIFFERENTIALS OR "PRESSURE GRADIENTS"

There is little argument about the significance of the established pressure gradients which have been recorded by many workers between the supratentorial and infratentorial compartments or between the infratentorial space and the spinal cord. The compression and distortion of neuraxial structures, either at midbrain or medullary level, clearly carries a grave prognosis and, indeed, the experience of neurosurgery in general indicates that this is the method of termination of the majority of space-occupying lesions left untreated.

More recently, Ng and Nimmannitya[36] have shown the frequency with which such tentorial hernias are associated with fatal cerebral infarction, and it seems that any severe brain swelling will carry in its train the risk of uncal or tonsillar herniation and that this gravely decreases the survival.

The debate and possibly the interest of pressure gradients, however, is not so much in those in which obstruction of the tentorial pathways and separation of the CSF spaces has already occurred but in those reports of pressure gradients in which the gradients clearly preceded the development of herniation and in which those who propound the significance of pressure gradients would maintain that differences in pressure have produced the herniation. The significance of these gradients in tissue pressure is probably best considered in relation to their effect on the local vasculature. Weinstein et al.[28] were the first to show that inflation of a subdural balloon diminished the perfusion of brain immediately subjacent to the balloon, as evidenced by its failure to fill at a terminal injection with Evans' blue. More recently, Symon et al.[1] have shown that differential pressures between the two hemispheres are associated with premature exhaustion of the autoregulatory capacity in the maximally compressed hemisphere and reduction of blood flow in the area of high pressure. It is well known from the work of Häggendal[37] and Zwetnow,[38] among others, that the capacity of the brain to maintain its blood flow in the face of rising intracranial pressure has many of the characteristics of the autoregulatory mechanisms to reduced perfusion pressure from falling systemic arterial pressure. Indeed, Symon et al.[39] have suggested that the close correspondence of pressure levels at which the autoregulatory mechanism to raised intracranial pressure and the autoregulatory mechanism to diminished systemic arterial pressure fail suggests that the two mechanisms are the same, although a more general view is that autoregulation to raised intracranial pressure will be successful in maintaining perfusion to somewhat lower levels of perfusion pressure than in the case of falling systemic arterial pressure. Be that as it may, however, the likely mechanism of maintenance of blood flow is a phasic relaxation of the resistance vessels within the brain; autoregulation fails when this relaxation reaches its maximum and the vascular bed then becomes pressure-passive in the "vasoparalysis" of Langfitt.[40]

The progressive exhaustion of the autoregulatory capacity has been suggested[41] to be responsible for the increase in intracranial pulsation which is well known in states of raised intracranial pressure and which was attributed by Foldes and Arrowood[42] to diminished damping effect of the arterial wall. Local measurements of pulse transmission between artery and vein in the middle cerebral cortex, however, have indicated that using this as an index of resistance, relaxation of the resistance vessels appears to occur in an orderly fashion during the compensatory phase of increasing intracranial pressure, but that a breakpoint in pulse transmission occurs at around the level at which autoregulation would be expected to fail. Beyond this point, very small increases in pressure are associated with very marked increases in the transmission of pulse from artery to vein. At this point, it appears that there is an exhaustion of the vascular components of brain compliance. Under these circumstances of vasodilatation and exhausted autoregulation, the local circulation is certainly more exposed to systemic blood pressure changes, and the situation becomes not dissimilar to that demonstrated in the autoregulatory breakthrough at high intervascular pressures by Strandgaard[43] and others in systemic arterial hypertension. As a corollary of the transmission of intravascular pressure changes directly to the brain substance, the capillaries will become subjected to high fluxes of pressures, and it seems likely that this may result in the progressive formation of edema. Reulen[20] has shown that the high differential pressures established between an edematous expanding lesion, such as a cryogenic lesion in animals, results in the breakdown of brain resistance to the spread of edema and the expansion of the mass into the surrounding normal brain. The development of increasing local tissue pressure would be associated with progressive exhaustion of the autoregulatory capacity in this edge of the expanding lesion, and the whole vicious cycle would repeat itself. The details of this hypothesis are shown in Fig. 9.

The complete acceptance of such concepts is still hindered by our continued inability to measure tissue pressure with an accuracy sufficient to suppress all doubt. A certain amount of collateral evidence would suggest that such a state of changed reactivity in the cerebral circulation might provide the key to a state of critical exhaustion of compliance appearing focally, notably the work of Fitch and McDowell[44] in Leeds, who have

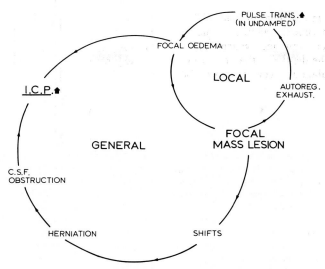

PULSE TRANS.▲
(IN UNDAMPED)

FOCAL OEDEMA

LOCAL

I.C.P.▲   AUTOREG.
                                             EXHAUST.

                         FOCAL
GENERAL   MASS LESION

C.S.F.
OBSTRUCTION

HERNIATION   SHIFTS

Fig. 9.   Schema of the theoretical extension of a focal mass lesion.

shown that the vasodilatation produced by halothane when superadded to a state of critical intracranial dynamics imposed by the inflation of an intracranial balloon, may result in the development of pressure gradients across the tentorium during the halothane inhalation, where none existed before. There can be little doubt that, under these circumstances, the vasodilatation of halothane superadded to a preexistent critical level of balloon inflation, had been sufficient to establish a pressure gradient, and, as a demonstration of the effect of this gradient, the pupil would dilate in response to the development of a pressure cone. It is particularly interesting that these experiments showed increases in supratentorial pressure produced by the halothane comparable to those in the previous work of Jennett and his associates,[45] who were among the first to point out the dangers of vasodilator anesthesia in states of critically balanced intracranial pressure-volume relationships.

The increased intracranial pulsation, which is likely to be associated with such regions of focally raised intracranial pressure besides involving the capillary bed in excessive pulsation and damage to the blood-brain barrier, may be responsible for the bony changes which are so typically seen in the region of a very slowly growing intracranial mass. It is general surgical experience that a pulsating mass produces damage to bone very readily, while steady pressure from an expanding lesion is much less prone to do so. Thus, for example, any aortic aneurysm or an intracranial aneurysm produces destruction of the bone very readily in virtue of its pulsatile component. Focally raised intracranial pulsation in association with a large temporal cyst, for example, may well explain the thinning of the bone which so typically occurs in such lesions.

This review cannot at this stage present conclusive evidence that intracranial tissue gradients exist or that differential pressures between the two halves of the supratentorial compartment or between one portion of a hemisphere and another are the inevitable concomitant of an expanding lesion. Nor can it indicate clearly what range of differential pressures might be expected under various circumstances. It seems clear, however, that the fact that differential pressure measurements have now been made by a number of investigators indicates that their significance cannot be underestimated. It also seems clear that CSF space measurements may be predicted with confidence not to show differential pressures until the subarachnoid space becomes obstructed. Measurements actually within the substance of the brain or, perhaps, epidural measurements, which, when the intracranial pressure is raised, bear many similarities to direct tissue pressure measurement, will be necessary to elucidate these interesting phenomena further. At the summary of a recent conference on intracranial pressure, there was general agreement that further fundamental work was necessary to continue the analysis of the relationship between local cerebral blood flow and local intracranial pressure. There are now elegant experimental methods (such as the hydrogen clearance method) which may be confidently used in the depths of the brain to enable blood flow circulation in very circumscribed areas,[46] but continuing experience is necessary in the use of methods such as the wick method to enhance our knowledge of comparable highly focal tissue pressure measurement.

REFERENCES

1. Symon L, Pasztor E, Branston NM, et al: Effect of supratentorial space-occupying lesions on regional intracranial pressure and local cerebral blood flow: An experimental study in baboons. J Neurol Neurosurg Psychiatry 37:617, 1974
2. Cushing H: Studies in Intracranial Physiology. London, Oxford University Press, 1929
3. Masserman JH: Cerebrospinal hydrodynamics IV. Clinical experimental studies. Arch Neurol Psychiatry 32:523, 1934
4. Merritt HH, Fremont-Smith F: The cerebrospinal fluid. Philadelphia, WB Saunders, 1937
5. Ayer JB: Cerebrospinal fluid pressure from the clinical point of view. Res Publ Assoc Res Nerv Ment Dis 4:159, 1924
6. Ruch TC, Patton HD: Physiology and Biophysics (ed 19). Philadelphia, WB Saunders, 1960, p 5
7. Bradley KC: Cerebrospinal fluid pressure. J Neurol Neurosurg Psychiatry 33:387, 1970
8. Loman A: Components of cerebrospinal fluid pressure as affected by changes in posture. Arch Neurol Psychiatry 31:679, 1934
9. Symon L: Regional cerebrovascular responses to acute ischemia in normocapnia and hypercapnia: an experimental study in baboons. J Neurol Neurosurg Psychiatry 33:756, 1970
10. Symon L: A comparative study of cerebral arterial pressure in dogs and macaques. J Physiol 191:449, 1967
11. Bakay L, Sweet WH: Cervical and intracranial intraarterial pressure with and without vascular occlusion. Surg Gynecol Obstet 96:67, 1952
12. Stromberg DD, Fox JR: Primate pial arterial pressure responses to changes in inspired CO_2 and systemic arterial pressure. Abstracts of 6th International CBF Symposium on Cerebral Circulation and Metabolism, Philadelphia, 1973. Stroke 4: 327, 1973
13. Symon L: Regional vascular reactivity in the middle cerebral arterial distribution: An experimental study in baboons. J Neurosurg 33:532, 1970
14. Rowan JO, Johnston IH, Harper AM et al: Perfusion pressure in intracranial hypertension, in Brock M, Dietz H (eds): Intracranial Pressure. Berlin, Springer, 1972, p 164
15. Shulman K, Yarnell P, Ransohoff J: Dural sinus pressure in normal and hydrocephalic dogs. Arch Neurol (Chic) 10:575, 1964
16. Brock M, Pöll W, Furuse M, Dietz H: Der "docht-Katheter." Acta Neurochirurg 28:201, 1973
17. Pöll W, Brock M, Markakis E, et al: Brain tissue pressure, in Brock M, Dietz, H (eds): Intracranial Pressure. Berlin, Springer, 1972, p 188
18. Shulman K, Marmarou A, Weitz S: Induced tissue pressure gradients in experimental brain compression and swelling. Proc 2nd Int Symp Intracranial Pressure, Lund, 1974 (in press)
19. Halsey JH, Capper NF, Clark RM: Intracranial pressure gradients in experimental cerebral infarction. Proc 2nd Int Symp Intracranial Pressure, Lund, 1974 (in press)
20. Reulen HJ, Graham R, Klatzo I: Development of pressure gradients within brain tissue during the formation of vasogenic brain edema. Proc 2nd Int Symp Intracranial Pressure, Lund, 1974 (in press)
21. Brodersen P, Højgaard K, Lassen NA: Measurement of "interstitial fluid" pressure in the brain in dogs, in Brock M, Dietz H (eds): Intracranial Pressure. Berlin, Springer, 1972, p 185
22. Schettini A, McKay L, Majors R, et al: Experimental approach for monitoring surface brain pressure. J Neurosurg 34:38, 1971
23. Smythe GE, Henderson WR: Observations on the cerebrospinal fluid pressure on simultaneous ventricular and lumbar punctures. J Neurol Neurosurg Psychiatry 1:226, 1938
24. Kaufmann GE, Clark K: Continuous simultaneous monitoring of intraventricular and cervical subarachnoid cerebrospinal fluid pressure to indicate development of cerebral or tonsillar herniation. J Neurosurg 33:145, 1970
25. Soni SR: Continuous measurement of differential CSF pressures across the tentorium. Proc Soc Br Neurol Surg, May 1974. J Neurol Neurosurg Psychiatry 37:1283, 1974
26. Symon L, Dorsch NWC: Use of long-term intracranial pressure measurement to assess hydrocephalic patients prior to shunt preparation. J Neurosurg 42:258, 1975
27. Langfitt TW, Weinstein JD, Kassell NF, et al: Transmission of increased intracranial pressure. I. Within the craniospinal axis. J Neurosurg 21:989, 1964
28. Weinstein JD, Langfitt TW, Bruno L, et al: Experimental study of patterns of brain distortion and

ischaemia produced by an intracranial mass. J Neurosurg 28:513, 1968

29. Johnston IH, Rowan JO: Intracranial pressure gradients in cerebral hemisphere. Blood flow differences during expansion of unilateral supratentorial mass lesions in primates. Abstr 6th Int CBF Symp Cerebral Circulation and Metabolism, Philadelphia, 1973. Stroke 4:347, 1973

30. Dorsch NWC, Stephens RJ, Symon L: An intracranial pressure transducer. Bio-Med Eng 5:452, 1971

31. Brock M, Beck J, Markakis E et al: Intracranial pressure gradients associated with experimental cerebral embolism. Stroke 3:123, 1972

32. O'Brien MD, Waltz AG: Intracranial pressure changes during experimental cerebral infarction, in Brock M, Dietz H (eds): Intracranial Pressure. Berlin, Springer, 1972, p 105

33. Dorsch NWC, Symon L: Intracranial pressure changes in acute ischemic regions of the primate hemisphere, in Brock M, Dietz H (eds): Intracranial Pressure. Berlin, Springer, 1972

34. Brock M, Furuse M, Faber R, et al: Brain tissue pressure gradients. Proc 2nd Int Symp Intracranial Pressure, Lund, 1974 (in press)

35. Tulleken CAF, Meyer JS, Ott EO: Brain tissue pressure gradients and experimental infarction recorded by multiple wick type transducers. Proc 2nd Int Symp Intracranial Pressure, Lund, 1974 (in press)

36. Ng LKK, Nimmannitya J: Massive cerebral infarction with severe brain swelling. Stroke 1:158, 1970

37. Häggendal E, Löfgren J, Nilsson NJ, et al: Die gehirndurchblüteng bei experimentalen liquor-druck anderungen. Verhandel Int. Neurokirurgen Kongres Bad Durkheim, 1966

38. Zwetnow N: Cerebral blood flow autoregulation to blood pressure and intracranial pressure variations. Scan J Clin Lab Invest Suppl 102:5A, 1968

39. Symon L, Pasztor E, Dorsch NWC, et al: Physiological responses of local areas of the cerebral circulation in experimental primates determined by the method of hydrogen clearance. Stroke 4:632, 1973

40. Langfitt TW, Kassell NF, Weinstein JD: Cerebral vasomotor paralysis produced by intracranial hypertension. Neurology 15:622, 1965

41. Symon L, Crockard HA, Juhasz J: Some aspects of cerebrovascular resistance in raised intracranial pressure: an experimental study. Proc 2nd Int Symp Intracranial Pressure, Lund, 1974 (in press)

42. Foldes FF, Arrowood JG: Changes in cerebrospinal fluid pressure under the influence of continuous subarachnoidal infusion of normal saline. J Clin Invest 27:346, 1948

43. Strandgaard W, Olesen J, Skinhøj E, Lassen NA: Autoregulation of brain circulation in severe arterial hypertension. Br Med J 1:507, 1973

44. Fitch W, McDowell DG: Effect of Halothane on intracranial pressure gradients in the presence of intracranial space-occupying lesions. Br J Anaesthes 43:904, 1971

45. Jennett WB, Barker J, Fitch W, et al: Effects of anaesthesia on intracranial pressure in patients with space-occupying lesions. Lancet 1:61, 1969

46. Pasztor E, Symon L, Dorsch NWC, et al: The hydrogen clearance method in assessment of blood flow in cortex, white matter and deep nuclei of baboons. Stroke 4:556, 1973

Open Discussion

DR. LANGFITT: It seems to me there is clear evidence now that differences in pressure do occur across the supratentorial space in response to expansion of a mass lesion. The best evidence for this is shifts and distortions of the brain tissue.

One important point is that although pressure differences may occur, the volume of the shift is a function of the volume of the mass as independent of pressure. The rate at which the shift occurs may well be due to the difference in pressure across the tissue, but the final volume of the shift is a function of the volume of the mass and independent of pressure.

Furthermore, when the mass stops expanding, I believe there is very good evidence that the pressure differences dissipate. This has been shown by Waltz and perhaps by a number of other people. It follows, then, that if the mass is slowly expanding even over a matter of days, the difference in pressure across the supratentorial space to produce that shift may be measurable by our techniques, in contrast to most of our experimental work which has been done in acute situations.

In the experiments we did a number of years ago, in which we rapidly expanded a balloon over the frontal pole of a cat, we saw a pressure difference across the brain. After sacrificing these animals, one could see actual shift downward to the brain stem. This would occur over a period of several minutes, and as soon as the pressure difference across the brain stopped, the shift of the brain stopped. (The movement of the brain that occurred dissipating the pressure difference is due to plastic creep.)

Finally, when brain distortion and shift are present, any dysfunction that results is related to the shift or distortion and not to any pressure difference that caused the shift in the first place. In other words, except in the most rapidly expanding intracranial lesions, such as in acute intracerebral hematoma, pressure differences across the supratentorial space contribute nothing to the pathophysiology of the process.

MR. SYMON: When Tom Langfitt got up, I thought it couldn't be true that we have converted him, but as he went on, it became clear that his conversion was incomplete. The problem is that the intracranial pressure is never a static entity. It is always a dynamic entity because we always have to contend with constantly changing pressures due to pulsations, coughing, sneezing, lying down, standing up, etc.

I think the important thing we have to concentrate on is the exhaustion of compliance predominantly in the vascular compartment. In McDowell's experiments, it is quite clear that although you may not be able to show pressure gradients in a situation of almost exhausted compliance, a very small further load on the vascular compartment at this stage will produce very marked pressure gradients, even perhaps tentorial herniation.

I know this, of course is evidence between supra- and infratentorial compartment, but I submit there is no theoretical reason why the same concepts cannot apply to exhaustion of vascular compliance focally.

I think the problem we have to face is that until we can measure with great accuracy focal intracranial pressure measurements, we will never be able to get around this problem, and this is where we need a methodological advance such as Dr. Taylor and Dr. Marmarou were talking about.

Aubrey E. Taylor, Ph.D.
Harris J. Granger, Ph.D.

36

Interstitial Fluid Pressure—Basic Concepts

Until recently, most physiologists felt that tissue fluid pressure was positive (0 − +2 mm Hg) and not responsive to small changes in capillary filtration forces. In the early 1960s, Guyton[10] and later Scholander[21] measured subatmospheric pressures in subcutaneous tissue; moreover, the pressure was highly responsive to changes in tissue hydration. Subsequently, many investigators have used the implanted capsule technique of Guyton and the wick method of Scholander to study fluid dynamics in a variety of experimental models (Snashall et al.,[22] Ladegaard-Pedersen et al.,[14] Prather et al.,[20] Calnan et al.,[5] Meyer et al.,[16] Aukland et al.,[2] Kirsch et al.,[13] and Gibson[7]).

Since this portion of the symposium deals with fluid pressures in brain tissue, we will discuss the various techniques used to measure tissue fluid pressure, the theory relating the various pressures in the tissues, and the application of these techniques and concepts to the problem of measuring cerebral interstitial fluid pressure.

GUYTON'S CAPSULE METHOD

Guyton implanted hollow, perforated spheres into subcutaneous muscle and lung tissues. One month after implanting the capsule, both the interior and exterior of the capsule were covered with dense connective tissue. In the center of the capsule was a small pocket of fluid. Pressure was measured by inserting a needle through a performation into the fluid pocket (Fig. 1). Many modifications of this technique have been used to measure interstitial fluid pressure in subcutaneous tissue; even plastic hair curlers (called tissue cages) have been used.[5] In all instances, the pressure measured within the capsule has been

negative, averaging about −6 mm Hg. Tissue fluid pressure measurements in lung and muscle have also been negative; but this does not mean that fluid pressures in all tissues are negative.[1,16] Capsules implanted in kidney tissues have measured positive pressure.[18] Therefore, tissue pressure must be investigated in each capillary bed, for it is well known that each capillary bed has different capillary pressures, capillary permeabilities, and capillary densities than do other capillary beds; so it is not unreasonable to assume that different tissue fluid pressures can also exist in different capillary beds. Also, it is important to realize that the tissue pressures measured by this and following techniques measure some functional or average tissue fluid pressure and that different areas even with the same tissue may be gaining or losing fluid.

SCHOLANDER'S WICK METHOD

Basically, cotton fibers are pulled into a small polyethylene catheter and the wick is boiled in saline in order to wet the cotton wick. The wick is then threaded through a needle. The needle can then be placed into the tissue and the surrounding needle withdrawn, which leaves the cotton wick and catheter within the tissue (Fig. 2). The wick has several advantages over the capsule procedure in that no healing time is required, and measurements can be made in animals or organs too small for capsule implantation. However, the wick is not as sensitive as are the larger capsules to tissue hydration and the absolute value of the pressures measured with the wicks are always less negative than the corresponding capsular pressures. Also, the wick pressures do not stabilize for 20 to 40

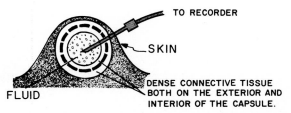

Fig. 1. Schematic representation of the Guyton capsule technique. The small perforated capsules are implanted and allowed to heal for 4 to 8 weeks. Dense connective tissue surrounds both the inside and outside of the capsule. A hyperdermic needle, connected to a stiff catheter system, is inserted into the fluid interior of the capsule.

minutes after insertion into the tissues, and, frequently, bleeding occurs during the needle puncture.

Both of these techniques have been used in brain tissue to estimate brain interstitial fluid pressure and we will discuss these findings in a later section of this paper.

TOTAL TISSUE PRESSURE, SOLID TISSUE PRESSURE, AND THE RELATIONSHIP TO INTERSTITIAL FLUID PRESSURE

When interstitial fluid pressure was demonstrated to be subatmospheric, several vigorous arguments arose concerning how this pressure was related to pressure measurements made with balloons or needles placed into the tissues, for both methods had measured positive

tissue pressures (+1 to +4 mm Hg). Both the balloons and needles were measuring another type of pressure: *total tissue pressure,* or the pressure tending to collapse blood vessels, lymphatics vessels, etc.

The total tissue pressure is equal to the sum of the tissue fluid pressure and the contact pressure (solid tissue pressure) caused by tissues exerting pressure on other tissue structures.

Total Tissue Pressure = Interstitial Fluid Pressure + Solid Tissue Pressure

When a pressure cuff is inflated around a limb, some fluid will move out of the tissues directly under the cuff and all of the cuff pressure will not be transmitted into the fluid. An analogy is pushing against a wall; the pressure at point of contact at the wall can be great, but the surrounding air pressure has not been altered by this

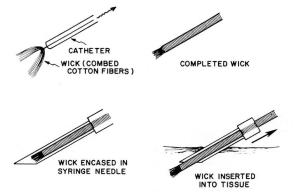

Fig. 2. Schematic representation of the preparation and usage of the Sholander wick method. The wicks are prepared by pulling combed cotton into catheters of a size to easily slip into a given sized hypodermic needle. After pulling the cotton into the catheter, the wick is boiled in isotonic saline or Tyrode's solution. The wick is then encased in the needle and placed into the tissue by inserting the needle. The needle is then withdrawn, leaving the wick in the tissues. Twenty to 30 minutes are usually required for the wick pressure measurements to stabilize.

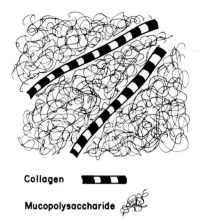

Collagen ▰▰▰

Mucopolysaccharide

Fig. 3. Schematic structure of the extracellular matrix. Dense coils of mucopolysaccharides are cross-linked to collagen and no free fluid channels actually exist. The fluid is within the gel in very small "equivalent pores" of 250–300 A°.

procedure. At normal tissue hydrations, the solid tissue pressure is +9 mm Hg in subcutaneous tissue because of cell, gel, and fiber contact points, but as the tissues become edematous the contact points are pushed apart and no solid pressure exists and total tissue pressure equals tissue fluid pressure.[12]

FREE FLUID VERSUS BOUND FLUID

The interstitial space is not just a watery phase but is composed of mucopolysaccharides, collagen, and fluid. There are normally no pools of free fluid, but the fluid is in a gel-collagen network in small channels of fluid of about 300 A° radius as schematically represented in Fig. 3. Only when the tissues become edematous do large pools of free fluid begin to appear. This composition of the interstitium allows the subatmospheric pressures to exist, for the gel can exist in the tissues at a low hydration state.

For a complete review of the physics and physiology of the interstitial spaces, the reader is referred to Granter et al.,[8] Guyton et al.,[11] and Granger et al.[9]

MEASUREMENT OF TISSUE PRESSURE IN BRAIN TISSUE

Table 1 shows the results obtained by various investigators who have attempted to measure interstitial fluid pressure by either capsules or wicks implanted into brain tissue. The work of Brodersen et al.[4] is the most complete, for it relates wick pressures to cerebrospinal fluid pressures at different hydration states. If the cerebrospinal fluid pressure is considered as the total tissue pressure, then

$$10 = \text{Solid Tissue Pressure} \times 6.5$$
or
$$\text{Solid Tissue Pressure} = 16.5 \text{ mm Hg}$$

In fact, for all measurements except Brock's[3] in Table 1, the interstitial fluid pressure is less than cerebrospinal fluid pressure, which is the reference pressure in this fluid system. Also, at

Table 1
Tissue Pressure Measurements in Brain Tissue

Condition	P_T (mm Hg)	P_{CSF} (mm Hg)	Method and Reference
Normal	−6.5	+10.0	Wick (Brodersen et al.)
Increased P_{CSF}(1)	−6.5	+50.0	
2 liters H_2O	+5.0	....	
Increased P_{CSF}(2)	+10.0	+50.0	
	+5.4	+6.1	Wick (Pöll et al.)
	+5.6	....	
	+5.0	+5.0	Wick (Brock et al.)
	+4.8	....	Capsule (Adachi et al.)
20% Mannitol			
(max. press.)	−6.0	−7.5	Capsule (Matsuo)
After 6 hrs.	−6.0	+3.6	

normal hydrations, changes in CSF pressure did not change the tissue pressure. However, after the brain tissue was made edematous by infusion of 2 liters of water into the experimental animal, increases in CSF caused an increase in interstitial fluid pressure. This finding is analogous to observation made with implanted capsule in subcutaneous tissue. In dehydrated tissues, most of the applied pressure is transmitted through solid elements and not through fluid elements. Once the tissues become edematous, applied pressure is easily transmitted to the fluid elements.

The data of Pöll et al.[19] indicate that P_T and P_{CSF} differ by only 1 mm Hg, and Brock's[3] data indicate that P_T and P_{CSF} are equivalent. There is really no apparent reason why these measurements are so different, except the possibility that Pöll's and Brock's wicks may communicate with the subarachnoid spaces.

The Japanese group have implanted Guyton capsules into brain tissue; unfortunately they did not simultaneously measure CSF pressure. However, one of their experiments has some very interesting data; a 20 percent mannitol solution was intravenously administered, and capsular and cerebrospinal fluid pressures were measured. Both pressures decreased to negative values, capsular pressure to −6.0 mm Hg and cerebrospinal fluid pressure to −7.5 mm Hg maximally, and at the end of 6 hours, tissue pressure was still negative (−5 mm Hg) and cerebrospinal fluid pressure had increased to +3.6. These authors hypothesized that brain tissue pressure and cerebrospinal fluid pressure are not identical pressures. The capsule implants in brain tissue are very interesting and do seem to yield pressures similar to the wick pressure measurements with this one exception; however, the protein content of the capsular fluid was very high (2 to 3 g%) which certainly is far too high for brain tissue fluid protein concentrations.

POSSIBLE MODEL OF FLUID EXCHANGE IN BRAIN TISSUE

Figure 4 is a schematic representation of cerebrospinal fluid pressure (CSF), brain interstitial tissue, and the capillary exchange system for the conditions of a negative interstitial fluid

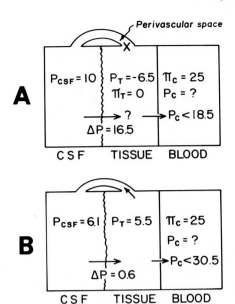

Fig. 4. Schematic representation of the relationship between cerebrospinal fluid pressure (P_{CFS}), brain tissue pressure (P_T), capillary pressure (P_C), tissue colloid osmotic pressure (π_T), and plasma colloid osmotic pressure (π_C) when tissue preparation is negative (*a*) or positive (*b*). ΔP refers to pressure head between CSF and tissue, and the values shown for P_C are those values for which the capillary is absorbing.

pressure (*a*) and for a positive interstitial fluid pressure (*b*). Even with this oversimplified model, it becomes readily apparent that if interstitial fluid pressure is negative in brain tissue, then no fluid flow is possible through the perivascular spaces, and there is a very high gradient for flow between cerebrospinal fluid and brain tissue. At the capillary membrane, the capillary would be an absorbing capillary only for values <18.5 mm Hg. Panel *b* shows the case for a positive interstitial fluid pressure. Only a small pressure head exists between CSF and tissue, but more importantly, the capillary will be an absorbing capillary at pressures <30.5 mm Hg which is 12 mm Hg higher than the negative fluid pressure case. Also, if the capillary does filter, then the possibility exists that P_T could increase and fluid could move out of the tissues into the CSF by bulk flow or by way of the perivascular spaces.

This model is certainly a gross oversimplification of the real brain tissue fluid system, but it does indicate that a small positive interstitial fluid pressure may allow the capillary pressure to vary from moment to moment without causing serious tissue edema.* Since the filtration coefficient (volume flow/mm Hg gradient-min-100 g) is extremely low for brain capillaries, then a large gradient could exist between brain tissue and capillary without large fluid shifts occurring.

Obviously, much more investigative work must be done on this complex system before a more meaningful physiological model can be formulated.

Since the tissue pressure measurements in brain tissue do not agree, then several basic experimental approaches are necessary to answer the question, What is brain tissue pressure? And how is it related to cerebrospinal fluid pressure and alterations in capillary pressures and/or permeabilities? A few possible approaches are the following: (1) the relationship between P_{CSF} and P_T must be measured for many different states of tissue hydration; (2) other methods of measuring tissue pressures must be employed such as the small styrofoam blocks as used by Ott[17]; (3)

measurements of the amount of edema formation at different venous pressures must be measured. Perhaps some isovolumetric preparation similar to Fenstermacher's technique[6] can be employed to study the overall brain edema problem, and tissue volume change can be compared to measurements of tissue and cerebrospinal fluid pressure; (4) the relationship between cerebrospinal fluid and tissue pressure can be measured by varying cerebrospinal fluid pressure. Not only should the steady state pressures be measured, but the transients should also be evaluated; (5) finally, the permeability of the brain capillaries should be studied during elevation of venous pressures.

The exchange of fluid between CSF, tissue, and brain tissue capillaries poses both a very difficult and exciting problem. The technique utilized to study fluid dynamics in other beds, or some modification, should yield new and valuable information concerning the regulation of brain interstitial volume.

---

*For this analysis, only plasma colloid osmotic pressure has been used to calculate plasma osmotic pressure; however, the brain capillaries are unique among capillary beds in that small solutes other than proteins can exert considerable osmotic pressure across the membranes of brain capillaries. The effective osmotic pressure of any solute across a membrane is defined as the reflection coefficient times the Van't Hoff osmotic pressure, where the reflection coefficient is equal to one for an impermeable species and is equal to zero for a freely permeable species (i.e., the velocity of solute in the membrane is identical to the velocity of the solvent). Fenstermacher and Johnson (6) obtained reflection coefficients in brain capillaries of 0.44, 0.89, 0.98 and 1 for urea, glucose, sucrose and raffinose respectively; therefore, any gradient of small molecules between brain and tissue fluid can potentially produce large osmotic pressures.

REFERENCES

1. Adachi C, Mihara H, Matsuo O: Analysis of fluid in capsules implanted into dog brain. Jap J Physiol 24:59–71, 1974

2. Aukland K, Fanes HO: Protein concentration of interstitial fluid collected from rat skin by a wick method. Acta Physiol Scand 88:350–358, 1973

3. Brock M, Winkelmuller W, Pöll W, et al: Measurement of brain-tissue pressure. Lancet 1:595–596, 1972

4. Brodersen P, Hojgaard K, Lassen NA: Measurement of "interstitial fluid" pressure in the brain in dogs, in Brock M, Dietz H (eds): Intracranial Pressure, Experimental and Clinical Aspects. Berlin, Springer, 1972, pp 185–187

5. Calnan JS, Ford PM, Holt PLJ, et al: Implanted tissue cages. Br J Plastic Surg 25:164–174, 1972

6. Fenstermacher JD, Johnson JA: Filtration and reflection coefficients of the rabbit blood-brain barrier. Am J Physiol 211:341–346, 1966

7. Gibson WH: Dynamics of lymph flow, tissue pressure and protein exchange in subcutaneous tissue. Dissertation, Univ of Miss Med Ctr, 1974

8. Granger HJ: Transcapillary exchanges and their regulation, in Reneau DD, Dekker M (eds): Systems Analyses of Biomedical Transport. New York, Marcel Dekker, (in press)

9. Granger HJ, Chen D, Chen HI: Structure and function of the interstitium, in Sgouris JT, Rene A (eds): Proceedings: NIH Symposium on Albumin, Bethesda, MD, National Institute of Health, 1975

10. Guyton AC: A concept of negative interstitial pressure based on pressures in implanted perforated capsules. Circ Res 12:399–414, 1963

11. Guyton AC, Granger HJ, Taylor AE: Interstitial fluid pressure. Physiol Rev 51:527–563, 1971

12. Guyton AC, Taylor AE, Granger HJ: Analysis of types of pressure in the pulmonary interstitial spaces—interstitial fluid pressure, solid tissue pressure, and total tissue pressure, in Angela GC (ed): Control Hemodynamics and Gas Exchange. Torino, Italy, Edizioni Minerva Medica, 1971, pp 4–45

13. Kirsch K, Rafflenbeul W, Roedel H: Untersuchungen zuy Ursache des negativen interstitiellen Gewebsdruckes (Guyton-Kapsel). Pfluger Arch 328:193–204, 1971

14. Ladegaard-Pedersen HJ: Measurement of interstitial pressure in subcutaneous tissue in dogs. Circ Res 62:765–770, 1960

15. Matsuo O: Variations in brain capsule pressure with the administration of hypertonic solutions. Kobe J Med Sci 19:39–49, 1973

16. Meyer BJ, Meyer A, Guyton AC: Interstitial fluid pressure. V Negative pressure in the lungs. Circ Res 22:263–271, 1968

17. Ott CE, Haas JA, Cuche JL et al: Effect of increased peritubule protein concentration on proximal tubule reabsorption in the presence and absence of extracellular volume expansion (in press)

18. Ott CE, Navar LG, Guyton AC. Pressures in static and dynamic states from capsules implanted in the kidney. Am J Physiol 221:394–400, 1971

19. Pöll W, Brock M, Markakis E et al: Brain tissue pressure, in Brock M, Dietz H (eds): Intracranial Pressure, Experimental and Clinical Aspects, Berlin, Springer, 1972, pp 188–194

20. Prather JW, Bowes DN, Warrell DA: Comparison of capsule and wick techniques for measurement of interstitial fluid pressure. J Appl Physiol 31:942–945, 1971

21. Scholander PF, Hargens AR, Miller SL: Negative pressure in the interstitial fluid of animals. Science 161:321–328, 1968

22. Snashall PD, Lucas J, Guz A et al: Measurement of interstitial fluid pressure by means of a cotton wick in man and animals: An analysis of the origin of the pressure. Clin Sci 41:35–53, 1971

Open Discussion

DR. OMMAYA: We have heard this morning about some of the dangers of high intracranial pressure, and I think some of the data we have had recently bring out the importance of recognizing the dangers of normal intracranial pressure and low intracranial pressure. I think it reemphasizes again what Dr. Miller points out, that measurements of brain compliance is extremely important.

We have paid particular interest to the rate of dependence of the pressure-volume measurement and have come to the conclusion that in order to interpret the intracranial pressure recording, you have to know what the compliance is. Intracranial pressure measurements are therefore very important when the compliance is normal or decreasing. It is probably not so useful when compliance is increasing, but it will warn you that the normal or low intracranial pressure under increased compliance may be dangerous.

We studied the effects of rapid inflation of extradural balloons in a monkey on ICP, SAP and pressures in the pial arteries and veins. We found the classic Cushing response to this high rate of inflation with gradients falling in the pial artery and veins. With slow infusion, there is a very different response, the degree of the Cushing response is much less, the gradients are different. However, there is still a gradient difference according to time.

The key point I want to make is that although there are differences, the gradient in the capillaries at the time of brain death at both infusion rates crosses between the arteries and veins, although the intracranial pressure measurements are vastly different. In other words, the intracranial pressure measurement in itself is a gross reflection of the actual critical pressure gradient pressure measurement which is across the capillaries, and that is why brain death occurs irrespective of the level of intracranial pressure.

DR. TAYLOR: I believe there is a whole physiology of pressure related to other than large arteries and resistance vessels. There is a whole relationship of pressure to veins, and there is probably in the ECF space a pressure related to capillary pressure.

The brain must relate in elevating its pressure—a vascular pressure. I am quite certain intuitively that this must not at all times be large arterial pressure. There is a physiology of this linkage at the capillary level and perhaps even below this.

Our concept of compliance, of complaint changes, indeed, do not reside with any changes in resistance vessels. Our concept is that this change occurs in the compliance vessels of the venous side of the system. What remains to be done now is to correlate tissue pressures with wedge pressures, under circumstances where we can dissociate tissue pressure from CSF pressure.

DR. MILLER: The whole argument is one of theory versus practice. I agree totally that if you change volume you are going to change tissue pressure. The question is, if you try to do it in the manner in which he is discussing, then as the fluid moves away, or if there is any stressful relaxation within the tissues, mucopolysaccharides expand and take up room resulting in little change in pressure.

DR. RAPOPORT: This is what appears to happen with the white matter, from the discussions today.

DR. MILLER: I think you can get different compliance curves. There is a very simple experiment which can be done and that is to have two pressure monitors next to each other. Through one monitor, volume can be removed so that there is volume flowing between a measured distance, then conductance can be measured through the tissues. Then, this artifact can be removed as a portion of the change in the compliance. Actual compliance can then be calculated.

I would like to say one thing about Dr. Bruce's talk when he discussed mucopolysaccharides. Dr. Cook in our laboratory found a tremendous amount of mucopolysaccharide and little acid in the gray matter. In the white matter, there is very little mucopolysaccharide. These differences can really affect the conductance. The flow from the capillary is now a function like adding up resistances in parallel, so the conductance will be less than any one of the conductances, and conductance is a function of half distance. As a result there is a very low conductance through this whole system according to how far it has to flow away.

Dr. Rapoport then followed this discussion with a lengthy discussion of a mathematical model to explain the possible formation of edema. This discussion has been summarized by Dr. Rapoport as an addendum to his paper in this book.

Robert G. Grossman, M.D.
Aleksandr I. Seregin, Ph.D.

37

Effects of Traumatically Induced Edema on Membrane Potentials of Cortical Glial Cells and Neurons

Trauma to a localized area of the brain frequently produces progressive impairment of function of a surrounding zone of cerebral tissue which is associated with tissue swelling.[3] Cold injury of the cerebral cortex has been used as a model of traumatically induced edema by many investigators to study the factors involved in the spread of injury-induced edema.[1,11] The predominant type of edema associated with the early stages of a cold-induced lesion of the brain is vasogenic and is related to the extracellular spread of protein and fluid from injured capillaries.[8] Although the spread of edema into the areas surrounding the site of trauma has been well studied by using a variety of tracer substances, the mechanisms producing progressive neural dysfunction and eventual glial reaction to the spread of the edema fluid have not been completely clarified. There are number of possible mechanisms that might produce neural dysfunction in an area into which edema fluid spreads.

1. Mechanical disruption of extracellular clefts and interference with intercellular communication;
2. Ischemia due to compression of the vasculature;
3. Effects of substances leaking from capillaries and cells, whose permeability has been altered by the injury, on the electrophysiological activity of neurons and glia.

An additional point of clinical interest is the question of what cellular factors limit the spread of edema and the mechanisms which restore the tissue to a normal state.

The present experiments were designed to investigate the sequence of events that occur at the cellular level in neurons and glia in the immediate area surrounding a cold injury of the cerebral cortex. Experiments were carried out in 11 adult cats anesthetized with pentobarbital. The intracellular recording techniques used have been described previously.[7] Cold injury of the sensorimotor cortex was produced by applying a brass cannister, 8 mm in diameter, filled with dry ice, to the cortex for 30 seconds. A cold injury of this severity produced hyperemia and slight swelling of the cortex in an area which was sharply circumscribed within 10 minutes. Intracellular recording was then carried out by making vertical puncture with micropipettes at 21 positions, starting rostral to the lesion, traversing the lesion, and passing caudal to the lesion. The first 7 positions were in the cortex surrounding the rostral pole of the injury, the next 7 positions were in the lesion, and the last 7 positions were again in the cortex surrounding the injury. Recordings were carried out in the lesion, and then in the surrounding tissue into which edema was spreading for up to 12 hours. The extent of spread of edema was studied by the IV injection of Evans blue dye, and perfusing the animal one-half hour after dye injection. In all cases, the edema had penetrated at least 3 mm from the circumscribed edge of the original lesion site into the surrounding gray matter.

Previous studies have established the criteria for the electrophysiological identification of cortical glial cells, and have adduced evidence that the highest membrane potential cells that are penetrated superficially in the cortex or at the external

273

limiting membrane are astrocytes. The modal membrane potential for such cells is −80 to −90 mV. In some cases, cells with membrane potentials of −100 mV are penetrated.[6,7,9]

In addition, in normal cortex at least 25 percent of cells identified as glial cells respond to the firing of adjacent neurons during synchronized electrocortical activity during barbiturate-induced spindle bursts with slow depolarizing potentials.[5] In contrast to the glia, stable neuronal membrane potentials in lightly anesthetized cat cortex range from −55 to −75 mV, and on occasion a neuron with a membrane potential of −80 mV may be penetrated.[6]

Immediately following injury, the spontaneous extracellularly recorded potentials of the electrocorticogram of the directly injured cortex became smaller in amplitude, and spindle bursts became less well defined. The deterioration of the spontaneous electrical activity progressed in some cases to amorphous, low-amplitude slow waves over a period of several hours. The spontaneous electrical activity of the surrounding cortex also deteriorated as edema spread into the surrounding cortex. Intracellular recording in the circumscribed lesion area revealed that no intracellular potentials could be recorded in the first 12 hours after injury.

Recovery of potentials of some glia and of at least a few neurons within lesions of this severity occur, as shown by a previous study of such lesions carried out 4 to 43 days after similar injuries. However, in the present study, our primary interest was in the electrophysiological effects of the spread of edema into the cortex surrounding the traumatically induced lesion. The effect of the spread of edema, as judged by the penetration of cellular elements, was to slightly increase the numbers of glia penetrated at each cortical position but to decrease the numbers of neurons penetrated, when compared to the control data established for each position in a similar penetration prior to making the cold lesion. Data for a typical experiment are given in Table 1. The probability of penetration of a cell depends on the size of a cell, and certain characteristics of its membrane, such as its fragility, and the maintenance of a membrane potential which can be recorded as the sign of penetration. The simplest explanation of larger numbers of glia in cortex into which edema is spreading is that the glia are undergoing swelling. The interpretation of the reduction of numbers of neurons penetrated in edematous cortex is more difficult. Neurons do not appear to swell as

Table 1
Experiment 4

	Glial Cells	
	Total	MP > − 70 mV
Before Lesion	73	19 (26%) av MP −83 mV, Range −90–70 mV
After Lesion	39	12 (30%) av MP −76 mV, Range −86–70 mV

	Neurons	
	Total	MP > −50 mV
Before Lesion	108	8 (7%) av MP −57 mV
After Lesion	31	1 (3%) MP −55 mV

much as glia in osmotically induced cerebral edema.[4,10] It is possible that the volume of neurons in the edematous area is decreased by expansion of the extracellular clefts and by glial swelling. Alternatively, if the injury changes the permeability of the neural membrane sufficiently to depolarize the neuron, then fewer neuronal membrane potentials will be recorded. The average membrane potential of the glia in the cortex that was becoming edematous was greatly changed, at least in this early stage of edema. Cells with membrane potentials as high as −92 mV were penetrated. However, no ultrahigh potential cells (−100 mV) were penetrated. The comparatively few neurons that were penetrated in the edematous cortex had membrane potentials which were at the lower limits of normal. Although the glial membrane potentials recorded were in the normal range in edematous cortex, no glia were penetrated that exhibited the normal glial response of slow depolarization in association with spindle burse activity of the cortex. Although the intensity of synchronized electrocortical activity was decreased in the edematous cortex, some activity was present, and the absence of any slow glial depolarization during synchronized electrocortical waves suggests that the normal neural-glial spatial relationships which allow neurally released substances to depolarize glia are disturbed in the cortex, perhaps by simple edematous expansion of the extracellular clefts.

The experiments suggest that the infiltration of fluid and proteins from injured capillaries into the extracellular clefts of the cortex does not injure glia, at least in the early stages of the development of edema, by damaging their membranes to the point of lowering their membrane potentials. The glial response to the injury appears to be one of swelling. Neurochemical studies have shown that exposure of glial cells to increased levels of K+, which might be expected to occur if neurons depolarize and release their intracellular K+, results in glial swelling and a sequestration of extracellular electrolytes within the glia.[2] It is possible that glial swelling around a focal injury is a homeostatic mechanism to sequester edema fluid.

REFERENCES

1. Blakemore WF: The ultrastructural appearance of astrocytes following thermal lesion of the rat cortex. J Neurol Sci 12:319–332, 1971
2. Bourke RS, Nelson KM, Naumann RA, Young OM: Studies of the production and subsequent reduction of swelling in primate cerebral cortex under isosmotic conditions in vivo. Exp Brain Res 10:427–446, 1970
3. Cavanaugh JB: The proliferation of astrocytes around a needle wound in the rat brain. J Anat 106:471–487, 1970
4. Dila CJ, Pappius HM: Cerebral water and electrolytes. An experimental model of inappropriate secretion of antidiuretic hormone. Arch Neurol 26:85–90, 1972
5. Grossman RG, Hampton T: Depolarization of cortical glial cells during electrocortical activity. Brain Res 11:316–324, 1968

6. Grossman RG, Lynch L, Shires GT: Ionic content and membrane potentials of cortical neurons and glia. Neurology 18:292, 1968
7. Grossman, RG, Rosman LJ: Intracellular potentials of inexcitable cells in epileptogenic cortex undergoing fibrillary gliosis after a local injury. Brain Res 28:181–201, 1971
8. Klatzo I: Neuropathological aspects of brain edema. J Neuropathol Exp Neurol 26:1–14, 1967
9. Pape LG, Katzman R: Response of glia in cat sensorimotor cortex to increased extracellular potassium. Brain Res 38:71–92, 1972
10. Wasterlain CG, Torach RM: Cerebral edema and water intoxication: II. An ultrastructural study. Arch Neurol 19:79–87, 1968
11. Van Der Veen PH, Go KG, Zuiderveen I, et al: Electrical impedance of cat brain with cold-induced edema. Exp Neurol 40:615–682, 1973

Open Discussion

CHAIRMAN BECKER: Dr. Bruce, the first day you warned all of us that brain edema cannot be correlated with neurological dysfunction. I am wondering what you would think about that now in relation to what has been presented.

DR. BRUCE: I think Dr. Miller's example of the patient with pseudotumor cerebri, having intracranial pressures of 90 mm Hg and brain edema, who could perform perfectly well is pertinent.

CHAIRMAN BECKER: Do you think there are different kinds of edema, and in pseudotumor, that is actually a specific type of edema?

DR. BRUCE: I do. Protein edema versus hydrostatic edema makes a great difference on neurological effects.

With regards to the tissue pressure question, we may have half the data already—Dr. Marmarou's and Dr. Shulman's presentations of the way the tissue changes occur in 1 to 2 hours, and that by 4 hours, the pressure gradients are essentially dissipated. [Dr. Symon] has the data to tell us at what point the hydrogen flows are lowest in the edematous areas and in the normal areas. If the low flows don't correlate with the highest tissue pressure gradients, then it is highly suggestive that the tissue pressure gradients are not responsible for the low flows. Also, it would be interesting to follow the progress of the neurological deficit, because if it correlates better with the low flow than it does with the tissue pressure, then I think we may have the answer to what we are searching for.

DR. DILA: To Dr. Bruce's comment on cerebral edema and function—patients with brain tumors show a resolution of edema around the tumor on CAT scan coinciding with preoperative steroid treatment. At the same time we see improvement in neurological status. One may speculate on the potential steroid effect that is being cleared up.

DR. RANSOHOFF: I do think there is very good evidence for the statement that you cannot correlate edema to brain dysfunction. I think Bob Grossman's experiments today have really demonstrated quite well that some of the cells in the area of the edema are functioning in terms of their potassium capacity extremely well.

Certainly, the correlation in some of the spinal cord studies where function returns far ahead of any change in the water content of the tissue demonstrates that once the glial or vascular membranes are functioning, the function of the tissue returns, and that the secondary clearance of the edema really has almost nothing to do with the function. Indeed, if you look at the CAT scan after massive steroid doses when the patient's response is extremely rapid, the early CAT scan will show no change in the edema.

DR. O'CONNER: There are several types of edema, as everyone has alluded to. The point I would like to make is that there is a type of edema (gray matter?) that might have neurological function and cause neurological dysfunction, whereas other types of edema (white matter edema?) may not cause any neurologic dysfunction.

With regard to Dr. Grossman's data on the edema that he saw surrounding the freeze lesion, he spoke of two methods of clearing up potassium: potassium may be moved by the sodium pump or by a passive mechanism. In the normal cortex, there is no good evidence that active uptake or a very vigorous sodium pump is present in glial cells. Therefore, reuptake of potassium must be via a passive mechanism. Experiments showing massive stimulation of metabolism by potassium occur in reactive glial cells. The reactive glial cells may function to clear up the edema and affect the neurological effects that may occur in gray matter edema.

K. Shulman, M.D.
A. Marmarou, Ph.D.
K. Shapiro, M.D.

38

Brain Tissue Pressure and Focal Pressure Gradients

Certain observations in the course of neurosurgery suggest that local areas of the brain can swell, and during these times of tissue expansion, there is an increase in the pressure of such tissue. In these regions the cortical gyri are expanded with an obliteration of sulci; incisions of the pia arachnoid cause extrusion of gray and white matter. Further clinical observations seem to indicate that the more rapid the onset of the focal process, the more pronounced is regional expansion. This may mean that one is dealing with a transient process and that with time areas of focal brain edema spread and, in so doing, diffuse into neighboring regions. This report, by measuring brain tissue pressure, attempts to elucidate the biomechanics of the brain extracellular fluid space in the production and resolution of brain tissue pressure gradients. Like the CSF space of the brain, the extracellular fluid space will have a pressure which is determined by the compliance and outflow resistance of that tissue space. These parameters are more difficult to characterize than the CSF biomechanics because of our limited understanding of the geometry of the extracellular fluid space and of the precise mechanisms of fluid ingress and outflow from this space. Finally, brain tissue pressure may be elevated and tissue pressure gradients with the CSF space and with adjacent brain areas may exist in specific brain pathology and be absent in another pathological process. The experimental model used to study brain tissue pressure, therefore, must be carefully selected.

The object of the present series of experiments was to study the magnitude and time course of short-term (4 to 6 hours) intracompartmental (supratentorial) tissue pressure gradients. Intercompartmental pressure gradients associated with tentorial herniation have been studied but are not included.

MATERIALS AND METHODS

Cats weighing 2.5–4.5 kg were anesthetized with sodium pentobarbital (Nembutal, 30 mg/kg i.p.). Femoral vessels were cannulated and arterial blood pressure measured with a pressure transducer. All animals were tracheostomized and mechanically ventilated with a conventional Starling pump. The acid base status was checked periodically and the animals were kept at a $PACO_2$ of 30 to 40 mm Hg with a pO_2 of greater than 95 mm Hg. The head was fixed in the stereotaxic frame.

In series A (saline infusion and balloon expansion), cotton wick brain tissue probes encased in Pe 50 polyethylene tubing were introduced through a stainless steel needle, one into the left hemisphere and two into the right. The cotton wick fibers offer a resistance to volume change. This resistance is a function of the packing density D/A and fiber length L, so that resistance is proportional to (DxL)/A. The catheter resistance acts only to retard flow and at equilibrium does not affect the volume change in the strain gauge chamber. Thus the static properties of the wick gauge tissue pressure system are determined solely by the strain gauge characteristics and are independent of wick resistance.[7] Frequency response of the tissue pressure wick system is limited so that the reflection of the arterial pulsation of brain are not seen, but respiratory fluctuations are regularly seen and are an indication of a functional system. CSF space pressure was

This research was supported in part by NIH Training Grant 5 T01 NS05511-09.

measured either in the lateral ventricle (LVP) or in the cisterna magna (CMP). Two series of experiments were performed in the same animals; first artificial CSF (Elliot's B solution) was infused through a 23-gauge needle directly into left hemisphere white matter approximately 8 mm from the ipsilateral tissue pressure catheter at a slow rate of 1.5 ml/hr. In another group of animals, an epidural balloon was inflated over the left hemisphere.

In the more recent series (B), tissue pressure was measured using glass micropipettes with cotton wick packing, making it unnecessary to use a needle as a guide for introduction of the wick catheter. The glass pipette O.D. was 0.7 mm. Two glass-clad cotton wick catheters were placed in the left hemisphere and one in the right. CSF pressure was monitored in the cisterna magna or lateral ventricles. A freeze lesion was made at the extreme of the left frontal lobe by applying a cannister containing liquid nitrogen via 0.8 cm burr hole for a period of 5 minutes. All pressures were then continuously measured for a period of 4 hours. Prior to sacrifice, Evans blue (2 mg/kg) was given intravenously to demonstrate the extent of the edematous area. The brain was removed and fixed in formalin for later sectioning.

RESULTS

Steady-State Brain Tissue Pressure

The resting brain tissue pressure (BTP) measured 1 hour after insertion of the wick probe was within the pressure envelope of either the CMP or LVP. Prior to stabilization, BTP tends to pass through a negative pressure phase before approaching a resting pressure slightly less than the CMP or LVP. BTP in 13 animals was +14.0 mm Hg (gauge refers to right atrium) and was not different from CMP or LVP. There was no pressure difference between multiple tissue pressure probes. Addition of volume to the cistern causes a rise of BTP and CMP with an identical time course. Fluctuations of BTP catheters were synchronous with respiratory rate.

Balloon Compression

Epidural balloon compression causes brain compaction and a rise of VFP beginning 35 to 40 minutes after start of inflation (Fig. 1). Tissue pressure increases in both hemispheres but does not exceed VFP. Further compaction leads to dissociation of VFP and CMP (balloon volume > .75 ml) and development of tissue pressure gradients. The magnitude of BTP of both hemispheres remains bounded by the compartmental CSF pressures.

Tissue Pressure after White Matter Infusion (Direct Edema)

Infusion of artificial CSF into the white matter of the brain produces a type of white matter edema associated with enlargement of the left hemisphere with compression of the left lateral ventricle. The fluid seems to pass along the association fiber bundles of the ipsilateral hemisphere rather than in commissural fibers, such as the corpus callosum, and can be demonstrated by Evans blue placed in the infusate. No fluid cavity or hemorrhage is seen at the tip of the needle if the infusion rate is slow. Microscopically, there is myelin separation and enlargement of the ECF space quite similar to the microscopic picture of edema adjacent to the freeze lesion (vasogenic edema). Pressure in the ipsilateral tissue pressure catheter increases greater than CMP or contralateral tissue pressure (Fig. 2); as the infusion continues, the gradient is gradually lost.

Focal Freeze Lesion

A left frontal freeze lesion causes focal hemisphere edema with associated blue staining of the white matter. The amount of Evans blue is not as great as the increase in the white matter, the blue staining underestimating the degree of edema. The amount of edema varied from animal to animal despite the same freeze insult.

Animals with considerable expansion of white matter developed a VFP to CMP gradient ranging from 10 to 30 mm Hg approximately 1 hour following application of the cold probe. Transient BTP elevations exceeding VFP were seen but not sustained (Fig. 3). Gradients between proximal and remote wick probes ranged from 4–14 mm Hg in animals with raised VFP. In a single animal in which there was gross hemorrhagic insult directly adjacent to the site of the tissue pressure catheter, the BTP increased to a maximum of 40 mm Hg (Fig. 4). In animals with proportionately less expansion of white matter, no dissociation of supratentorial to infratentorial pressures occurs and tissue pressures remain within the range of the CMP.

DISCUSSION

Placement of the polyethylene-clad or glass-clad cotton wick catheter in subcutaneous tissue results in a stable negative pressure ranging from -1 to -4 mm Hg. In brain tissue, a positive pressure is measured, and under steady-state conditions, the BTP is not different from CSF pressure. The wick pressure measures an interstitial fluid pressure; this pressure plus a solid tissue pressure is equal to total tissue pressure.[3] Since our data show that BTP equals CSF pressure, we assume that for the brain this is total tissue pressure; the solid tissue pressure in the resting steady state must be negligible. Tight fluid junctions do not exist in the ependymal walls of the ventricles as shown by Brightman and Reese,[1] and under steady-state conditions, there is fluid communication between the ECF space and ventricle, perhaps explaining the steady-state concordance

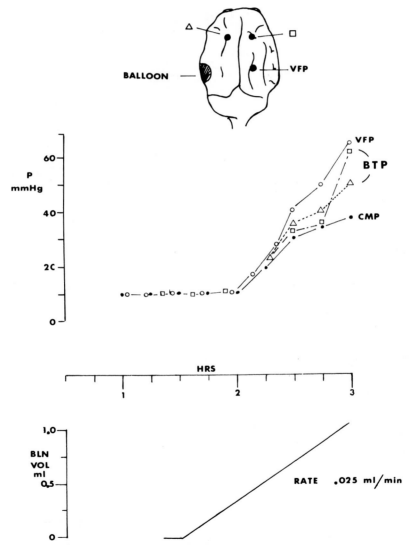

Fig. 1. Response of brain tissue to inflation of epidural balloon. Resting BTP prior to balloon expansion is close to steady-state CSF pressure. As brain is compressed, both CSF and BT pressures rise. With further compression, CSF pressures dissociate and brain tissue pressure gradients develop. The absolute magnitude of BTP remains bounded by VFP and CMP.

of pressures. All brain tissue pressures are thus equal at steady state, either because of direct tissue ECF link or via ECF to CSF linkage.

The demonstration of brain tissue pressure gradients is an attempt to show nonsteady-state conditions. With an extradural compressive mass, it is our concept that the brain ECF space is compacted as is the CSF space, and since these are in some communication, the BTP rises along with LVP, without much of a pressure gradient. The data seem to demonstrate this. The BTP in the hemisphere contralateral to the compression also rises. This elevation of BTP may reflect direct transmission of the compressing force through the brain and ventricle. An alternate explanation is that the force may cause deformation of the ven-

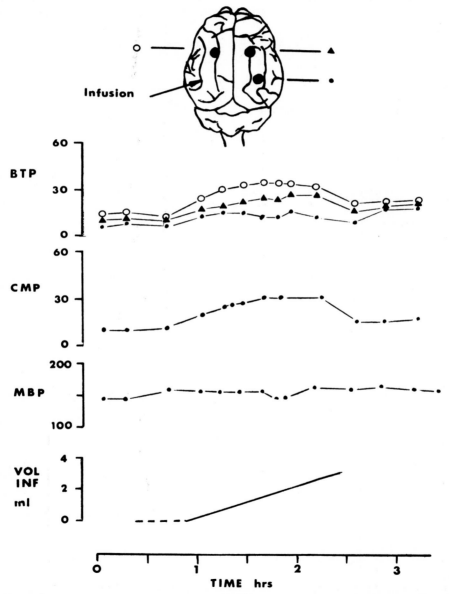

Fig. 2. Response of brain interstitial fluid pressure (BTP) to direct infusion of isotonic solution into white matter (.025 ml/min). BTP in the ipsilateral hemisphere increases greater than BTP at remote sites. As the infusion continues, the gradient is gradually lost.

tricular system with a rise of LVP and a transependymal egress of CSF to elevate contralateral BTP.

This introduces the notion that BTP will be elevated, perhaps to a similar degree, when the ECF is either compressed by an outside force or distended by a fluid force primarily within the ECF. A rapid change in the volume of the ECF space leads to a "tightness," and the brain tissue pressure rises. If the driving force (increased fluid addition) to the space ceases, tissue pressure falls, for now fluid leaves the space faster than it enters in the region of the tissue pressure catheter, and

the brain tissue pressure comes to lie roughly within the CSF pressure envelope (its basic reference pressure). A model which is designed so that the independent variable is an expansion of the ECF space should, by these concepts of the ECF space biomechanics, show a primary rise of the tissue pressure closest to the pathology, a secondary rise of adjacent brain tissue pressures, and a later rise of CSF pressure. In the model of infusion of artificial CSF into the left hemisphere, brain tissue pressure in this hemisphere did increase. However, it did not increase to a high level, and this level of elevation did not last for a

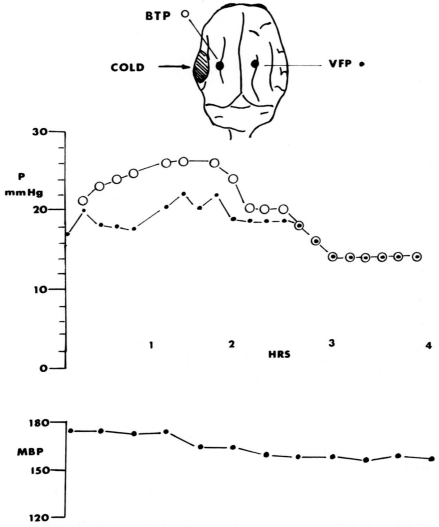

Fig. 3. Response of brain tissue pressure (BTP) to cold lesion in central area. Tissue pressure rises to a maximum of 28 mm Hg. Gradient (6 mm Hg) between tissue and VFP was not sustained.

prolonged period. This suggests that the compliance of the space is such that it is fairly easily increased and that a fair amount of fluid can be infused without a large rise in pressure; 1.5 cc/hr (0.025 ml/min) produces a rise of only 15 mm Hg. These figures are comparable to CSF formation and absorption rates in the cat. The final brain tissue pressure then reflects both the compliance and the outflow resistance of the interstitial fluid space. To the infusion model, the outflow of mixed electrolyte solutions was relatively rapid.

In the cold-injury model, there is a local increase in vascular permeability with an outpour-

ing of plasmalike fluid into the ECF space.[6] Once in the tissue, this fluid has the ability to spread throughout the extracellular channels of the white matter. This spread of fluid is easiest along the fiber tracts that is following the long association fibers of one hemisphere and is therefore directional. In our animals with the freeze lesion and with the infusion of CSF, this restriction of fluid movement to one hemisphere was constant in both models. The edema of the freeze lesion expands the ECF space by what is estimated to be about 30 percent.[2,10] Errors in the method caused by the colloid osmotic effect of the extravasated plasma

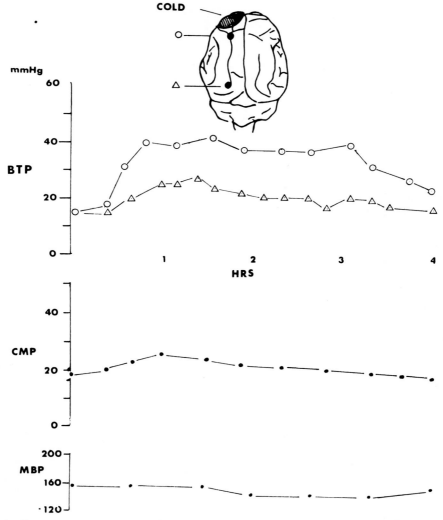

Fig. 4. Response of brain interstitial fluid pressure (BTP) to a focal freeze lesion. Gross hemorrhagic necrosis at the lesion site coincided with a higher rise of BTP at wick adjacent to the lesion than in other experiments where a more gradual rise was observed.

protein can be excluded in using the wick catheter, since it has been shown by Scholander and others that the wick technique measures a hydrostatic pressure uninfluenced by osmotic or colloidal osmotic forces.[5,9] In our concept, the wick catheter sees the wave of spreading edema. As the leading front approaches the wick catheter adjacent to the lesion, the ECF space is distended, elevating the pressure in this catheter. With continued distension of the ECF space, the brain tissue pressure does not rise further and gradients between tissue pressure catheters decrease because of increased brain tissue pressure in adjacent catheters or decrease in the reference catheter. Data on this point are not clear at the present time. The rate of capillary extravasation into the ECF also may vary, but we provide no new data on this important point. These factors eventually limit the spread of edema. The possibility exists, then, that the ECF space will be distended and contain increased fluid volume at a time when the BTP measured in that space will be relatively low, with only a small or no gradient to adjacent spaces. It is our concept, then, that the initial rise of BTP is not the cause but rather the effect of the edema in the case of the freeze lesion and is due to extravasation of a high protein fluid and limited fluid flow through the ECF. However, the spread of the edema is enhanced by the elevation of brain tissue pressure.

Our data differs from Reulen and Dreysch[8] in that we show no progressive elevations of tissue pressure with time. Excluding animal experiments complicated by intracranial parenchymal hemor-rhage, our studies of the freeze lesion show brain tissue pressure gradients that seem to be real but which do not exceed 30 to 35 mm Hg. This pressure approximates that found in the terminal arteriolar tree. This concordance of ECF pressure and a vascular pressure suggests that the generator of edema in the cold lesion model may be the pressure head from the capillary and precapillary vasculature. Klatzo has demonstrated that the spread of cold edema (vasogenic edema) is related to the level of blood pressure.[4] Our data would suggest further that in and around the area of the cold lesion, an elevation of blood pressure elevates capillary pressure, increasing this fluid extravasation. We expect that in the uncomplicated cold lesion model, the tissue pressure will not exceed its generating force and will passively reflect the perfusion pressure in the vascular tree, the extent of blood-brain barrier damage, and the biomechanics of the ECF space, that is, its compliance and resistance to outflow of this additional fluid. We therefore cannot support the progressive elevations of tissue pressure described by Reulen and Kreysch.

These studies demonstrate some of the pathophysiologic changes accounting for the spread of fluid through the ECF space. We have attempted to define the fluid transmission characteristics of this space and show its relations to other compartments of the brain using a biophysical approach. The importance of elevated brain tissue pressure upon capillary hemodynamics and capillary transport remains to be studied.

REFERENCES

1. Brightman MS, Reese TS: Junctions between intimately apposed cell membranes in the vertebrate brain. J Cell Biol 40:648, 1969
2. Fenske A, Samii M, Reulen JH, et al: Extracellular space and electrolyte distribution in cortex and white matter of dog brain in cold induced oedema. Acta Neurochir 28:81, 1973
3. Guyton AC, Granger HJ, Taylor AE: Interstitial fluid pressure. Physiol Rev 51:527, 1971
4. Klatzo I, Wisniewski H, Steinwall O, Streicher E: Dynamics of cold injury edema, in Klatzo I, Seitelberger F (eds): Brain Edema. New York, Springer, 1967, pp 554–563
5. Ladegard-Pedersen HJ: Measurement of the interstitial pressure in subcutaneous tissue in dogs. Circ Res 26:765, 1970
6. Lee JC, Bakay L: Ultrastructural changes in the edematous cerebral nervous system. II. Cold induced edema. Arch Neurol 14:36, 1966
7. Marmarou A, Shulman K: An evaluation of static and dynamic properties of tissue pressure catheters. Second Int Symp Intracranial Pressure, Lund, Sweden, 1974
8. Reulen HJ, Kreysch HG: Measurement of brain tissue pressure in cold induced cerebral oedema. Acta Neurochir 29:29–40, 1973
9. Scholander PF, Hargens AR, Miller St L: Negative pressure in the interstitial fluid of animals. Science 161:321, 1968
10. Streicher EP, Ferrit PJ, Prokop JD, et al: Brain volume and thiocynate space in local cold injury. Arch Neurol 11:444, 1964

Open Discussion

DR. SYMON: I support this concept of Dr. Shulman's. The driving pressure in the end must predominantly be an intravascular pressure. The question is whether or not there is an interaction not only between vascular pressure and tissue pressure but also in the reverse way, so increasing tissue pressure as a result produces increasing capillary pressure from an exhaustion of autoregulation.

Whether you need to involve in this concept a change in the compliance vessels as well is another matter. I have no personal evidence on that. Nevertheless, I think it is possible to see a linkage between rising tissue pressure, rising capillary pressure, and thereby a progressive potential further rise in tissue pressure.

Romas Sakalas, M.D., Editor

Summary—Pressure-Volume Relationship Section

The topic in this section was pressure-volume relationships in the intracranial cavity and in brain tissue itself. The concepts in these areas that have been developed have important scientific implications that ultimately relate to patient management.

The first part of the program developed basic concepts of intracranial pressure-volume relationships, and Dr. Miller and Dr. Symon defined applications of these concepts and their significance in patient management and scientific investigation.

As our understanding of these areas has advanced, the importance of defining brain tissue pressure has become apparent. These pressures and the state of the interstitial compartment relate to capillary flow and cellular metabolism and function.

The papers presented in this part have attempted to clarify some issues concerning basic physiology and pathophysiology of pressure-volume relationships. The discussions have centered on three issues: (1) the evaluation and determinaton of compliance, elastance, and outflow resistance—their role in intracranial pressure and their usefulness in clinical application; (2) the study of the components of intracranial pressure—brain tissue pressure, capillary bed pressure, and CSF pressure, in the normal and injured state; (3) the production of tissue pressure gradients following focal brain injury and the response of individual cells to this injury.

It appears that the major components which determine both the steady-state and transient characteristics of intracranial pressure are compliance and outflow resistance. Dr. Marmarou studied both of these parameters. He has de-termined that when pressure data are plotted on a logarithmic axis against changes in volume, the resulting curve approximates a straight line. The shape of this line is the pressure-volume index (PVI). Compliance can now be determined by $C = .4343$ PVI/P. Using his data along with other work, Dr. Marmarou has determined that two-thirds of the compliance is in the intracranial compartment and the remaining one-third in the spinal compartment.

He was able to calculate outflow resistance by determining the rate of absorption following an injected volume. Thus, by determining via the PVI and calculating outflow resistance, the dynamic changes occurring in intracranial pressure can be easily followed.

Intracranial pressure monitoring has provided a tremendous amount of information concerning the pathophysiology of brain injury. The importance of intracranial pressure measurements in the clinical setting, particularly in trauma patients, was reviewed by Dr. Miller. He points out that continuous monitoring of intracranial pressure is not sufficient because it does not yield information about what point a patient is at in the volume-pressure curve. Dr. Miller has developed the volume-pressure response test which does. As the test is presently performed, a pressure response of > 2 mm Hg to a 1 cc volume injection denotes a state of high elastance. High pressure elastance is at a critical position on the volume-pressure curve where additional volumetric increases cannot be tolerated. Dr. Miller found this to be especially true in those patients with brain shifts, where apparently all compensatory mechanisms have been exhausted and a critical stage is reached. Knowledge of ICP and elastance, as gauged by the VPR test, provides the necessary information for appropriate therapy and/or diagnostic procedures to be undertaken by the clinician.

An excellent review of recent work on the components comprising intracranial pressure—CSF pressure, vascular pressure, and brain tissue pressure—was presented by Dr. Symon. He also discussed the relationship of intracranial pressure and intracranial brain shifts. He reviewed the evidence for intracompartmental pressure gradients and intercompartmental tissue gradients in response to injury. His own work with extradural balloons demonstrated that pressure gradients exist between hemispheres. Based on these data and work of others, the evidence is accumulating that brain shifts are a result of tissue pressure gradients. The mechanism by which brain shifts occur as a result of pressure gradients may be via exhaustion of autoregulation in the injured area. In this circumstance, the local circulation is more liable to be influenced by the systemic blood pressure changes which may result in progressive formation of edema.

Dr. Shulman attempted to study the biomechanics of brain tissue pressure gradients by the wick method in response to a variety of methods of increasing ICP. This group showed that gradients rapidly disappeared in infusion models, whereas freeze models and balloon models did maintain pressure gradients. He, also, feels that pressure gradients in the cold lesion model could be the result of edema due to an increased pressure level from the capillary and precapillary vasculature.

It, therefore, becomes increasingly evident from Dr. Symon's and Dr. Shulman's presentations that the vascular bed and microcirculatory pressure dynamics play an extremely important part in ICP and brain compliance. Dr. Taylor has addressed his paper to this particular area. He argues that there certainly must be relationships between CSF pressure, tissue pressure, and capillary pressure. In spite of some conflicting work with regard to positive and negative brain tissue pressures, it appears, based on Dr. Taylor's model, that there is a positive interstitial fluid pressure rather than a negative interstitial fluid pressure, since only a positive state allows for minor changes in capillary pressure without the development of edema in the normal state.

When edema does develop, such as in the cold-injury model, how is function interfered with? Dr. Grossman, in an elegant study, attempted to clarify glial reaction to the spread of the edema fluid. His data show that glial membrane potentials are in the normal range but that normal slow glial depolarization to synchronized electrocortical waves was not present, suggesting disturbed normal neural-glial spatial relationships. This suggests the neural dysfunction in an edematous area may be the result of mechanical disruption of extracellular clefts and interference of intercellular communication.

HEAD INJURIES

Index